Re
Phys

Look for these other volumes in the *Mosby Physiology Monograph Series:*

Renal Physiology

FIFTH EDITION

BRUCE M. KOEPPEN, MD, PhD

Dean
Frank H. Netter MD School of Medicine
Quinnipiac University
Hamden, Connecticut

BRUCE A. STANTON, PhD

Professor of Microbiology and Immunology, and of Physiology
Andrew C. Vail Memorial Professor
The Geisel School of Medicine at Dartmouth
Hanover, New Hampshire

1600 John F. Kennedy Blvd.
Ste 1800
Philadelphia, PA 19103-2899

RENAL PHYSIOLOGY, FIFTH EDITION

ISBN: 978-0-323-08691-2

Notices

Knowledge and best practice in this field are constantly changing. As new research and experience broaden our understanding, changes in research methods, professional practices, or medical treatment may become necessary.

Practitioners and researchers must always rely on their own experience and knowledge in evaluating and using any information, methods, compounds, or experiments described herein. In using such information or methods they should be mindful of their own safety and the safety of others, including parties for whom they have a professional responsibility.

With respect to any drug or pharmaceutical products identified, readers are advised to check the most current information provided (i) on procedures featured or (ii) by the manufacturer of each product to be administered, to verify the recommended dose or formula, the method and duration of administration, and contraindications. It is the responsibility of practitioners, relying on their own experience and knowledge of their patients, to make diagnoses, to determine dosages and the best treatment for each individual patient, and to take all appropriate safety precautions.

To the fullest extent of the law, neither the Publisher nor the authors, contributors, or editors, assume any liability for any injury and/or damage to persons or property as a matter of products liability, negligence or otherwise, or from any use or operation of any methods, products, instructions, or ideas contained in the material herein.

ISBN: 978-0-323-08691-2

Content Development Strategist: William Schmidt
Content Development Specialist: Lisa Barnes
Publishing Services Manager: Patricia Tannian
Project Manager: Carrie Stetz
Design Direction: Steven Stave

Printed in China

Last digit is the print number: 9 8 7 6 5 4 3 2 1

This book is dedicated to
our family, friends, colleagues, and, most especially, our students.

PREFACE

When we wrote the first edition of *Renal Physiology* in 1992, our goal was to provide a clear and concise overview of the function of the kidneys for health professions students who were studying the topic for the first time. The feedback we have received over the years has affirmed that we met our goal, and that achievement has been a key element to the book's success. Thus, in this fifth edition we have adhered to our original goal, maintaining all the proven elements of the last four editions.

Since 1992, much has been learned about kidney function at the cellular, molecular, and clinical level. Although this new information is exciting and provides new and greater insights into the function of the kidneys in health and disease, it can prove daunting to first-time students and in some cases may cause them to lose the forest for the trees. In an attempt to balance the needs of the first-time student with our desire to present some of the latest advances in the field of renal physiology, we have updated the highlighted text boxes, titled "At the Cellular Level" and "In the Clinic," to supplement the main text for students who wish additional detail. The other features of the book, which include clinical material that illustrates important physiologic principles, multiple-choice questions, self-study problems, and integrated case studies, have been retained and updated. To achieve our goal of keeping the book concise, we have removed some old material as new material was added. We hope that all who use this book find that the changes have made it an improved learning tool and a valuable source of information.

To the instructor: This book is intended to provide students in the biomedical and health sciences with a basic understanding of the workings of the kidneys. We believe that it is better for the student at this stage to master a few central concepts and ideas rather than to assimilate a large array of facts. Consequently, this book is designed to teach the important aspects and fundamental concepts of normal renal function. We have emphasized clarity and conciseness in presenting the material. To accomplish this goal, we have been selective in the material included. The broader field of nephrology, with its current and future frontiers, is better learned at a later time and only after the "big picture" has been well established. For clarity and simplicity, we have made statements as assertions of fact even though we recognize that not all aspects of a particular problem have been resolved.

To the student: As an aid to learning this material, each chapter includes a list of objectives that reflect the fundamental concepts to be mastered. At the end of each chapter, we have provided a summary and a list of key words and concepts that should serve as a checklist while working through the chapter. We have also provided a series of self-study problems that review the central principles of each chapter. Because these questions are learning tools, answers and explanations are provided in Appendix D. Multiple-choice questions are presented at the end of each chapter. Comprehensive clinical cases are included in other appendixes. We recommend working through the clinical cases in Appendix A only after completing the book. In this way, they can indicate where additional work or review is required.

We have provided a highly selective bibliography that is intended to provide the next step in the study of the kidney; it is a place to begin to add details to the subjects presented here and a resource for exploring other aspects of the kidney not treated in this book.

We encourage all who use this book to send us your comments and suggestions. Please let us know what we have done right as well as what needs improvement.

Bruce M. Koeppen
Bruce A. Stanton

ACKNOWLEDGMENTS

We thank our students at the University of Connecticut School of Medicine and School of Dental Medicine and at the Geisel School of Medicine at Dartmouth, who continually provide feedback on how to improve this book. We also thank our colleagues and the many individuals from around the world who have contacted us with thoughtful suggestions for this as well as for previous editions. Special thanks go to Drs. Peter Aronson, Dennis Brown, Gerald DiBona, Gerhard Giebisch, Orson Moe, and R. Brooks Robey whose insights and suggestions on the fifth edition have been invaluable.

Finally, we thank Laura Stingelin, Lisa Barnes, Carrie Stetz, Elyse O'Grady, William Schmidt, and the staff at Elsevier for their support and commitment to quality.

CONTENTS

CHAPTER **4**

RENAL TRANSPORT MECHANISMS: NaCl AND WATER ABSORPTION ALONG THE NEPHRON 45

CHAPTER **5**

REGULATION OF BODY FLUID OSMOLALITY: REGULATION OF WATER BALANCE 73

CHAPTER **6**

REGULATION OF EXTRACELLULAR FLUID VOLUME AND NaCl BALANCE 93

APPENDIX E

APPENDIX F

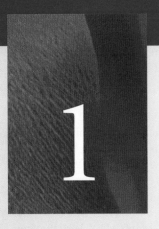

1

PHYSIOLOGY OF BODY FLUIDS

OBJECTIVES

Upon completion of this chapter, the student should be able to answer the following questions:

1. How do body fluid compartments differ with respect to their volumes and their ionic compositions?

2. What are the driving forces responsible for movement of water across cell membranes and the capillary wall?

3. How do the volumes of the intracellular and extracellular fluid compartments change under various pathophysiologic conditions?

In addition, the student should be able to define and understand the following properties of physiologically important solutions and fluids:

1. Molarity and equivalence
2. Osmotic pressure
3. Osmolarity and osmolality
4. Oncotic pressure
5. Tonicity

One of the major functions of the kidneys is to maintain the volume and composition of the body's fluids constant despite wide variation in the daily intake of water and solutes. In this chapter, the volume and composition of the body's fluids are discussed to provide a background for the study of the kidneys as regulatory organs. Some of the basic principles, terminology, and concepts related to the properties of solutes in solution also are reviewed.

PHYSICOCHEMICAL PROPERTIES OF ELECTROLYTE SOLUTIONS

Molarity and Equivalence

The amount of a substance dissolved in a solution (i.e., its concentration) is expressed in terms of either **molarity** or **equivalence**. Molarity is the amount of a substance relative to its molecular weight. For example, glucose has a molecular weight of 180 g/mol. If 1 L of water contains 1 g of glucose, the molarity of this glucose solution would be determined as:

$$\frac{1 g/L}{180 \ g/mol} = 0.0056 \ mol/L \ or \ 5.6 \ mmol/L \qquad (1\text{-}1)$$

For uncharged molecules, such as glucose and urea, concentrations in the body fluids are usually expressed in terms of molarity.* Because many of the substances of biologic interest are present at very low concentrations, units are more frequently expressed in the millimolar range (mmol/L).

The concentration of solutes, which normally dissociate into more than one particle when dissolved in solution (e.g., sodium chloride [NaCl]), is usually expressed in terms of equivalence. Equivalence refers to the stoichiometry of the interaction between cation and anion and is determined by the valence of these ions. For example, consider a 1 L solution containing 9 g of NaCl (molecular weight = 58.4 g/mol). The molarity of this solution is 154 mmol/L. Because NaCl dissociates into Na^+ and Cl^- ions, and assuming complete dissociation, this solution contains 154 mmol/L of Na^+ and 154 mmol/L of Cl^-. Because the valence of these ions is 1, these concentrations also can be expressed as milliequivalents (mEq) of the ion per liter (i.e., 154 mEq/L for Na^+ and Cl^-, respectively).

For univalent ions such as Na^+ and Cl^-, concentrations expressed in terms of molarity and equivalence are identical. However, this is not true for ions having valences greater than 1. Accordingly, the concentration of Ca^{++} (molecular weight = 40.1 g/mol and valence = 2) in a 1 L solution containing 0.1 g of this ion could be expressed as:

$$\frac{0.1 \ g/L}{40.1 \ g/mol} = 2.5 \ mmol/L \qquad (1\text{-}2)$$
$$2.5 \ mmol/L \times 2 \ Eq/mol = 5 \ mEq.$$

*The units used to express the concentrations of substances in various body fluids differ among laboratories. The International System of Units (SI) is used in most countries and in most scientific and medical journals in the United States. Despite this convention, traditional units are still widely used. For urea and glucose, the traditional unit of concentration is mg/dL (milligrams per deciliter, or 100 mL), whereas the SI unit is mmol/L (millimoles per liter). Similarly, electrolyte concentrations are traditionally expressed as mEq/L (milliequivalents per liter), whereas the SI unit is mmol/L (see Appendix B).

Although some exceptions exist, it is customary to express concentrations of ions in milliequivalents per liter (mEq/L).

Osmosis and Osmotic Pressure

The movement of water across cell membranes occurs by the process of **osmosis**. The driving force for this movement is the osmotic pressure difference across the cell membrane. Figure 1-1 illustrates the concept of osmosis and the measurement of the osmotic pressure of a solution.

Osmotic pressure is determined solely by the number of solute particles in the solution. It is not dependent on factors such as the size of the solute particles, their mass, or their chemical nature (e.g., valence). Osmotic pressure (π), measured in atmospheres (atm), is calculated by **van't Hoff's law** as:

$$\pi = nCRT \qquad (1\text{-}3)$$

where n is the number of dissociable particles per molecule, C is total solute concentration, R is gas constant, and T is temperature in degrees Kelvin (°K).

For a molecule that does not dissociate in water, such as glucose or urea, a solution containing 1 mmol/L of these solutes at 37° C can exert an osmotic pressure of 2.54×10^{-2} atm as calculated by equation 1-3 using the following values: n is 1, C is 0.001 mol/L, R is 0.082 atm L/mol, and T is 310° K.

Because 1 atm equals 760 mm Hg at sea level, π for this solution also can be expressed as 19.3 mm Hg. Alternatively, osmotic pressure is expressed in terms of osmolarity (see the following discussion). Thus a solution containing 1 mmol/L of solute particles exerts an osmotic pressure of 1 milliosmole/L (1 mOsm/L).

For substances that dissociate in a solution, n of equation 1-3 has a value other than 1. For example, a 150 mmol/L solution of NaCl has an osmolarity of 300 mOsm/L because each molecule of NaCl dissociates into a Na^+ and a Cl^- ion (i.e., $n = 2$). If dissociation of a substance into its component ions is not complete, n is not an integer. Accordingly, osmolarity for any solution can be calculated as:

$$\begin{aligned} Osmolarity &= Concentration \times Number \ of \\ &\quad dissociable \ particles \\ mOsm/L &= mmol/L \times number \ of \\ &\quad particles/mol \end{aligned} \qquad (1\text{-}4)$$

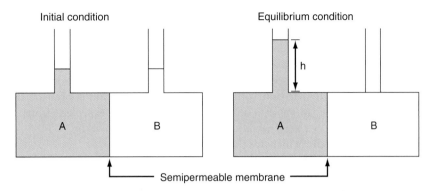

FIGURE 1-1 ■ Schematic representation of osmotic water movement and the generation of an osmotic pressure. Compartment A and compartment B are separated by a semipermeable membrane (i.e., the membrane is highly permeable to water but impermeable to solute). Compartment A contains a solute, and compartment B contains only distilled water. Over time, water moves by osmosis from compartment B to compartment A. (Note: This water movement is driven by the concentration gradient for water. Because of the presence of solute particles in compartment A, the concentration of water in compartment A is less than that in compartment B. Consequently, water moves across the semipermeable membrane from compartment B to compartment A down its gradient). This movement raises the level of fluid in compartment A and decreases the level in compartment B. At equilibrium, the hydrostatic pressure exerted by the column of water (h) stops the movement of water from compartment B to A. This pressure is equal and opposite to the osmotic pressure exerted by the solute particles in compartment A.

Osmolarity and Osmolality

Osmolarity and **osmolality** are frequently confused and incorrectly interchanged. Osmolarity refers to the number of solute particles per 1 L of solvent, whereas osmolality is the number of solute particles in 1 kg of solvent. For dilute solutions, the difference between osmolarity and osmolality is insignificant. Measurements of osmolarity are temperature dependent because the volume of solvent varies with temperature (i.e., the volume is larger at higher temperatures). In contrast, osmolality, which is based on the mass of the solvent, is temperature independent. For this reason, osmolality is the preferred term for biologic systems and is used throughout this and subsequent chapters. Osmolality has the units of Osm/kg H_2O. Because of the dilute nature of physiologic solutions and because water is the solvent, osmolalities are expressed as milliosmoles per kilogram of water (mOsm/kg H_2O).

Table 1-1 shows the relationships among molecular weight, equivalence, and osmoles for a number of physiologically significant solutes.

Tonicity

The **tonicity** of a solution is related to its effect on the volume of a cell. Solutions that do not change the volume of a cell are said to be **isotonic**. A **hypotonic**

	TABLE 1-1		
Units of Measurement for Physiologically Significant Substances			
SUBSTANCE	ATOMIC/ MOLECULAR WEIGHT	EQUIVALENTS/ MOL	OSMOLES/ MOL
Na^+	23.0	1	1
K^+	39.1	1	1
Cl^-	35.4	1	1
HCO_3^-	61.0	1	1
Ca^{++}	40.1	2	1
Phosphate (P_i)	95.0	3	1
NH_4^+	18.0	1	1
NaCl	58.4	2*	2†
$CaCl_2$	111	4‡	3
Glucose	180	—	1
Urea	60	—	1

$CaCl_2$, Calcium chloride; HCO_3^-, bicarbonate; *NaCl,* sodium chloride; NH_4^+, ammonium.
*One equivalent each from Na^+ and Cl^-.
†NaCl does not dissociate completely in solution. The actual Osm/mol volume is 1.88. However, for simplicity, a value of 2 often is used.
‡Ca^{++} contributes two equivalents, as do the Cl^- ions.

solution causes a cell to swell, whereas a **hypertonic** solution causes a cell to shrink. Although it is related to osmolality, tonicity also takes into consideration the ability of the solute to cross the cell membrane.

Consider two solutions: a 300 mmol/L solution of sucrose and a 300 mmol/L solution of urea. Both solutions have an osmolality of 300 mOsm/kg H_2O and therefore are said to be **isosmotic** (i.e., they have the same osmolality). When red blood cells (which, for the purpose of this illustration, also have an intracellular fluid osmolality of 300 mOsm/kg H_2O) are placed in the two solutions, those in the sucrose solution maintain their normal volume, but those placed in urea swell and eventually burst. Thus the sucrose solution is isotonic and the urea solution is hypotonic. The differential effect of these solutions on red cell volume is related to the permeability of the plasma membrane to sucrose and urea. The red blood cell membrane contains uniporters for urea (see Chapter 4). Thus urea easily crosses the cell membrane (i.e., the membrane is **permeable** to urea), driven by the concentration gradient (i.e., extracellular [urea] > intracellular [urea]). In contrast, the red blood cell membrane does not contain sucrose transporters, and sucrose cannot enter the cell (i.e., the membrane is **impermeable** to sucrose).

To exert an osmotic pressure across a membrane, a solute must not permeate that membrane. Because the red blood cell membrane is impermeable to sucrose, it exerts an osmotic pressure equal and opposite to the osmotic pressure generated by the contents of the red blood cell (in this case, 300 mOsm/kg H_2O). In contrast, urea is readily able to cross the red blood cell membrane, and it cannot exert an osmotic pressure to balance that generated by the intracellular solutes of the red blood cell. Consequently, sucrose is termed an **effective osmole** and urea is termed an **ineffective osmole**.

To take into account the effect of a solute's membrane permeability on osmotic pressure, it is necessary to rewrite equation 1-3 as:

$$\pi = \sigma(nCRT) \tag{1-5}$$

where σ is the **reflection coefficient** or **osmotic coefficient** and is a measure of the relative ability of the solute to cross a cell membrane.

For a solute that can freely cross the cell membrane (such as urea in this example), $\sigma = 0$, and no effective osmotic pressure is exerted. Thus urea is an ineffective

osmole for red blood cells. In contrast, $\sigma = 1$ for a solute that cannot cross the cell membrane (i.e., sucrose). Such a substance is said to be an effective osmole. Many solutes are neither completely able nor completely unable to cross cell membranes (i.e., $0 < \sigma < 1$) and generate an osmotic pressure that is only a fraction of what is expected from the total solute concentration.

Oncotic Pressure

Oncotic pressure is the osmotic pressure generated by large molecules (especially proteins) in solution. As illustrated in Figure 1-2, the magnitude of the osmotic pressure generated by a solution of protein does not conform to van't Hoff's law. The cause of this anomalous relationship between protein concentration and osmotic pressure is not completely understood but appears to be related to the size and shape of the protein molecule. For example, the correlation to van't Hoff's law is more precise with small, globular proteins than with larger protein molecules.

The oncotic pressure exerted by proteins in human plasma has a normal value of approximately 26 to 28 mm Hg. Although this pressure appears to be small when considered in terms of osmotic pressure (28 mm Hg $\approx$ 1.4 mOsm/kg H_2O), it is an important force involved in fluid movement across capillaries (details of this topic are presented in the following section on fluid exchange between body fluid compartments).

Specific Gravity

The total solute concentration in a solution also can be measured as **specific gravity**. Specific gravity is defined as the weight of a volume of solution divided by the weight of an equal volume of distilled water. Thus the specific gravity of distilled water is 1. Because biologic fluids contain a number of different substances, their specific gravities are greater than 1. For example, normal human plasma has a specific gravity in the range of 1.008 to 1.010.

VOLUMES OF BODY FLUID COMPARTMENTS

Water makes up approximately 60% of the body's weight, with variability among individuals being a

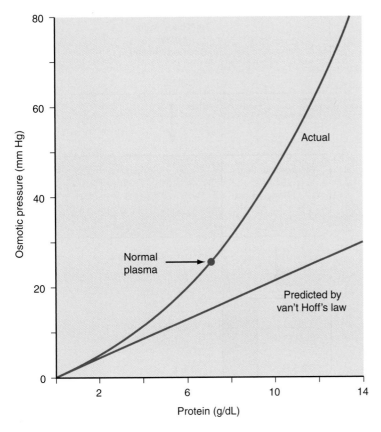

FIGURE 1-2 ■ Relationship between the concentration of plasma proteins in solution and the osmotic pressure (oncotic pressure) they generate. Protein concentration is expressed as grams per deciliter. Normal plasma protein concentration is indicated. Note that the actual pressure generated exceeds that predicted by van't Hoff's law.

function of the amount of adipose tissue that is present. Because the water content of adipose tissue is lower than that of other tissue, increased amounts of adipose tissue reduce the fraction of total body weight attributed to water. The percentage of body weight attributed to water also varies with age. In newborns, it is approximately 75%. This percentage decreases to the adult value of 60% by 1 year of age.

As illustrated in Figure 1-3, **total body water** is distributed between two major compartments, which are divided by the cell membrane.* The **intracellular fluid** (ICF) compartment is the larger compartment and contains approximately two thirds of the total body water. The remaining one third of the body water is contained in the **extracellular fluid** (ECF) compartment. Expressed as percentages of body weight, the volumes of total body water, ICF, and ECF are:

$$\text{Total body water} = 0.6 \times (\text{body weight})$$
$$\text{ICF} = 0.4 \times (\text{body weight})$$
$$\text{ECF} = 0.2 \times (\text{body weight})$$

(1-6)

---

*In these and all subsequent calculations, it is assumed that 1 L of fluid (e.g., ICF and ECF) has a mass of 1 kg. This assumption allows conversion from measurements of body weight to volume of body fluids.

IN THE CLINIC

The specific gravity of urine is sometimes measured in clinical settings and used to assess the concentrating ability of the kidney. The specific gravity of urine varies in proportion to its osmolality. However, because specific gravity depends on both the number of solute particles and their weight, the relationship between specific gravity and osmolality is not always predictable. For example, patients who have been injected with radiocontrast dye (molecular weight >500 g/mol) for radiographic studies can have high values of urine-specific gravity (1.040 to 1.050) even though the urine osmolality is similar to that of plasma (e.g., 300 mOsm/kg H_2O).

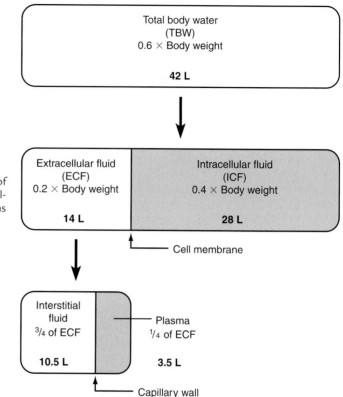

FIGURE 1-3 ■ Relationship between the volumes of the major body fluid compartments. The actual values shown are calculated for a person who weighs 70 kg.

The ECF compartment is further subdivided into **interstitial fluid** and **plasma**, which are separated by the capillary wall. The interstitial fluid surrounds the cells in the various tissues of the body and constitutes three fourths of the ECF volume. The ECF includes water contained within the bone and dense connective tissue, as well as the cerebrospinal fluid. Plasma represents the remaining one fourth of the ECF. Under some pathologic conditions, additional fluid may accumulate in what is referred to as a "**third space.**" Third space collections of fluid are part of the ECF and include, for example, the accumulation of fluid in the peritoneal cavity (**ascites**) of persons with liver disease.

COMPOSITION OF BODY FLUID COMPARTMENTS

Sodium is the major cation of the ECF, and Cl^- and bicarbonate (HCO_3^-) are the major anions. The ionic composition of the plasma and interstitial fluid compartments of the ECF is similar because they are separated only by the capillary endothelium, a barrier that is freely permeable to small ions. The major difference between the interstitial fluid and plasma is that the latter contains significantly more protein. This differential concentration of protein can affect the distribution of cations and anions between these two compartments (i.e., the Donnan effect) because plasma proteins have a net negative charge that tends to increase the cation concentrations and reduce the anion concentrations in the plasma compartment. However, this effect is small, and the ionic compositions of the interstitial fluid and plasma can be considered identical. Because of its abundance, Na^+ (and its attendant anions, primarily Cl^- and HCO_3^-) is the major determinant of ECF osmolality. Accordingly, a rough estimate of the ECF osmolality can be obtained by simply doubling the sodium concentration [Na^+]. For example, if the plasma [Na^+] is 145 mEq/L, the osmolality of plasma and ECF can be estimated as:

$$\text{Plasma osmolality} = 2(\text{plasma } [Na^+]) \tag{1-7}$$
$$= 290 \text{ mOsm/kg } H_2O$$

Because water is in osmotic equilibrium across the capillary endothelium and the plasma membrane of cells, measurement of the plasma osmolality also provides a measure of the osmolality of the ECF and ICF.

IN THE CLINIC

In clinical situations, a more accurate estimate of the plasma osmolality is obtained by also considering the contribution of glucose and urea to the plasma osmolality. Accordingly, plasma osmolality can be estimated as:

$$\text{Plasma osmolality} =$$
$$2(\text{plasma}[Na^+]) + \frac{[\text{glucose}]}{18} + \frac{[\text{urea}]}{2.8} \tag{1-8}$$

The glucose and urea concentrations are expressed in units of mg/dL (dividing by 18 for glucose and 2.8 for urea* allows conversion from the units of mg/dL to mmol/L and thus to mOsm/kg H_2O). This estimation of plasma osmolality is especially useful when dealing with patients who have an elevated plasma [glucose] level as a result of diabetes mellitus and patients with chronic renal failure whose plasma [urea] level is elevated.

---

*The [urea] in plasma is measured as the nitrogen in the urea molecule, or blood urea nitrogen.

In contrast to the ECF, where the $[Na^+]$ is approximately 145 mEq/L, the $[Na^+]$ of the ICF is only 10 to 15 mEq/L. K^+ is the predominant cation of the ICF, and its concentration is approximately 150 mEq/L. This asymmetric distribution of Na^+ and K^+ across the plasma membrane is maintained by the activity of the ubiquitous sodium–potassium–adenosine triphosphatase (Na^+-K^+-ATPase) mechanism. By its action, Na^+ is extruded from the cell in exchange for K^+. The anion composition of the ICF differs from that of the ECF. For example, Cl^- and HCO_3^- are the predominant anions of the ECF, and organic molecules and the negatively charged groups on proteins are the major anions of the ICF.

FLUID EXCHANGE BETWEEN BODY FLUID COMPARTMENTS

Water moves freely and rapidly between the various body fluid compartments. Two forces determine this movement: hydrostatic pressure and osmotic pressure. Hydrostatic pressure from the pumping of the heart (and the effect of gravity on the column of blood in the vessel) and osmotic pressure exerted by plasma proteins (oncotic pressure) are important determinants of fluid movement across the capillary wall. By contrast, because hydrostatic pressure gradients are not present across the cell membrane, only osmotic pressure differences between ICF and ECF cause fluid movement into and out of cells.

Capillary Fluid Exchange

The movement of fluid across a capillary wall is determined by the algebraic sum of the hydrostatic and oncotic pressures (the so-called **Starling forces**) as expressed by the following equation:

$$\text{Filtration rate} = K_f[(P_c - P_i) - \sigma(\pi_c - \pi_i)] \tag{1-9}$$

where the filtration rate is the volume of fluid moving across the capillary wall (expressed in units of either volume/capillary surface area or volume/time) and where K_f is the filtration coefficient of the capillary wall, P_c is hydrostatic pressure within the capillary lumen, π_c is oncotic pressure of the plasma, P_i is hydrostatic pressure of the interstitial fluid, π_i is oncotic pressure of the interstitial fluid, and σ is the reflection coefficient for proteins across the capillary wall.

The Starling forces for capillary fluid exchange vary between tissues and organs. They also can change in a given capillary bed under physiologic conditions (e.g., exercising muscle) and pathophysiologic conditions (e.g., congestive heart failure). Figure 1-4 illustrates these forces for a capillary bed located in skeletal muscle at rest.

The capillary filtration coefficient (K_f) reflects the intrinsic permeability of the capillary wall to the movement of fluid, as well as the surface area available for

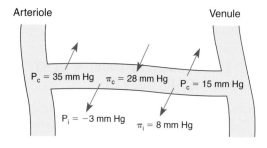

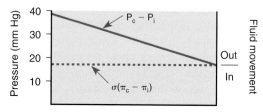

FIGURE 1-4 ■ *Top,* Schematic representation of the Starling forces responsible for the filtration and absorption of fluid across the wall of a typical skeletal muscle capillary. Note that P_c decreases from the arteriole end to the venule end of the capillary, whereas all the other Starling forces are constant along the length of the capillary. Some of the fluid filtered into the interstitium returns to the circulation via postcapillary venules, and some is taken up by lymphatic vessels and returned to the vascular system (not shown). *Bottom,* Graph of hydrostatic and oncotic pressure differences along the capillary (in this example, σ = 0.9). Net fluid movement across the wall of the capillary also is indicated. Note that fluid is filtered out of the capillary except at the venous end, where the net driving forces are zero. P_c, Capillary hydrostatic pressure; P_i, interstitial hydrostatic pressure; π_c, capillary oncotic pressure; π_i, interstitial oncotic pressure.

filtration. The K_f varies among different capillary beds. For example, the K_f of glomerular capillaries in the kidneys is approximately 100 times greater in magnitude than that of skeletal muscle capillaries. This difference in K_f accounts for the large volume of fluid filtered across glomerular capillaries compared with the amount filtered across skeletal muscle capillaries (see Chapter 3).

The hydrostatic pressure within the lumen of a capillary (P_c) is a force promoting the movement of fluid from the lumen into the interstitium. Its magnitude depends on arterial pressure, venous pressure, and precapillary (arteriolar) and postcapillary

(venular and small vein) resistances. An increase in the arterial or venous pressures results in an increase in P_c, whereas a decrease in these pressures has the opposite effect. P_c increases with either a decrease in precapillary resistance or an increase in postcapillary resistance. Likewise, an increase in precapillary resistance or a decrease in postcapillary resistance decreases P_c. For virtually all capillary beds, precapillary resistance is greater than postcapillary resistance, and thus the precapillary resistance plays a greater role in determining P_c. An important exception is the glomerular capillaries, where both precapillary and postcapillary resistances modulate P_c (see Chapter 3). The magnitude of P_c varies not only among tissues, but also among capillary beds within a given tissue; it also is dependent on the physiologic state of the tissue.

Precapillary sphincters control not only the hydrostatic pressure within an individual capillary, but also the number of perfused capillaries in the tissue. For example, in skeletal muscle at rest, not all capillaries are perfused. During exercise, relaxation of precapillary sphincters allows perfusion of more capillaries. The increased number of perfused capillaries reduces the diffusion distance between the cells and capillaries and thereby facilitates the exchange of O_2 and cellular metabolites (e.g., carbon dioxide [CO_2] and lactic acid).

The hydrostatic pressure within the interstitium (P_i) is difficult to measure, but in the absence of edema (i.e., abnormal accumulation of fluid in the interstitium), its value is near zero or slightly negative. Thus under normal conditions it causes fluid to move out of the capillary. However, when edema is present, P_i is positive and it opposes the movement of fluid out of the capillary (see Chapter 6).

The oncotic pressure of plasma proteins (π_c) retards the movement of fluid out of the capillary lumen. At a normal plasma protein concentration, π_c has a value of approximately 26 to 28 mm Hg. The degree to which oncotic pressure influences capillary fluid movement depends on the permeability of the capillary wall to the protein molecules. If the capillary wall is highly permeable to protein, σ is near zero and the oncotic pressure generated by plasma proteins plays little or no role in capillary fluid exchange. This situation is seen in the capillaries of the liver (i.e., hepatic sinusoids), which are highly permeable to proteins. As a result, the protein concentration of the interstitial fluid is essentially the same as that of plasma. In the capillaries of skeletal muscle, σ is approximately 0.9, whereas in the glomeruli of the kidneys the value is essentially 1. Therefore plasma protein oncotic pressure plays an important role in fluid movement across these capillary beds.

The protein that leaks across the capillary wall into the interstitium exerts an oncotic pressure (π_i) and promotes the movement of fluid out of the capillary lumen. In skeletal muscle capillaries under normal conditions, π_i is small and has a value of only 8 mm Hg.

As depicted in Figure 1-4, the balance of Starling forces across muscle capillaries causes fluid to leave the lumen (filtration) along its entire length. Some of this filtered fluid reenters the vasculature across the postcapillary venule where the Starling forces are reversed (i.e., the net driving force for fluid movement is into the vessel). The remainder of the filtered fluid is returned to the circulation through the lymphatics. The sinusoids of the liver also filter along their entire length. In contrast, during digestion of a meal, the balance of forces across capillaries of the gastrointestinal tract results in the net uptake of fluid into the capillary.

Normally, 8 to 12 L/day of fluid moves across capillary beds throughout the body and are collected by lymphatic vessels. This lymphatic fluid flows first to lymph nodes, where most of the fluid is returned to the circulation. Fluid not returned to the circulation at the lymph nodes (1 to 4 L/day) reenters the circulation through the thoracic and right lymphatic ducts. However, under conditions of increased capillary filtration, such as that which occurs in persons with congestive heart failure, thoracic and right lymphatic duct flow can increase 10-fold to 20-fold.

Cellular Fluid Exchange

Osmotic pressure differences between ECF and ICF are responsible for fluid movement between these compartments. Because the plasma membrane of cells contains water channels (aquaporins [AQPs]), water can easily cross the membrane. Thus a change in the osmolality of either ICF or ECF results in rapid movement (i.e., in minutes) of water between these

compartments. Thus, except for transient changes, the ICF and ECF compartments are in osmotic equilibrium.

AT THE CELLULAR LEVEL

Water movement across the plasma membrane of cells occurs through a class of integral membrane proteins called **aquaporins** (AQPs). Although water can cross the membrane through other transporters (e.g., an Na^+-glucose symporter), AQPs are the main route of water movement into and out of the cell. To date, 13 AQPs have been identified. These AQPs can be divided into two subgroups. One group, which includes the AQP involved in the regulation of water movement across the apical membrane of renal collecting duct cells by arginine vasopressin (AQP-2) (see Chapter 5), is permeable only to water. The second group is permeable not only to water but also to low-molecular-weight substances, including gases and metalloids. Because glycerol can cross the membrane via this group of aquaporins, they are termed aquaglyceroporins. AQPs exist in the plasma membrane as a homotetramer, with each monomer functioning as a water channel (see Chapter 4).

In contrast to the movement of water, the movement of ions across cell membranes is more variable from cell to cell and depends on the presence of specific membrane transport proteins. Consequently, as a first approximation, fluid exchange between the ICF and ECF under pathophysiologic conditions can be analyzed by assuming that appreciable shifts of ions between the compartments do not occur.

A useful approach for understanding the movement of fluids between the ICF and the ECF is outlined in Box 1-1. To illustrate this approach, consider what happens when solutions containing various amounts of NaCl are added to the ECF.*

---

*Fluids usually are administered intravenously. When electrolyte solutions are infused by this route, rapid equilibration occurs (i.e., within minutes) between plasma and interstitial fluid because of the high permeability of the capillary wall to water and electrolytes. Thus these fluids essentially are added to the entire ECF.

BOX 1-1
PRINCIPLES FOR ANALYSIS OF FLUID SHIFTS BETWEEN ICF AND ECF

The volumes of the various body fluid compartments can be estimated in a healthy adult as shown in Figure 1-3.

- All exchanges of water and solutes with the external environment occur through the extracellular fluid (ECF) (e.g., intravenous infusion and intake or loss via the gastrointestinal tract). Changes in the intracellular fluid (ICF) are secondary to fluid shifts between the ECF and the ICF. Fluid shifts occur only if the perturbation of the ECF alters its osmolality.

- Except for brief periods of seconds to minutes, the ICF and the ECF are in osmotic equilibrium. A measurement of plasma osmolality provides a measure of both the ECF and the ICF osmolality.

- For the sake of simplification, it can be assumed that equilibration between the ICF and the ECF occurs only by movement of water and not by movement of osmotically active solutes.

- Conservation of mass must be maintained, especially when considering either addition or removal of water and/or solutes from the body.

membrane of all cells. Therefore no net movement of the infused NaCl into the cells occurs.

IN THE CLINIC

Neurosurgical procedures and cerebrovascular accidents (strokes) often result in the accumulation of interstitial fluid in the brain (i.e., edema) and swelling of the neurons. Because the brain is enclosed within the skull, edema can raise intracranial pressure and thereby disrupt neuronal function, leading to coma and death. The blood-brain barrier, which separates the cerebrospinal fluid and brain interstitial fluid from blood, is freely permeable to water but not to most other substances. As a result, excess fluid in brain tissue can be removed by imposing an osmotic gradient across the blood-brain barrier. Mannitol can be used for this purpose. Mannitol is a sugar (molecular weight = 182 g/mol) that does not readily cross the blood-brain barrier and membranes of cells (neurons as well as other cells in the body). Therefore mannitol is an effective osmole, and intravenous infusion results in the movement of fluid from the brain tissue by osmosis.

Example 1: Addition of Isotonic NaCl to ECF

The addition of an isotonic NaCl solution (e.g., intravenous infusion of 0.9% NaCl: osmolality $\approx$290 mOsm/kg H_2O to a patient)* to the ECF increases the volume of this compartment by the volume of fluid administered. Because this fluid has the same osmolality as ECF and therefore also has the same osmolality as ICF, no driving force for fluid movement between these compartments exists, and the volume of ICF is unchanged. Although Na^+ can cross cell membranes, it is effectively restricted to the ECF by the activity of Na^+-K^+-ATPase, which is present in the plasma

Example 2: Addition of Hypotonic NaCl to ECF

The addition of a hypotonic NaCl solution to the ECF (e.g., intravenous infusion of 0.45% NaCl: osmolality <145 mOsm/kg H_2O to a patient) decreases the osmolality of this fluid compartment, resulting in the movement of water into the ICF. After osmotic equilibration, the osmolalities of ICF and ECF are equal but lower than before the infusion, and the volume of each compartment is increased. The increase in ECF volume is greater than the increase in ICF volume.

Example 3: Addition of Hypertonic NaCl to ECF

The addition of a hypertonic NaCl solution to the ECF (e.g., intravenous infusion of 3% NaCl: osmolality $\approx$1000 mOsm/kg H_2O to a patient) increases the osmolality of this compartment, resulting in the movement of water out of cells. After osmotic equilibration, the osmolalities of ECF and ICF are equal but higher than before the infusion. The volume of the ECF is increased, whereas that of the ICF is decreased.

---

*A 0.9% NaCl solution (0.9 g NaCl/100 mL) contains 154 mmol/L of NaCl. Because NaCl does not dissociate completely in solution (i.e., 1.88 Osm/mol), the osmolality of this solution is 290 mOsm/kg H_2O, which is very similar to that of normal ECF.

IN THE CLINIC

Fluid and electrolyte disorders often are seen in clinical practice (e.g., in patients with vomiting and/or diarrhea). In most instances these disorders are self-limited, and correction of the disorder occurs without need for intervention. However, more severe or prolonged disorders may require fluid replacement therapy. Such therapy may be administered orally with special electrolyte solutions, or intravenous fluids may be administered.

Intravenous solutions are available in many formulations (see Table 1-2). The type of fluid administered to a particular patient is dictated by the patient's need. For example, if an increase in the patient's vascular volume is necessary, a solution containing substances that do not readily cross the capillary wall is infused (e.g., 5% albumin solution). The oncotic pressure generated by the albumin molecules retains fluid in the vascular compartment, expanding its volume. Expansion of extracellular fluid (ECF) is accomplished most often by using isotonic saline solutions (e.g., 0.9% sodium chloride [NaCl]).

As already noted, administration of an isotonic NaCl solution does not result in the development of an osmotic pressure gradient across the plasma membrane of cells. Therefore the entire volume of the infused solution remains in the ECF. Patients whose body fluids are hyperosmotic need hypotonic solutions. These solutions may be hypotonic NaCl (e.g., 0.45% NaCl or 5% dextrose in water [D5W]). Administration of D5W is equivalent to infusion of distilled water because the dextrose is metabolized to CO_2 and water. Administration of these fluids increases the volumes of both the intracellular fluid (ICF) and ECF. Finally, patients whose body fluids are hypotonic need hypertonic solutions, which typically are solutions that contain NaCl (e.g., 3% and 5% NaCl). These solutions expand the volume of the ECF but decrease the volume of the ICF. Other constituents, such as electrolytes (e.g., K^+) or drugs, can be added to intravenous solutions to tailor the therapy to the patient's fluid, electrolyte, and metabolic needs.

TABLE 1-2
Intravenous Solutions

SOLUTION	Na+ (mEq/L)	Cl− (mEq/L)	K+ (mEq/L)	Ca++ (mEq/L)	LACTATE (mmol/L)	GLUCOSE	OSMOLALITY (mOsm/kg H2O)	OTHER
0.45% NaCl (½NSS)	77	77	0	0	0	0	154	0
0.9% NaCl (NSS)	154	154	0	0	0	0	308	0
3.0% NaCl (hypertonic saline solution)	513	513	0	0	0	0	1024	0
Lactated Ringer's solution	130	109	4	3	28*	0	275	
D5W	0	0	0	0	0	50 g/L†	280	0
Dextrose (½ NSS)	77	77	0	0	0	50 g/L†	406	0
5% albumin in NSS	145	145	<1	0	0	0	309	50 g/L albumin

D5W, 5% dextrose in water; *NaCl*, sodium chloride; *NSS*, normal saline solution.
*Metabolized to HCO_3^-.
†Metabolized to CO_2 and H_2O.

SUMMARY

1. Water, which is a major constituent of the human body, accounts for 60% of the body's weight. Body water is divided between two major compartments: ICF and ECF. Two thirds of the water is in the ICF, and one third is in the ECF. Osmotic pressure gradients between ICF and ECF drive water movement between these compartments. Because the plasma membrane of most cells is highly permeable to water, ICF and ECF are in osmotic equilibrium.

2. The ECF is divided into a vascular compartment (plasma) and an interstitial fluid compartment. Starling forces across capillaries determine the exchange of fluid between these compartments.

3. Sodium is the major cation of ECF, and potassium is the major cation of the ICF. This asymmetric distribution of Na^+ and K^+ is maintained by the activity of Na^+-K^+-ATPase.

KEY WORDS AND CONCEPTS

- Molarity
- Equivalence
- Osmosis
- Osmotic pressure
- van't Hoff's law
- Osmolarity
- Osmolality
- Tonicity (isotonic, hypotonic, and hypertonic)
- Effective osmole
- Ineffective osmole
- Reflection coefficient
- Osmotic coefficient
- Oncotic pressure
- Specific gravity
- Total body water
- Intracellular fluid (ICF)
- Extracellular fluid (ECF)
- Interstitial fluid
- Plasma
- Capillary wall
- Starling forces
- Capillary filtration coefficient (K_f)
- Aquaporin (AQP)

SELF-STUDY PROBLEMS

1. Calculate the molarity and osmolality of a 1 L solution containing the following solutes. Assume complete dissociation of all electrolytes.

	Molarity (mmol/L)	Osmolality (mOsm/kg H_2O)
9 g NaCl	_____	_____
72 g Glucose	_____	_____
22.2 g $CaCl_2$	_____	_____
3 g Urea	_____	_____
8.4 g $NaHCO_3$	_____	_____

2. The intracellular contents of a cell generate an osmotic pressure of 300 mOsm/kg H_2O. The cell is placed in a solution containing 300 mmol/L of a solute (x). If solute x remains as a single particle in solution and has a reflection coefficient of 0.5, what happens to the volume of the cell in this solution? What would be the composition of an isotonic solution (i.e., a solution that does not cause a change in the volume of the cell) containing substance x?

3. A person's plasma [Na^+] is measured and found to be 130 mEq/L (normal = 145 mEq/L). What is the person's estimated plasma osmolality? What effect does the lower than normal plasma [Na^+] have on water movement across cell plasma membranes and across the capillary endothelium?

4. Figure 1-4 illustrates the normal values for the Starling forces involved in fluid movement across a typical skeletal muscle capillary. Draw the new hydrostatic ($P_c - P_i$) and oncotic $\sigma(\pi_c - \pi_i)$ pressure curves if P_c at the venous end of the capillary was increased to 20 mm Hg. What effect would this increase have on fluid exchange across the capillary wall?

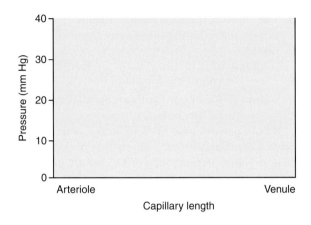

Pressure (mm Hg) vs Capillary length (Arteriole to Venule)

Note: For questions 5 through 8, for ease of calculation, the composition and osmolality of infused solutions that are provided are slightly different from the solutions used clinically (see Table 1-2).

5. A healthy volunteer (body weight = 50 kg) is infused with 1 L of a 5% dextrose and water solution (D5W: osmolality ~290 mOsm/kg H_2O). What would be the immediate and long-term effects (i.e., several hours after the dextrose has been metabolized) of this infusion on the following parameters? Assume an initial plasma $[Na^+]$ of 145 mEq/L and, for simplicity, no urine output.

Immediate effect:
ECF volume: _____ L
ICF volume: _____ L
Plasma $[Na^+]$: _____ mEq/L

Long-term effect:
ECF volume: _____ L
ICF volume: _____ L
Plasma $[Na^+]$: _____ mEq/L

Based on these effects of D5W on the volumes and compositions of the body fluids, how would this solution be used clinically?

6. A second healthy volunteer (body weight = 50 kg) is infused with 1 L of a 0.9% NaCl solution (isotonic saline: osmolality ~290 mOsm/kg H_2O). What would be the immediate and long-term effects (i.e., several hours) of this infusion on the following parameters? Assume an initial

plasma $[Na^+]$ of 145 mEq/L and, for simplicity, no urine output.

Immediate effect:
ECF volume: _____ L
ICF volume: _____ L
Plasma $[Na^+]$: _____ mEq/L

Long-term effect:
ECF volume: _____ L
ICF volume: _____ L
Plasma $[Na^+]$: _____ mEq/L

Based on these effects of the NaCl solution on the volumes and compositions of the body fluids, how would this solution be used clinically?

7. A person who weighs 60 kg has an episode of gastroenteritis with vomiting and diarrhea. Over a 2-day period this person loses 4 kg of body weight. Before becoming ill, this individual had a plasma $[Na^+]$ of 140 mEq/L, which was unchanged by the illness. Assuming the entire loss of body weight represents the loss of fluid (a reasonable assumption), estimate the following values:

Initial conditions (before gastroenteritis):
Total body water: _____ L
ICF volume: _____ L
ECF volume: _____ L
Total body osmoles: _____ mOsm
ICF osmoles: _____ mOsm
ECF osmoles: _____ mOsm

New equilibrium conditions (after gastroenteritis):
Total body water: _____ L
ICF volume: _____ L
ECF volume: _____ L
Total body osmoles: _____ mOsm
ICF osmoles: _____ mOsm
ECF osmoles: _____ mOsm

8. A person who weighs 50 kg with a plasma $[Na^+]$ of 145 mEq/L is infused with 5 g/kg of mannitol (molecular weight of mannitol = 182 g/mol) to reduce brain swelling after a stroke. After equilibration, estimate the following values, assuming mannitol is restricted to the ECF compartment, no excretion occurs, and the infusion volume of the mannitol solution is negligible (i.e., total body water is unchanged):

Initial conditions (before mannitol infusion):

Total body water:	_____ L
ICF volume:	_____ L
ECF volume:	_____ L
Total body osmoles:	_____ mOsm
ICF osmoles:	_____ mOsm
ECF osmoles:	_____ mOsm

New equilibrium conditions (after mannitol infusion):

Total body water:	_____ L
ICF volume:	_____ L
ECF volume:	_____ L
Total body osmoles:	_____ mOsm
ICF osmoles:	_____ mOsm
ECF osmoles:	_____ mOsm
Plasma osmolality:	_____ mOsm/kg H_2O
Plasma Na^+:	_____ mEq/L

9. Two healthy persons (body weight = 60 kg) excrete the following urine output over the same period.

Subject A: 1 L of urine with an osmolality of 1000 mOsm/kg H_2O

Subject B: 4 L of urine with an osmolality of 400 mOsm/kg H_2O

If both persons have no fluid intake, what is their plasma osmolality? Hint: Assume that both persons have an initial plasma $[Na^+]$ of 145 mEq/L and thus a plasma osmolality of approximately 290 mOsm/kg H_2O.

Subject A: _____

Subject B: _____

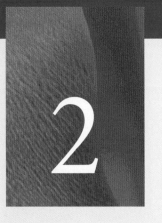

STRUCTURE AND FUNCTION OF THE KIDNEYS

OBJECTIVES

Upon completion of this chapter, the student should be able to answer the following questions:

1. Which structures in the glomerulus are filtration barriers to plasma proteins?

2. What is the physiologic significance of the juxtaglomerular apparatus?

3. Which blood vessels supply the kidneys?

4. Which nerves innervate the kidneys?

In addition, the student should be able to describe the following:

1. The location of the kidneys and their gross anatomic features

2. The different parts of the nephron and their locations within the cortex and medulla

3. The components of the glomerulus and the cell types located in each component

S tructure and function are closely linked in the kidneys. Consequently, an appreciation of the gross anatomic and histologic features of the kidneys is a prerequisite for an understanding of their function.

STRUCTURE OF THE KIDNEYS

Gross Anatomy

The kidneys are paired organs that lie on the posterior wall of the abdomen behind the peritoneum on either side of the vertebral column. In the adult human, each kidney weighs between 115 and 170 g and is approximately 11 cm long, 6 cm wide, and 3 cm thick.

The gross anatomic features of the human kidney are illustrated in Figure 2-1, *A*. The medial side of each kidney contains an indentation, through which pass the renal artery and vein, nerves, and pelvis. If a kidney were cut in half, two regions would be evident: an outer region called the **cortex** and an inner region called the **medulla**. The cortex and medulla are composed of **nephrons** (the functional units of the kidney), blood vessels, lymphatics, and nerves. The medulla in the human kidney is divided into conical masses called **renal pyramids**. The base of each pyramid originates at the corticomedullary border, and the apex terminates in a papilla, which lies within a **minor calyx**. Minor calyces collect urine from each papilla. The numerous minor calyces expand into two or three open-ended pouches, which are the major calyces. The **major calyces** in turn feed into the **pelvis**. The pelvis represents the

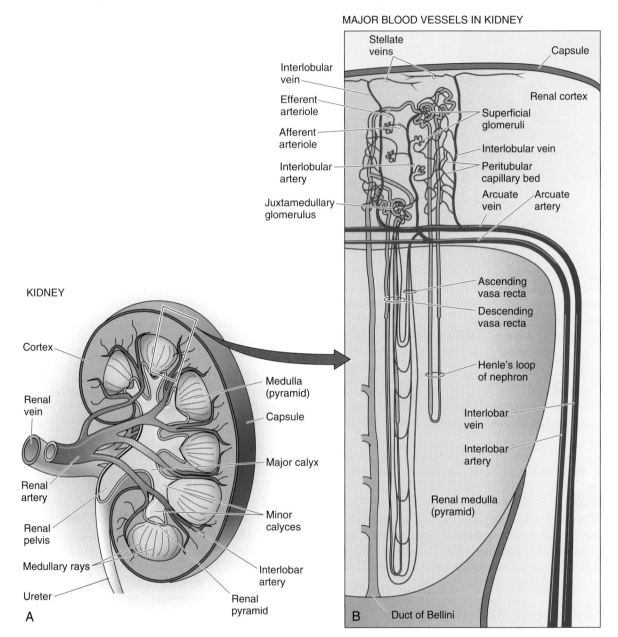

MAJOR BLOOD VESSELS IN KIDNEY

FIGURE 2-1 ■ Structure of a human kidney, cut open to show the internal structures. *(Modified From Boron WF, Boulpaep EL: Medical physiology, ed 2, Philadelphia, 2009, Saunders Elsevier.)*

upper, expanded region of the **ureter**, which carries urine from the pelvis to the urinary bladder. The walls of the calyces, pelvis, and ureters contain smooth muscle that contracts to propel the urine toward the **urinary bladder**.

The blood flow to the two kidneys is equal to about 25% (1.25 L/min) of the cardiac output in resting individuals. However, the kidneys constitute less than 0.5% of total body weight. As illustrated in Figure 2-1, the **renal artery** branches progressively to form the **interlobar artery**, the **arcuate artery**, the **interlobular artery**, and the **afferent arteriole**, which leads into the **glomerular capillaries**. The glomerular capillaries come together to form the **efferent arteriole**, which leads into a second capillary network, the **peritubular capillaries**, which supply blood to the nephron. The vessels of the venous system run parallel to the arterial vessels and progressively form the **interlobular vein, arcuate vein, interlobar vein**, and **renal vein**, which courses beside the ureter.

Ultrastructure of the Nephron

The functional unit of the kidneys is the nephron. Each human kidney contains approximately 1.2 million nephrons, which are hollow tubes composed of a single cell layer. The nephron consists of a **renal corpuscle, proximal tubule, loop of Henle, distal tubule**, and **collecting duct system** (Figure 2-2).* The **renal corpuscle** consists of glomerular capillaries and **Bowman's capsule**.† The proximal tubule initially forms several coils, followed by a straight piece that descends toward the medulla. The next segment is the loop of Henle, which is composed of the straight part of the proximal tubule, the descending thin limb (which ends in a hairpin turn), the ascending thin limb (only in nephrons with long loops of Henle), and the thick ascending limb. Near the end of the thick ascending limb, the nephron passes between the afferent and efferent arterioles of the same nephron. This short segment of the thick ascending limb that touches the glomerulus is called the **macula densa** (see Figure 2-2). The distal tubule begins a short distance beyond the macula densa and extends to the

point in the cortex where two or more nephrons join to form a cortical collecting duct. The **cortical collecting duct** enters the medulla and becomes the outer **medullary collecting duct** and then the **inner medullary collecting duct**.

Each nephron segment is made up of cells that are uniquely suited to perform specific transport functions. Proximal tubule cells have an extensively amplified apical membrane (the urine side of the cell) called the **brush border**, which is present only in the proximal tubule of the nephron. The basolateral membrane (the blood side of the cell) is highly invaginated. These invaginations contain many mitochondria. In contrast, the descending and ascending thin limbs of Henle's loop have poorly developed apical and basolateral surfaces and few mitochondria. The cells of the thick ascending limb and the distal tubule have abundant mitochondria and extensive infoldings of the basolateral membrane.

The collecting duct is composed of two cell types: principal cells and intercalated cells. **Principal cells** have a moderately invaginated basolateral membrane and contain few mitochondria. Principal cells play an important role in sodium chloride (NaCl) reabsorption (see Chapters 4 and 6) and K^+ secretion (see Chapter 7). **Intercalated cells**, which play an important role in regulating acid-base balance, have a high density of mitochondria. One population of intercalated cells secretes H^+ (i.e., reabsorbs bicarbonate $[HCO_3^-]$) and a second population of intercalated cells secretes HCO_3^- (see Chapter 8). The final segment of the nephron, the inner medullary collecting duct, is composed of inner medullary collecting duct cells. Cells of the inner medullary collecting duct have poorly developed apical and basolateral surfaces and few mitochondria.

Except for intercalated cells, all cells in the nephron have in the apical plasma membrane a single nonmotile primary cilium that protrudes into tubule fluid (Figure 2-3). Primary cilia are mechanosensors (i.e., they sense changes in the flow rate of tubule fluid) and chemosensors (i.e., they sense or respond to compounds in the surrounding fluid), and they initiate Ca^{++}-dependent signaling pathways, including those that control kidney cell function, proliferation, differentiation, and apoptosis (i.e., programmed cell death).

---

*The organization of the nephron is actually more complicated than presented here. However, for simplicity and clarity of presentation in subsequent chapters, the nephron is divided into five segments. For details on the subdivisions of the five nephron segments, consult Seldin and Giebisch's *The Kidney: Physiology and Pathophysiology*, edition 4 (see Additional Reading). The collecting duct system is not actually part of the nephron. However, for simplicity, we consider the collecting duct system part of the nephron.

†Although the renal corpuscle is composed of glomerular capillaries and Bowman's capsule, the term *glomerulus* commonly is used to described the renal corpuscle.

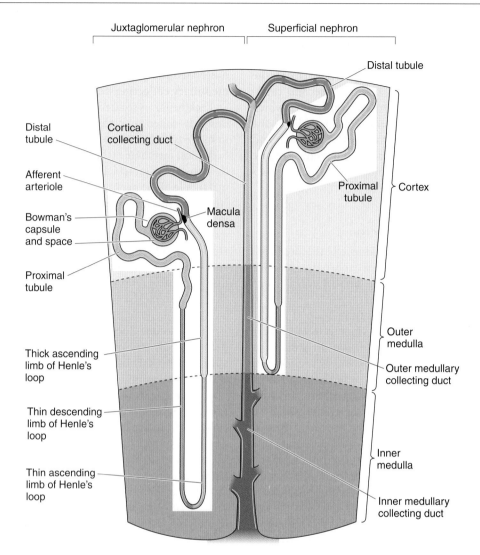

FIGURE 2-2 ▪ Diagram of a juxtaglomerular nephron (*left*) and a superficial nephron (*right*). *(Modified From Boron WF, Boulpaep EL: Medical physiology, ed 2, Philadelphia, 2009, Saunders Elsevier.)*

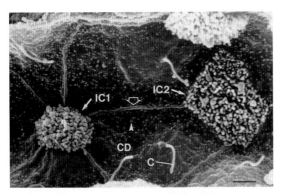

FIGURE 2-3 ▪ Scanning electron micrograph illustrating primary cilia (*C*) in the apical plasma membrane of principal cells within the cortical collecting duct. Note that intercalated cells (*IC1* and *IC2*) do not have cilia. Primary cilia are approximately 2 to 30 μm long and 0.5 μm in diameter. Collecting duct (*CD*) principal cells have short microvilli (*arrowhead*). The straight ridges (*open arrowhead*) represent the cell borders between principal cells. *(From Kriz W, Kaissling B: Structural organization of the mammalian kidney. In Seldin DW, Giebisch G, editors:* The kidney: physiology and pathophysiology, *ed 3, Philadelphia, 2000, Lippincott Williams & Wilkins.)*

IN THE CLINIC

Autosomal dominant polycystic kidney disease (ADPKD), which is the most common inherited kidney disease, occurs in 1 in 1000 people. Approximately 12.5 million people worldwide have ADPKD, which is caused primarily by mutations in the genes *PKD1* (85% of cases) and *PKD2* (~15% of cases). The major phenotype of ADPKD is enlargement of the kidneys related to the presence of hundreds to thousands of renal cysts that can be as large as 20 cm in diameter. Cysts also are seen in the liver and other organs. About 50% of patients with ADPKD progress to renal failure by the age of 60 years. Although it is not clear how mutations in *PKD1* and *PKD2* cause ADPKD, renal cyst formation results from defects in Ca^{++} uptake that lead to alterations in Ca^{++}-dependent signaling pathways, including those that control kidney cell proliferation, differentiation, and apoptosis.

AT THE CELLULAR LEVEL

Polycystin 1 (encoded by the *PKD1* gene) and polycystin 2 (encoded by the *PKD2* gene) are expressed in the membrane of primary cilia, and the *PKD1/PKD2* complex mediates the entry of Ca^{++} into cells. *PKD1* and *PKD2* are thought to play an important role in flow-dependent K^+ secretion by principal cells of the collecting duct (see Chapter 7). As described in more detail in Chapter 7, increased flow of tubule fluid in the collecting duct is a strong stimulus for K^+ secretion. Increased flow bends the primary cilium in principal cells, which activates the *PKD1/PKD2* Ca^{++} conducting channel complex, allowing Ca^{++} to enter the cell and increase intracellular $[Ca^{++}]$. The increase in $[Ca^{++}]$ activates K^+ channels in the apical plasma membrane, which enhances K^+ secretion from the cell into the tubule fluid.

Nephrons may be subdivided into superficial and juxtamedullary types (see Figure 2-2). The glomerulus of each superficial nephron is located in the outer region of the cortex. Its loop of Henle is short, and its efferent arteriole branches into peritubular capillaries that surround the nephron segments of its own and adjacent nephrons. This capillary network conveys oxygen and important nutrients to the nephron segments in the cortex, delivers substances to the nephron for secretion (i.e., the movement of a substance from the blood into the tubular fluid), and serves as a pathway for the return of reabsorbed water and solutes to the circulatory system. A few species, including humans, also possess very short superficial nephrons whose Henle's loops never enter the medulla.

The glomerulus of each **juxtamedullary nephron** is located in the region of the cortex adjacent to the medulla (see Figure 2-2). In comparison with the superficial nephrons, the juxtamedullary nephrons differ anatomically in two important ways: the loop of Henle is longer and extends deeper into the medulla, and the efferent arteriole forms not only a network of peritubular capillaries but also a series of vascular loops called the **vasa recta**.

As shown in Figure 2-1, *B*, the vasa recta descend into the medulla, where they form capillary networks that surround the collecting ducts and ascending limbs of the loop of Henle. The blood returns to the cortex in the ascending vasa recta. Although less than 0.7% of the blood enters the vasa recta, these vessels subserve important functions in the renal medulla, including (1) conveying oxygen and important nutrients to nephron segments, (2) delivering substances to the nephron for secretion, (3) serving as a pathway for the return of reabsorbed water and solutes to the circulatory system, and (4) concentrating and diluting the urine (urine concentration and dilution are discussed in more detail in Chapter 5).

Ultrastructure of the Glomerulus

The first step in urine formation begins with the passive movement of a plasma ultrafiltrate from the glomerular capillaries into **Bowman's space**. The term *ultrafiltration* refers to the passive movement of fluid that is similar is composition to plasma, except that the protein concentration in the ultrafiltrate is lower than that in the plasma, from the glomerular capillaries into Bowman's space. To appreciate the process of ultrafiltration, one must understand the anatomy of the glomerulus. The glomerulus consists of a network of capillaries supplied by the afferent arteriole and drained by the efferent arteriole (Figure 2-4). During embryologic development, the glomerular capillaries press into the closed end of the proximal tubule, forming **Bowman's capsule**. As the epithelial cells thin on the outside circumference of Bowman's

capsule, they form the parietal epithelium (Figure 2-5). The epithelia cells in contact with the capillaries thicken and develop into **podocytes**, which form the **visceral layer** of Bowman's capsule (see Figures 2-5 to 2-7). The space between the visceral layer and the parietal layer is Bowman's space, which at the urinary pole (i.e., where the proximal tubule joins Bowman's capsule) of the glomerulus becomes the lumen of the proximal tubule.

The endothelial cells of glomerular capillaries are covered by a basement membrane, which is surrounded by **podocytes** (see Figures 2-5 to 2-7). The capillary endothelium, basement membrane, and foot processes of podocytes form the so-called **filtration**

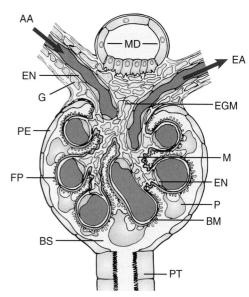

FIGURE 2-5 ■ Anatomy of the glomerulus and juxtaglomerular apparatus. The juxtaglomerular apparatus is composed of the macula densa (*MD*) region of the thick ascending limb, extraglomerular mesangial cells (*EGM*), and renin- and angiotensin II–producing granular cells (*G*) of the afferent arterioles (*AA*). *BM*, Basement membrane; *BS*, Bowman's space; *EA*, efferent arteriole; *EN*, endothelial cell; *FP*, foot processes of podocyte; *M*, mesangial cells between capillaries; *P*, podocyte cell body (visceral cell layer); *PE*, parietal epithelium; *PT*, proximal tubule cell. (*Modified from Kriz W, Kaissling B: Structural organization of the mammalian kidney. In Seldin DW, Giebisch G, editors: The kidney: physiology and pathophysiology, ed 2, New York, 1992, Raven.*)

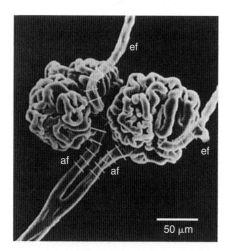

FIGURE 2-4 ■ Scanning electron micrograph of interlobular artery, afferent arteriole (*af*), efferent arteriole (*ef*), and glomerulus. The *white lines* on the afferent and efferent arterioles indicate that they are about 15 to 20 μm wide. (*From Kimura K, Hirata Y, Nanba S, et al: Effects of atrial natriuretic peptide on renal arterioles: morphometric analysis using microvascular casts, Am J Physiol 259:F936, 1990.*)

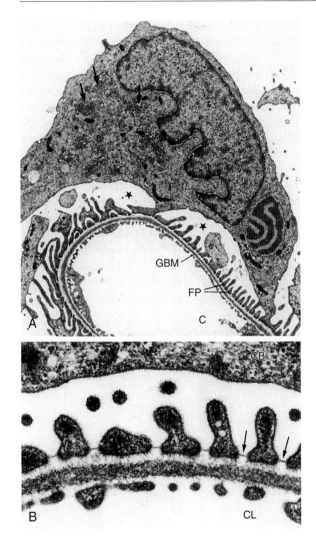

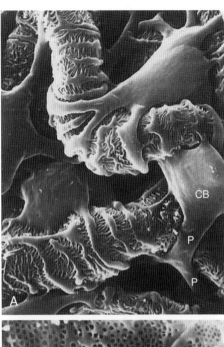

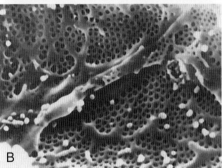

FIGURE 2-6 ■ **A,** Electron micrograph of a podocyte surrounding a glomerular capillary. The cell body of the podocyte contains a large nucleus with three indentations. Cell processes of the podocyte form the interdigitating foot processes (*FP*). The *arrows* in the cytoplasm of the podocyte indicate the well-developed Golgi apparatus, and the *asterisks* indicate Bowman's space. *C,* Capillary lumen; *GBM,* glomerular basement membrane. **B,** Electron micrograph of the filtration barrier of a glomerular capillary. The filtration barrier is composed of three layers: the endothelium, basement membrane, and foot processes of the podocytes. Note the filtration slit diaphragm bridging the floor of the filtration slits (*arrows*). *CL,* capillary lumen. *(From Kriz W, Kaissling B: Structural organization of the mammalian kidney. In Seldin DW, Giebisch G, editors:* The kidney: physiology and pathophysiology, *ed 2, New York, 1992, Raven.)*

FIGURE 2-7 ■ **A,** Scanning electron micrograph showing the outer surface of glomerular capillaries. This view would be seen from Bowman's space. Processes (*P*) of podocytes run from the cell body (*CB*) toward the capillaries, where they ultimately split into foot processes. Interdigitation of the foot processes creates the filtration slits. **B,** Scanning electron micrograph of the inner surface (blood side) of a glomerular capillary. This view would be seen from the lumen of the capillary. The fenestrations of the endothelial cells are seen as small 700-Å holes. The glycocalyx on the endothelial cells cannot be seen because it is removed during the process of tissue preparation. *(From Kriz W, Kaissling B: Structural organization of the mammalian kidney. In Seldin DW, Giebisch G, editors:* The kidney: physiology and pathophysiology, *ed 2, New York, 1992, Raven.)*

barrier (see Figures 2-5 to 2-7). The endothelium is fenestrated (i.e., it contains 700-Å holes where 1 Å = 10^{-10} m) and is freely permeable to water, small solutes (such as Na^+, urea, and glucose), and small proteins but is not permeable to large proteins, red blood cells, white blood cells, or platelets. Because endothelial cells express glycoproteins on their surface, they minimize the filtration into Bowman's space of albumin, the most abundant plasma protein, and small plasma proteins (see Chapter 3). In addition to their role as a barrier to filtration, the endothelial cells synthesize a number of vasoactive substances (e.g., nitric oxide, a vasodilator, and endothelin-1, a vasoconstrictor) that are important in controlling renal plasma flow (see Chapter 3).

The basement membrane, which is a porous matrix of negatively charged proteins, including type IV collagen, laminin, the proteoglycans agrin and perlecan, and fibronectin, is also an important filtration barrier to plasma proteins.

The podocytes have long fingerlike processes that completely encircle the outer surface of the capillaries (see Figures 2-6 and 2-7). The processes of the podocytes interdigitate to cover the basement membrane and are separated by apparent gaps called **filtration slits**. Each filtration slit is bridged by a thin diaphragm, the **filtration slit diaphragm**, which appears as a continuous structure when viewed by electron microscopy (see Figure 2-6). The filtration slit diaphragm is composed of several proteins including **nephrin, NEPH-1**, and **podocin**, along with intracellular proteins that associate with slit diaphragm proteins, including **CD2-AP** and **α-actinin 4** (ACTN4) (Figure 2-8). Filtration slits, which function primarily as a size-selective filter, minimize the filtration of proteins and macromolecules that cross the basement membrane from entering Bowman's space.

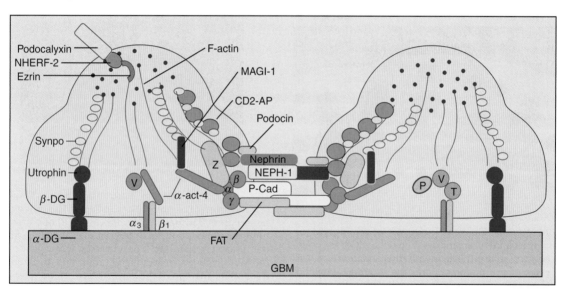

FIGURE 2-8 ■ Anatomy of podocyte foot processes. This figure illustrates the proteins that make up the slit diaphragm between two adjacent foot processes. Nephrin and NEPH-1 are membrane-spanning proteins that have large extracellular domains that interact. Podocin, also a membrane-spanning protein, organizes nephrin and NEPH-1 in specific microdomains in the plasma membrane, which is important for signaling events that determine the structural integrity of podocyte foot processes. Many of the proteins that comprise the slit diaphragm interact with adapter proteins inside the cell, including CD2-AP, bind to the filamentous actin (*F-actin*) cytoskeleton, which in turn binds either directly or indirectly to proteins such as α3β1 and MAGI-1 that interact with proteins expressed by the glomerular basement membrane (*GBM*). α-act-4, α-actinin 4; α3β1, α3β1 integrin; α-DG, α-dystroglycan; CD2-AP, an adapter protein that links nephrin and podocin to intracellular proteins; *FAT*, a protocadherin that organizes actin polymerization; *MAGI-1*, a membrane-associated guanylate kinase protein; *NHERF-2*, Na⁺-H⁺ exchanger regulatory factor 2; *P*, paxillin; *P-Cad*, p-cadherin; *Synpo*, synaptopodin; *T*, talin; *V*, vinculin; *Z*, zona occludens. (*Modified from Mundel P, Shankland SJ: Podocyte biology and response to injury,* J Am Soc Nephrol *13:3005-3015, 2002.*)

AT THE CELLULAR LEVEL

Nephrotic syndrome is produced by a variety of disorders and is characterized by an increase in the permeability of the glomerular capillaries to proteins and by a loss of normal podocyte structure, including effacement (i.e., thinning) of foot processes. The augmented permeability to proteins results in an increase in urinary protein excretion (**proteinuria**). Thus the appearance of proteins in the urine can indicate kidney disease. Hypoproteinemia often develops in persons with this syndrome as a result of the proteinuria. In addition, generalized edema commonly is seen in persons with the nephrotic syndrome (see Chapter 6). Mutations in several genes that encode slit diaphragm proteins (see Figure 2-8), including **nephrin, NEPH-1,** and **podocin,** along with intracellular proteins that associate with slit diaphragm proteins, including **CD2-AP** and **α-actinin 4** (ACTN4), or a knockout of these genes in mice, cause proteinuria and kidney disease. For example, mutations in the nephrin gene (*NPHS1*) lead to abnormal or absent slit diaphragms, causing massive proteinuria and renal failure (i.e., congenital nephrotic syndrome). In addition, mutations in the podocin gene (*NPHS2*) cause autosomal recessive, steroid-resistant nephrotic syndrome. These naturally occurring mutations and knockout studies in mice demonstrate that nephrin, NEPH-1, podocin, CD2-AP, and α-actinin 4 play key roles in podocyte structure and function.

IN THE CLINIC

Alport syndrome is characterized by hematuria (i.e., blood in the urine) and progressive glomerulonephritis (i.e., inflammation of the glomerular capillaries) and accounts for 1% to 2% of all cases of end-stage renal disease. Alport syndrome is caused by mutations in type IV collagen, a major component of the glomerular basement membrane. In about 80% of patients with Alport syndrome, the disease is X-linked with mutations in the *COL4A5* gene. Fifteen percent of patients also have mutations in type IV collagen genes (*COL4A3* and *COL4A4*); six have been identified, but the mode of inheritance is autosomal recessive. The remaining 5% of patients with Alport syndrome have autosomal dominant disease that arises from heterozygous mutations in the *COL4A3* or *COL4A4* genes. In persons with Alport syndrome the glomerular basement membrane becomes irregular in thickness and fails to serve as an effective filtration barrier to blood cells and protein.

Another important component of the renal corpuscle is the **mesangium**, which consists of **mesangial cells** and the **mesangial matrix** (Figure 2-9).

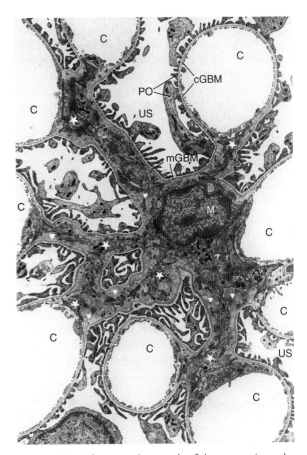

FIGURE 2-9 ■ Electron micrograph of the mesangium, the area between glomerular capillaries containing mesangial cells. *C,* Glomerular capillaries; *cGBM,* capillary glomerular basement membrane surrounded by foot processes of podocytes *(PO)* and endothelial cells; *mGBM,* mesangial glomerular basement membrane surrounded by foot processes of podocytes and mesangial cells; *M,* mesangial cell that gives rise to several processes, some marked by asterisks; *US,* urinary space. Note the extensive extracellular matrix surrounded by mesangial cells (marked by *arrowheads*). (Magnification ×4100.) *(From Kriz W, Kaissling B: Structural organization of the mammalian kidney. In Seldin DW, Giebisch G, editors:* The kidney: physiology and pathophysiology, *ed 2, New York, 1992, Raven.)*

AT THE CELLULAR LEVEL

Mesangial cells are involved in the development of **immune complex–mediated glomerular disease**. Because the glomerular basement membrane does not completely surround all glomerular capillaries (see Figure 2-9), some immune complexes can enter the mesangial area without crossing the glomerular basement membrane. Accumulation of immune complexes induces the infiltration of inflammatory cells into the mesangium and promotes the production of proinflammatory cytokines and autacoids by cells in the mesangium. These cytokines and autacoids enhance the inflammatory response. This inflammatory response can lead to cell death, scarring and eventually obliterating the glomerulus.

Mesangial cells, which possess many properties of smooth muscle cells, provide structural support for the glomerular capillaries, secrete the extracellular matrix, exhibit phagocytic activity that removes macromolecules from the mesangium, and secrete prostaglandins and proinflammatory cytokines. Because they also contract and are adjacent to glomerular capillaries, mesangial cells may influence the glomerular filtration rate (GFR) by regulating blood flow through the glomerular capillaries or by altering the capillary surface area (see Chapter 3). Mesangial cells located outside the glomerulus (between the afferent and efferent arterioles) are called **extraglomerular mesangial cells**.

Ultrastructure of the Juxtaglomerular Apparatus

The **juxtaglomerular apparatus** (JGA) is one component of an important feedback mechanism, the tubuloglomerular feedback mechanism, that is described in Chapter 3. The following structures make up the JGA (see Figure 2-5):

1. The **macula densa** of the thick ascending limb
2. The extraglomerular mesangial cells
3. The renin- and angiotensin II–producing **granular cells** of the afferent arteriole

The cells of the macula densa represent a morphologically distinct region of the thick ascending limb. This region passes through the angle formed by the afferent and efferent arterioles of the same nephron. The cells of the macula densa are in contact with the extraglomerular mesangial cells and the granular cells of the afferent arterioles. Granular cells of the afferent arterioles are derived from metanephric mesenchymal cells. They contain smooth muscle myofilaments and they manufacture, store, and release **renin**. Renin is involved in the formation of **angiotensin II** and ultimately in the secretion of **aldosterone** (see Chapters 4 and 6). The JGA is one component of the tubuloglomerular feedback mechanism that is involved in the autoregulation of renal blood flow and the GFR (see Chapter 3).

Innervation of the Kidneys

Renal nerves regulate renal blood flow, GFR, and salt and water reabsorption by the nephron. The nerve supply to the kidneys consists of sympathetic nerve fibers that originate in the celiac plexus. No parasympathetic innervation occurs. Adrenergic fibers that innervate the kidneys release norepinephrine. The adrenergic fibers lie adjacent to the smooth muscle cells of the major branches of the renal artery (the interlobar, arcuate, and interlobular arteries) and the afferent and efferent arterioles. Moreover, sympathetic nerves innervate the renin-producing granular cells of the afferent arterioles. Renin secretion is stimulated by increased sympathetic activity. Nerve fibers also innervate the proximal tubule, loop of Henle, distal tubule, and collecting duct; activation of these nerves enhances Na^+ reabsorption by these nephron segments.

SUMMARY

1. The functional unit of the kidneys is the nephron, which consists of a renal corpuscle (i.e., glomerulus), proximal tubule, Henle's loop, distal tubule, and collecting duct.
2. Cilia play an important role in mechanosensation and chemosensation in nephron cells. Mutations in *PKD1* and *PKD2*, which encode proteins that associate with the central cilium and mediate Ca^{++} entry into cells, cause polycystic kidney disease.
3. The first step in urine formation begins with the passive movement of a plasma ultrafiltrate from the glomerular capillaries into Bowman's space. The term *ultrafiltration* refers to the passive movement of a plasmalike fluid that has a very low concentration of proteins from the glomerular capillaries into Bowman's space. The endothelial cells of glomerular capillaries are covered by a glycocalyx and sit on a basement membrane, which is surrounded by podocytes. The capillary endothelium, basement membrane, and foot processes of podocytes form the so-called filtration barrier.
4. The filtration slit diaphragm between foot processes of podocytes is composed of several proteins, including nephrin, NEPH-1, podocin, and intracellular proteins that associate with slit diaphragm proteins, including podocin, CD2-AP, and α-actinin 4 (ACTN4). Mutations in these genes cause the nephrotic syndrome, which is associated with proteinuria and ultimately renal failure.
5. The JGA is one component of an important feedback mechanism (i.e., tubuloglomerular feedback) that regulates renal blood flow and the glomerular filtration rate. The structures that make up the JGA include the macula densa, extraglomerular mesangial cells, and renin-producing granular cells.
6. The kidneys are innervated by sympathetic nerves that regulate renal blood flow, GFR, and salt and water reabsorption by the nephron.

KEY WORDS AND CONCEPTS

- Cortex
- Medulla
- Nephrons
- Renal pyramids
- Calyx
- Pelvis
- Major calyces
- Minor calyces
- Urinary bladder
- Interlobar artery
- Arcuate artery
- Interlobular artery
- Afferent arteriole
- Glomerulus
- Efferent arteriole
- Renal corpuscle
- Bowman's capsule
- Proximal tubule
- Henle's loop
- Descending thin limb (of Henle)
- Ascending thin limb (of Henle)
- Thick ascending limb (of Henle)
- Macula densa
- Distal tubule
- Cortical collecting duct
- Outer medullary collecting duct
- Inner medullary collecting duct
- Brush border
- Principal cells
- Intercalated cells
- Superficial nephrons
- Juxtamedullary nephrons
- Vasa recta
- Collecting ducts
- Podocytes
- Visceral layer
- Parietal layer
- Bowman's space
- Filtration barrier
- Filtration slits
- Filtration slit diaphragm
- Nephrin
- NEPH-1
- Podocin
- CD2-AP
- α-actinin 4 (ACTN4)
- Mesangium

- Mesangial cells
- Mesangial matrix
- Extraglomerular mesangial cells (lacis cells)
- Juxtaglomerular apparatus (JGA)
- Proteinuria
- Nephrotic syndrome

SELF-STUDY PROBLEMS

1. Describe the gross anatomic features of the kidney.
2. Identify the five segments of the nephron.
3. Describe the blood supply to the kidneys.
4. What is the renal corpuscle?
5. Describe the structures that form the filtration barriers to plasma proteins in the glomerulus.
6. What structures are parts of the JGA?
7. What is the functional significance of the JGA?
8. What is the mesangium, and what is its functional significance?
9. Which nerves innervate the kidneys, and which functions are regulated by renal nerves?

3

GLOMERULAR FILTRATION AND RENAL BLOOD FLOW

OBJECTIVES

Upon completion of this chapter, the student should be able to answer the following questions:

1. How can the concepts of mass balance be used to measure the glomerular filtration rate?

2. Why can inulin clearance and creatinine clearance be used to measure the glomerular filtration rate?

3. Why is the plasma creatinine concentration used clinically to monitor the glomerular filtration rate?

4. What are the elements of the glomerular filtration barrier, and how do they determine how much protein enters Bowman's space?

5. What Starling forces are involved in the formation of the glomerular ultrafiltrate, and how do changes in each force affect the glomerular filtration rate?

6. What is autoregulation of renal blood flow and the glomerular filtration rate, and which factors and hormones are responsible for autoregulation?

7. Which hormones regulate renal blood flow?

8. Why do hormones influence renal blood flow despite autoregulation?

The first step in the formation of urine by the kidneys is the production of an ultrafiltrate of plasma across the filtration barrier. The process of glomerular filtration and regulation of the glomerular filtration rate (GFR) and renal blood flow (RBF) are discussed in this chapter. The concept of renal clearance, which is the theoretical basis for the measurements of GFR and RBF, also is presented.

RENAL CLEARANCE

The concept of **renal clearance** is based on the Fick principle (i.e., mass balance or conservation of mass).

Figure 3-1 illustrates the various factors required to describe the mass balance relationships of a kidney. The renal artery is the single input source to the kidney, whereas the renal vein and ureter constitute the two output routes. The following equation defines the mass balance relationship:

$$P_x^a \times RPF^a = (P_x^v \times RPF^v) + (U_x \times \dot{V}) \qquad (3\text{-}1)$$

where P_x^a and P_x^v are concentrations of substance x in the renal artery and renal vein plasma, respectively, RPF^a and RPF^v are **renal plasma flow** (RPF) rates in the artery and vein, respectively, U_x is the concentration of x in the urine, and $\dot{V}$ is the urine flow rate.

This relationship permits the quantification of the amount of x excreted in the urine versus the amount returned to the systemic circulation in the renal venous

27

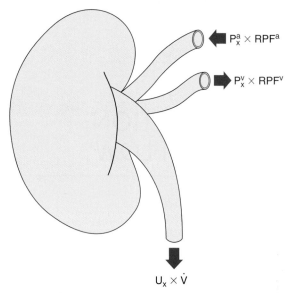

FIGURE 3-1 ■ Mass balance relationships for the kidney. P_x^a and P_x^v, Concentrations of substance x in the renal artery and renal vein plasma, respectively; RPF^a and RPF^v, renal plasma flow rates in the artery and vein, respectively; U_x, concentration of x in the urine; $\dot{V}$, urine flow rate.

blood. Thus for any substance that is neither synthesized nor metabolized by the kidneys, the amount that enters the kidneys is equal to the amount that leaves the kidneys in the urine plus the amount that leaves the kidneys in the renal venous blood.

The principle of renal clearance emphasizes the excretory function of the kidneys; it considers only the rate at which a substance is excreted into the urine and not its rate of return to the systemic circulation in the renal vein. Therefore in terms of mass balance (equation 3-1), the urinary excretion rate of x ($U_x \times \dot{V}$) is proportional to the plasma concentration of x (P_x^a):

$$P_x^a \propto U_x \times \dot{V} \qquad (3\text{-}2)$$

To equate the urinary excretion rate of x to its renal arterial plasma concentration, it is necessary to determine the rate at which x is removed from the plasma by the kidneys. This removal rate is the clearance (C_x).

$$P_x^a \times C_x = U_x \times \dot{V} \qquad (3\text{-}3)$$

If equation 3-3 is rearranged and the concentration of x in the renal artery plasma (P_x^a) is assumed to be identical to its concentration in a plasma sample from any peripheral blood vessel, the following relationship is obtained:

$$C_x = \frac{U_x \times \dot{V}}{P_x^a} \qquad (3\text{-}4)$$

Clearance has the dimensions of volume/time, and it represents a volume of plasma from which all the substance has been removed and excreted into the urine per unit time. The last point is best illustrated by considering the following example. If a substance is present in the urine at a concentration of 100 mg/mL and the urine flow rate is 1 mL/min, the excretion rate for this substance is calculated as follows:

$$\text{Excretion rate} = U_x \times \dot{V} = 100 \text{ mg/mL} \times (1 \text{ mL/min})$$
$$= 100 \text{ mg/min} \qquad (3\text{-}5)$$

If this substance is present in the plasma at a concentration of 1 mg/mL, its clearance according to equation 3-4 is as follows:

$$C_x = \frac{U_x \times \dot{V}}{P_x^a} = \frac{100 \text{ mg/min}}{1 \text{ mg/mL}} = 100 \text{ mL/min} \qquad (3\text{-}6)$$

In other words, 100 mL of plasma are completely cleared of substance x each minute. The definition of clearance as a volume of plasma from which all the substance has been removed and excreted into the urine per unit time is somewhat misleading because it is not a real volume of plasma; rather, it is an idealized volume.* The concept of clearance is important because it can be used to measure the GFR and RPF and determine whether a substance is reabsorbed or secreted along the nephron.

---

*For most substances cleared from the plasma by the kidneys, only a portion is actually removed and excreted in a single pass through the kidneys.

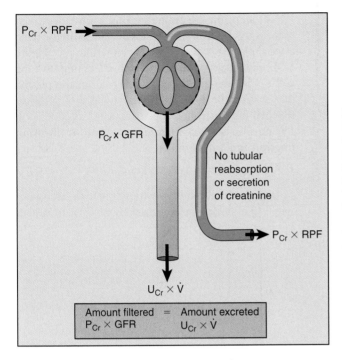

FIGURE 3-2 ■ Renal handling of creatinine. Creatinine is freely filtered across the filtration barrier and is, to a first approximation, not reabsorbed, secreted, or metabolized by the nephron. Note that not all the creatinine coming to the kidney in the renal artery is filtered (normally, 15% to 20% of plasma creatinine is filtered). The portion that is not filtered is returned to the systemic circulation in the renal vein. *GFR*, Glomerular filtration rate; P_{Cr}, plasma creatinine concentration; *RPF*, renal plasma flow; U_{Cr}, urinary concentration of creatinine; $\dot{V}$, urine flow rate.

Glomerular Filtration Rate

The GFR of the kidney is equal to the sum of the filtration rates of all functioning nephrons. Thus it is an index of kidney function. A decrease in GFR generally means that kidney disease is progressing, whereas movement toward a normal GFR generally suggests recuperation. Thus knowledge of the patient's GFR is essential in evaluating the severity and course of kidney disease.

Creatinine, which is a byproduct of skeletal muscle creatine phosphate metabolism, can be used to measure the GFR.* Creatinine is freely filtered across the glomerular filtration barrier into Bowman's space, and to a first approximation it is not reabsorbed, secreted, or metabolized by the cells of the nephron. Accordingly, the amount of creatinine excreted in the urine per minute equals the amount of creatinine filtered across the filtration barrier each minute (Figure 3-2):

$$\text{Amount filtered} = \text{Amount excreted}$$
$$\text{GFR} \times P_{Cr} = U_{Cr} \times \dot{V} \tag{3-7}$$

---

*Under experimental conditions GFR is usually measured using inulin, a polyfructose molecule (molecular weight ≈5000). However, because inulin is not produced by the body and must be infused, it is not used in most clinical situations.

where P_{Cr} is plasma concentration of creatinine, U_{Cr} is urine concentration of creatinine, and $\dot{V}$ is the urine flow rate.

If equation 3-7 is solved for the GFR:

$$\text{GFR} = \frac{U_{cr} \times \dot{V}}{P_{cr}} \tag{3-8}$$

This equation is the same form as that for clearance (equation 3-4). Thus the clearance of creatinine provides a means for determining the GFR. Clearance has the dimensions of volume/time, and it represents a volume of plasma from which all the substance has been removed and excreted into the urine per unit time.

Creatinine is not the only substance that can be used to measure the GFR. Any substance that meets the following criteria can serve as an appropriate marker for the measurement of GFR. The substance must:

1. Be freely filtered across the filtration barrier into Bowman's space
2. Not be reabsorbed or secreted by the nephron
3. Not be metabolized or produced by the kidney
4. Not alter the GFR

IN THE CLINIC

Creatinine is used to estimate GFR in clinical practice. It is synthesized at a relatively constant rate, and the amount produced is proportional to the muscle mass. However, creatinine is not a perfect substance for measuring GFR because it is secreted to a small extent by the organic cation secretory system in the proximal tubule (see Chapter 4). The error introduced by this secretory component is approximately 10%. Thus the amount of creatinine excreted in the urine exceeds the amount expected from filtration alone by 10%. However, the method used to measure the plasma creatinine concentration (P_{Cr}) overestimates the true value by 10%. Consequently, the two errors cancel, and in most clinical situations creatinine clearance provides a reasonably accurate measure of the GFR.

IN THE CLINIC

A decrease in GFR may be the first and only clinical sign of kidney disease. Thus measuring the GFR is important when kidney disease is suspected. A 50% loss of functioning nephrons reduces the GFR by only about 25%. The decline in GFR is not 50% because the remaining nephrons compensate. Because measurements of GFR are cumbersome, the National Institute of Diabetes and Digestive and Kidney Diseases, the National Kidney Foundation, and American Society of Nephrology all recommend estimating GFR from the plasma creatinine concentration (P_{Cr}), which is inversely related to the GFR (Figure 3-3). However, as Figure 3-3 shows, the GFR must decline substantially before an increase in the P_{Cr} can be detected in a clinical setting. For example, a decrease in GFR from 120 to 100 mL/min is accompanied by an increase in the P_{Cr} from 1.0 to 1.2 mg/dL. This situation does not appear to represent a significant change in the P_{Cr}, but the GFR actually has fallen by almost 20%. Figure 3-4 illustrates how a decrease in GFR by 50% causes a doubling of P_{Cr}. Initially, when GFR is reduced, the excretion of creatinine declines because the amount of creatinine that is filtered (i.e., GFR × P_{Cr}) and excreted (i.e., U_{cr} × $\dot{V}$) decreases. Because creatinine production is constant and its production transiently exceeds filtration and excretion, creatinine accumulates in the extracellular fluid until the amount filtered equals the amount produced (i.e., GFR × P_{Cr} = production). At this point, P_{Cr} remains stable but elevated.

Not all of the creatinine (or other substances used to measure the GFR) that enters the kidney in the renal arterial plasma is filtered at the glomerulus (see Figure 3-2). Likewise, not all of the plasma coming into the kidneys is filtered. Although nearly all of the plasma that enters the kidneys in the renal artery passes through a glomerulus, approximately 10% does not. The portion of filtered plasma is termed the **filtration fraction** and is determined as:

$$\text{Filtration fraction} = \text{GFR}/\text{RPF} \qquad (3\text{-}9)$$

Under normal conditions, the filtration fraction averages 0.15 to 0.20, which means that only 15% to 20% of

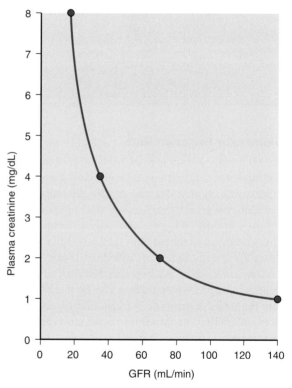

FIGURE 3-3 ■ Relationship between glomerular filtration rate (GFR) and plasma [creatinine] (P_{Cr}). The amount of creatinine filtered is equal to the amount excreted; thus GFR × P_{Cr} = U_{Cr} × $\dot{V}$, where U_{Cr} is urinary concentration of creatinine and $\dot{V}$ is urine flow rate. Because the production of creatinine is constant, excretion must be constant to maintain creatinine balance. Therefore if the GFR falls from 120 to 60 mL/min, the P_{Cr} must increase from 1 to 2 mg/dL to keep the filtration of creatinine and its excretion equal to the production rate.

the plasma that enters the glomerulus is actually filtered. The remaining 80% to 85% continues through the glomerular capillaries and into the efferent arterioles, peritubular capillaries, and the vasa recta. It is finally returned to the systemic circulation in the renal vein.

GLOMERULAR FILTRATION

The first step in the formation of urine is ultrafiltration of the plasma by the glomerulus. In healthy adults, the GFR ranges from 90 to 140 mL/min for men and from 80 to 125 mL/min for women. Thus in 24 hours as much as 180 L of plasma is filtered by the glomeruli. The plasma ultrafiltrate is devoid of cellular elements (i.e., red and white blood cells and platelets) and has a very low concentration of proteins. The concentrations of salts and of organic molecules, such as glucose and amino acids, are similar in the plasma and ultrafiltrate. Starling forces drive ultrafiltration across the glomerular capillaries, and changes in these forces alter the GFR. The GFR and RPF normally are held within very narrow ranges by a phenomenon called **autoregulation**. The next sections of this chapter review the composition of the glomerular filtrate, the dynamics of its formation, and the relationship between RPF and GFR. In addition, the factors that contribute to the autoregulation and regulation of GFR and RBF are discussed.

Determinants of Ultrafiltrate Composition

The glomerular filtration barrier determines the composition of the plasma ultrafiltrate. It restricts the filtration of molecules primarily on the basis of size. In general, molecules with a radius smaller than 20 Å are

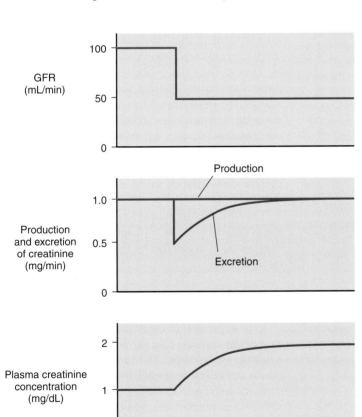

FIGURE 3-4 ▪ Effect of a 50% decrease in glomerular filtration rate (*GFR*) on plasma creatinine concentration. *(Modified from Boron W, Boulpaep EL: Textbook of medical physiology, ed 2, Philadelphia, 2009, Saunders Elsevier.)*

IN THE CLINIC

A reduction in GFR in disease states is most often due to decreases in the ultrafiltration coefficient (K_f) because of the loss of filtration surface area. The GFR also changes in pathophysiologic conditions because of changes in the hydrostatic pressure in the glomerular capillary (P_{GC}), oncotic pressure in the glomerular capillary (π_{GC}), and hydrostatic pressure in Bowman's space (P_{BS}).

1. Changes in K_f: An increased K_f enhances the GFR, whereas a decreased K_f reduces the GFR. Some kidney diseases reduce the K_f by decreasing the number of filtering glomeruli (i.e., diminished surface area). Some drugs and hormones that dilate the glomerular arterioles also increase the K_f. Similarly, drugs and hormones that constrict the glomerular arterioles also decrease the K_f.
2. Changes in P_{GC}: With decreased renal perfusion, the GFR declines because the P_{GC} decreases. As previously discussed, a reduction in the P_{GC} is caused by a decline in renal arterial pressure, an increase in afferent arteriolar resistance, or a decrease in efferent arteriolar resistance.
3. Changes in π_{GC}: An inverse relationship exists between the π_{GC} and the GFR. Alterations in the π_{GC} result from changes in protein synthesis outside the kidneys. In addition, protein loss in the urine caused by some renal diseases can lead to a decrease in the plasma protein concentration and thus in the π_{GC}.
4. Changes in P_{BS}: An increased P_{BS} reduces the GFR, whereas a decreased P_{BS} enhances the GFR. Acute obstruction of the urinary tract (e.g., a kidney stone occluding the ureter) increases the P_{BS}.

filtered freely, molecules larger than 42 Å are not filtered, and molecules between 20 and 42 Å are filtered to various degrees. For example, serum albumin, an anionic protein that has an effective molecular radius of 35.5 Å, is filtered poorly. Because the filtered albumin and other small proteins normally are reabsorbed avidly by the proximal tubule, almost no protein appears in the urine of persons with normal renal function.*

---

*Some studies suggest that the filtration of anionic proteins is affected by the presence of negatively charged glycoproteins on the surfaces of the glomerular filtration barrier. These charged glycoproteins repel similarly charged molecules. Because most plasma proteins are negatively charged, the negative charge on the filtration barrier may restrict the filtration of anionic proteins that have a molecular radius of 20 to 42 Å.

Dynamics of Ultrafiltration

The forces responsible for the glomerular filtration of plasma are the same as those in all capillary beds (see Chapter 1). Ultrafiltration occurs because the Starling forces (i.e., hydrostatic and oncotic pressures) drive fluid from the lumen of glomerular capillaries, across the filtration barrier, and into Bowman's space (Figure 3-5). The hydrostatic pressure in the glomerular capillary (P_{GC}) is oriented to promote the movement of fluid from the glomerular capillary into Bowman's space. Because the reflection coefficient (σ) for proteins across the glomerular capillary is essentially 1, the glomerular ultrafiltrate has a very low concentration of proteins, and the oncotic pressure in Bowman's space (π_{BS}) is near zero. Therefore P_{GC} is the only force that favors filtration. The hydrostatic pressure in Bowman's space (P_{BS}) and the oncotic pressure in the glomerular capillary (π_{GC}) oppose filtration.

As shown in Figure 3-5, a net ultrafiltration pressure (P_{UF}) of 17 mm Hg exists at the afferent end of the glomerulus, whereas at the efferent end, it is 8 mm Hg (where $P_{UF} = P_{GC} - P_{BS} - \pi_{GC}$). Two additional points concerning Starling forces and this pressure change are important. First, P_{GC} decreases slightly along the length of the capillary because of the resistance to flow. Second, π_{GC} increases along the length of the glomerular capillary. Because water is filtered and protein is retained in the glomerular capillary, the protein concentration in the capillary rises, and π_{GC} increases.

The GFR is proportional to the sum of the Starling forces that exist across the capillaries $[(P_{GC} - P_{BS}) - \sigma(\pi_{GC} - \pi_{BS})]$ multiplied by the ultrafiltration coefficient (K_f). That is:

$$\text{GFR} = K_f \left[(P_{GC} - P_{BS}) - \sigma(\pi_{GC} - \pi_{BS}) \right] \qquad (3\text{-}10)$$

K_f is the product of the intrinsic permeability of the glomerular capillary and the glomerular surface area available for filtration. The rate of glomerular filtration is considerably greater in glomerular capillaries than in systemic capillaries, mainly because K_f is approximately 100 times greater in glomerular capillaries. Furthermore, the P_{GC} is approximately twice as great as the hydrostatic pressure in systemic capillaries.

The GFR can be altered by changing K_f or by changing any of the Starling forces. In healthy

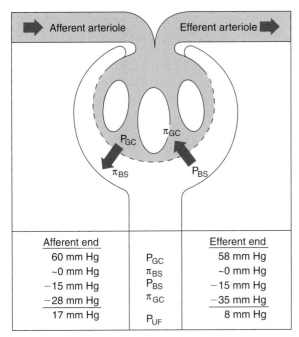

Afferent arteriole		Efferent arteriole

Afferent end		Efferent end
60 mm Hg	P_{GC}	58 mm Hg
~0 mm Hg	π_{BS}	~0 mm Hg
−15 mm Hg	P_{BS}	−15 mm Hg
−28 mm Hg	π_{GC}	−35 mm Hg
17 mm Hg	P_{UF}	8 mm Hg

FIGURE 3-5 ■ Idealized glomerular capillary and the Starling forces across it. The reflection coefficient (σ) for protein across the glomerular capillary is 1. P_{BS}, Hydrostatic pressure in Bowman's space; P_{GC}, hydrostatic pressure in the glomerular capillary; P_{UF}, net ultrafiltration pressure; π_{GC}, oncotic pressure in the glomerular capillary; π_{BS}, oncotic pressure in Bowman's space. The negative signs for P_{BS} and π_{GC} indicate that these forces oppose the formation of the glomerular filtrate.

persons, the GFR is regulated by alterations in the P_{GC} that are mediated mainly by changes in afferent or efferent arteriolar resistance. P_{GC} is affected in three ways:

1. *Changes in afferent arteriolar resistance*: a decrease in resistance increases the P_{GC} and GFR, whereas an increase in resistance decreases the P_{GC} and GFR.
2. *Changes in efferent arteriolar resistance*: a decrease in resistance reduces the P_{GC} and GFR, whereas an increase in resistance elevates the P_{GC} and GFR.
3. *Changes in renal artery pressure*: an increase in blood pressure transiently increases the P_{GC} (which enhances the GFR), whereas a decrease in blood pressure transiently decreases the P_{GC} (which reduces the GFR).

RENAL BLOOD FLOW

Blood flow (~1.25 L/min) through the kidneys serves several important functions. This blood flow:

1. Indirectly determines the GFR
2. Modifies the rate of solute and water reabsorption by the proximal tubule
3. Participates in the concentration and dilution of urine
4. Delivers oxygen, nutrients, and hormones to the cells of the nephron and returns carbon dioxide and reabsorbed fluid and solutes to the general circulation
5. Delivers substrates for excretion in the urine

Blood flow through any organ may be represented by the following equation:

$$Q = \frac{\Delta P}{R} \tag{3-11}$$

where Q is blood flow, ΔP is mean arterial pressure minus venous pressure for that organ, and R is resistance to flow through that organ.

Accordingly, RBF is equal to the pressure difference between the renal artery and the renal vein divided by the renal vascular resistance:

$$RBF = \frac{\text{Aortic pressure} - \text{Renal venous pressure}}{\text{Renal vascular resistance}} \tag{3-12}$$

The interlobular artery, afferent arteriole, and efferent arteriole are the major resistance vessels in the kidneys and determine renal vascular resistance. Like most other organs, the kidneys regulate their blood flow by adjusting the vascular resistance in response to changes in arterial pressure. As shown in Figure 3-6, these adjustments are so precise that blood flow remains relatively constant as arterial blood pressure fluctuates between 90 and 180 mm Hg. The GFR also is regulated over the same range of arterial pressures. The phenomenon whereby RBF and GFR are maintained at a relatively constant level, namely **autoregulation**, is achieved by changes in vascular resistance, mainly through the afferent arterioles of the kidneys. Because both the GFR and RBF are regulated over the same range of pressures and because RBF is an important determinant of GFR, it is not surprising that the same mechanisms regulate both flows.

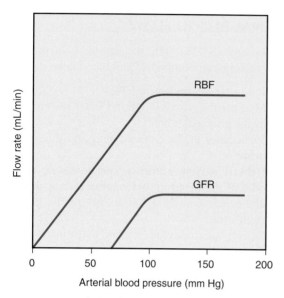

FIGURE 3-6 ■ Relationship between arterial blood pressure and renal blood flow (*RBF*) and between arterial blood pressure and glomerular filtration rate (*GFR*). Autoregulation maintains the GFR and RBF at a relatively constant level as blood pressure fluctuates between 90 and 180 mm Hg.

Chapter 2) and converted into a signal or signals that affect afferent arteriolar resistance and thus the GFR. When the GFR increases and causes the NaCl concentration of tubular fluid at the macula densa to rise, more NaCl enters macula densa cells. This process leads to an increase in the formation and release of adenosine triphosphate (ATP) and adenosine, a metabolite of ATP, by macula densa cells, which causes vasoconstriction of the afferent arteriole. Vasoconstriction of the afferent arteriole returns the GFR to normal levels. In contrast, when the GFR and NaCl concentration of tubule fluid decrease, less NaCl enters macula densa cells, and the production and release of ATP and adenosine decline. The decrease in ATP and adenosine causes vasodilation of the afferent arteriole, which returns the GFR to normal. Nitric oxide (NO), a vasodilator produced by the macula densa, attenuates tubuloglomerular feedback, whereas angiotensin II enhances tubuloglomerular feedback. Thus the macula densa may release both vasoconstrictors (e.g., ATP and adenosine) and a vasodilator (e.g., NO), which oppose each other's action at the level of the afferent arteriole. Production and release of

Two mechanisms are responsible for the autoregulation of RBF and GFR: one mechanism that responds to changes in arterial pressure and another that responds to changes in the sodium chloride (NaCl) concentration of tubular fluid. Both mechanisms regulate the tone of the afferent arteriole. The pressure-sensitive mechanism, the so-called **myogenic mechanism**, is related to an intrinsic property of vascular smooth muscle: the tendency to contract when it is stretched. Accordingly, when the arterial pressure rises and the renal afferent arteriole is stretched, the smooth muscle contracts. Because the increase in the resistance of the arteriole offsets the increase in pressure, RBF and therefore GFR remain constant (i.e., RBF is constant if $\Delta P/R$ is kept constant [see equation 3-11]).

The second mechanism responsible for the autoregulation of GFR and RBF is the NaCl concentration–dependent mechanism known as **tubuloglomerular feedback** (Figure 3-7). This mechanism involves a feedback loop in which the NaCl concentration of tubular fluid is sensed by the macula densa of the **juxtaglomerular apparatus** (JGA; see Figure 2-5 in

AT THE CELLULAR LEVEL

Tubuloglomerular feedback is absent in mice that do not express the adenosine receptor A1. This finding underscores the importance of adenosine signaling in tubuloglomerular feedback. Studies have shown that when GFR increases and causes NaCl concentration of tubular fluid at the macula densa to rise, more NaCl enters cells through the Na^+-K^+-$2Cl^-$ cotransporter (NKCC2) located in the apical plasma membrane (see Chapter 4). Increased intracellular [NaCl] in turn stimulates the release of adenosine triphosphate (ATP) through ATP-conducting ion channels located in the basolateral membrane of macula densa cells. In addition, adenosine production is enhanced. Adenosine binds to A1 receptors and ATP binds to P2X receptors located on the plasma membrane of smooth muscle cells in the afferent arteriole. Both hormones increase intracellular $[Ca^{++}]$, which causes vasoconstriction of the afferent artery and therefore a decrease in GFR. Although adenosine is a vasodilator in most other vascular beds, it constricts the afferent arteriole in the kidney.

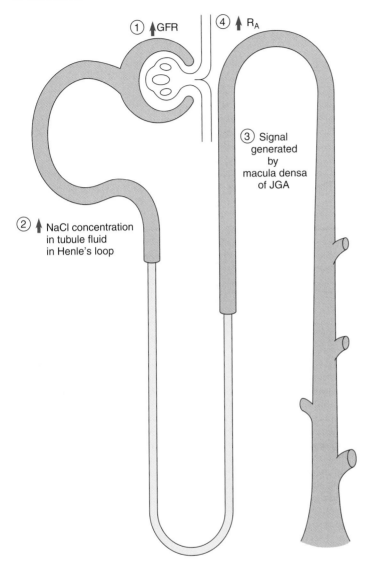

① ↑GFR

④ ↑R_A

③ Signal
generated
by
macula densa
of JGA

② ↑ NaCl concentration
in tubule fluid
in Henle's loop

FIGURE 3-7 ■ Tubuloglomerular feedback. An increase in the glomerular filtration rate (*GFR*) (*1*) increases sodium chloride (*NaCl*) concentration in tubule fluid in the loop of Henle (*2*), which is sensed by the macula densa and converted into a signal (*3*) that increases the resistance of the afferent arteriole (R_A) (*4*), which decreases the GFR. *JGA,* Juxtaglomerular apparatus. *(Modified from Cogan MG: Fluid and electrolytes: physiology and pathophysiology, Norwalk, CT, 1991, Appleton & Lange.)*

vasoconstrictors and vasodilators ensure exquisite control over tubuloglomerular feedback.

Figure 3-8 illustrates the role of the macula densa in controlling the secretion of renin by the granular cells of the afferent arteriole. This aspect of JGA function is considered in detail in Chapter 6.

Because animals engage in many activities that can change arterial blood pressure (e.g., changes in posture, mild to moderate exercise, and sleep), mechanisms that maintain RBF and GFR at relatively constant levels despite changes in arterial pressure are highly desirable. If the GFR and RBF were to rise or fall suddenly in proportion to changes in blood pressure, urinary excretion of fluid and solute also would change suddenly. Such changes in water and solute excretion without comparable changes in intake would alter the fluid and electrolyte balance (the reason for which is discussed in Chapter 6). Accordingly, autoregulation of the GFR and RBF provides an effective means for uncoupling renal function from arterial pressure, and

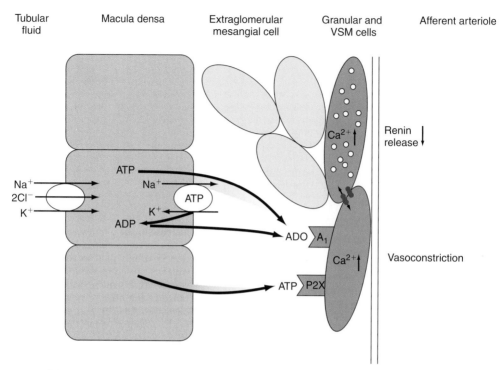

FIGURE 3-8 ■ Cellular mechanism whereby an increase in the delivery of sodium chloride (*NaCl*) to the macula densa causes vasoconstriction of the afferent arteriole of the same nephron (i.e., tubuloglomerular feedback). An increase in the glomerular filtration rate (GFR) elevates the [NaCl] in tubule fluid at the macula densa. This action in turn enhances NaCl uptake across the apical cell membrane of macula densa cells through the Na^+-K^+-$2Cl^-$ (NKCC2) symporter, which leads to an increase in adenosine triphosphate (*ATP*) and adenosine (*ADO*). ATP binds to P2X receptors and adenosine binds to adenosine A1 receptors in the plasma membrane of smooth muscle cells surrounding the afferent arteriole, both of which increase intracellular [Ca^{++}]. The rise in [Ca^{++}] induces vasoconstriction of the afferent arteriole, returning GFR to normal levels. Note that ATP and ADO also inhibit renin release by granular cells in the afferent arteriole. This action, too, results from an increase in intracellular [Ca^{++}] reflecting electrical coupling of the granular and vascular smooth muscle (*VSM*) cells. When GFR is reduced, [NaCl] in tubule fluid decreases, as does NaCl uptake into macula densa cells. This decrease in turn decreases ATP and ADO release, which decreases intracellular [Ca^{++}] and thereby increases GFR and stimulates renin release by granular cells. In addition, a decrease in NaCl entry into macula densa cells enhances the production of prostaglandin E_2, which also stimulates renin secretion by granular cells. As discussed in detail in Chapters 4 and 6, renin increases plasma angiotensin II, a hormone that enhances NaCl and water retention by the kidneys. *ADP*, adenosine diphosphate. (*Modified from Persson AEG, Ollerstam R, Liu R et al: Mechanisms for macula densa cell release of renin,* Acta Physiol Scand *181:471-474, 2004.*)

it ensures that fluid and solute excretion remain constant when the extracellular fluid volume is normal (see Chapter 1).

Three points concerning autoregulation should be noted:

1. Autoregulation is absent when arterial pressure is less than 90 mm Hg.
2. Autoregulation is not perfect; RBF and GFR do change slightly as the arterial blood pressure varies.

3. Despite autoregulation, RBF and GFR can be changed by certain hormones and by changes in sympathetic nerve activity (Table 3-1).

REGULATION OF RENAL BLOOD FLOW AND GLOMERULAR FILTRATION RATE

Several factors and hormones affect GFR and RBF (see Table 3-1). As discussed, the myogenic mechanism and tubuloglomerular feedback play key roles in

TABLE 3-1

Hormones that Influence Glomerular Filtration Rate and Renal Blood Flow

	STIMULUS	EFFECT ON GFR	EFFECT ON RBF
Vasoconstrictors			
Sympathetic nerves	↓ ECFV	↓	↓
Angiotensin II*	↓ ECFV	↓	↓
Endothelin	↑ Stretch, AII, bradykinin, epinephrine, ↓ ECFV	↓	↓
Vasodilators			
Prostaglandins (PGE$_1$, PGE$_2$, PGI$_2$)	↓ ECFV, ↑ shear	No change/↑	↑
Nitric oxide	Stress, AII ↑ shear stress, acetylcholine, histamine, bradykinin, ATP	↑	↑
Bradykinin	Prostaglandins, ↓ ACE	↑	↑
Natriuretic peptides (ANP, BNP)	↑ ECFV	↑	No change

*These effects of angiotensin II are evident with concentrations that constrict the afferent and efferent arterioles.
ACE, Angiotensin-converting enzyme; *AII,* angiotensin II; *ANP,* atrial natriuretic peptide; *ATP,* adenosine triphosphate; *BNP,* brain natriuretic peptide; *ECFV,* extracellular fluid volume; *GFR,* glomerular filtration rate; *PGE,* prostaglandin E; *PGI$_2$,* prostacyclin; *RBF,* renal blood flow.

IN THE CLINIC

Persons with **renal artery stenosis** (narrowing of the artery lumen) caused by atherosclerosis, for example, can have an elevated systemic arterial blood pressure mediated by stimulation of the renin-angiotensin system (see Chapter 6). Pressure in the renal artery proximal to the stenosis is increased, but pressure distal to the stenosis is normal or reduced. Autoregulation is important in maintaining RBF, hydrostatic pressure in the glomerular capillary (P_{GC}), and GFR in the presence of this stenosis. The administration of drugs to lower the systemic blood pressure also lowers the pressure distal to the stenosis; accordingly, the RBF, P_{GC}, and GFR decrease.

maintaining GFR and RBF at a constant level when the extracellular fluid volume is normal. In addition, sympathetic nerves and angiotensin II play major roles in regulating GFR and RBF. Although they are quantitatively less important than sympathetic nerves

and angiotensin II, prostaglandins, NO, endothelin, bradykinin, ATP, and adenosine also affect RBF and GFR. Figure 3-9 shows how changes in afferent and efferent arteriolar resistance, mediated by changes in the hormones listed in Table 3-1, modulate the GFR and RBF.

Sympathetic Nerves

The afferent and efferent arterioles are innervated by sympathetic neurons; however, sympathetic tone is minimal when the volume of extracellular fluid is normal (see Chapter 6). Sympathetic nerves release norepinephrine and dopamine, and circulating epinephrine (which is a catecholamine like norepinephrine and dopamine) is secreted by the adrenal medulla. Norepinephrine and epinephrine cause vasoconstriction by binding to α_1-adrenoceptors, which are located mainly on the afferent arterioles. Activation of α_1-adrenoceptors decreases GFR and RBF. Dehydration or strong emotional stimuli, such as fear and pain, activate sympathetic nerves and reduce GFR and RBF.

Renalase, a catecholamine-metabolizing hormone produced by kidneys, facilitates the degradation of catecholamines.

Angiotensin II

Angiotensin II is produced systemically and locally within the kidneys. It constricts the afferent and efferent arterioles* and decreases the RBF and GFR. Figure 3-10 shows how norepinephrine, epinephrine, and angiotensin II act together to decrease the RBF and GFR and thereby increase blood pressure and extracellular fluid (ECF) volume, as would occur, for example, with hemorrhage.

Prostaglandins

Prostaglandins do not play a major role in regulating RBF in healthy, resting people. However, during

*The efferent arteriole is more sensitive to angiotensin II than the afferent arteriole. Thus with low concentrations of angiotensin II, constriction of the efferent arteriole predominates, GFR increases, and RBF decreases. However, with high concentrations of angiotensin II, constriction of both afferent and efferent arterioles occurs and both GFR and RBF fall (see Figure 3-9).

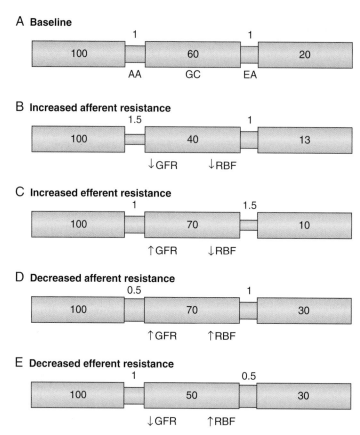

FIGURE 3-9 ▪Relationship between selective changes in the resistance of either the afferent arteriole or the efferent arteriole on renal blood flow (*RBF*) and glomerular filtration rate (*GFR*). Numbers in the bars refer to vascular pressure (mm Hg), and numbers above the bars refer to the resistance relative to baseline. Constriction of either the afferent or efferent arteriole increases resistance, and according to equation 3-11 ($Q = \Delta P/R$), an increase in resistance (R) decreases flow (Q) (i.e., RBF). Dilation of either the afferent or efferent arteriole increases flow (i.e., RBF). Baseline (**A**) and constriction of the afferent arteriole (**B**) decrease the hydrostatic pressure in the glomerular capillary (P_{GC}) because less of the arterial pressure is transmitted to the glomerulus, thereby reducing the GFR. RBF decreases because resistance increases. In contrast, constriction of the efferent arteriole (**C**) elevates the P_{GC} and thus increases the GFR. RBF decreases because resistance increases. Dilation of the afferent arteriole (**D**) increases the P_{GC} and thus increases the GFR. RBF increases because resistance decreases. Dilation of the efferent arteriole (**E**) decreases the P_{GC}, thereby decreasing the GFR. *AA*, Afferent arteriole; *GC*, glomerular capillary; *EA*, efferent arteriole. (*Modified from Boron W, Boulpaep EL: Textbook of medical physiology, ed 2, Philadelphia, 2009, Saunders Elsevier.*)

pathophysiologic conditions such as hemorrhage, prostaglandins (PGI$_2$, PGE$_1$, and PGE$_2$) are produced locally within the kidneys, and they increase RBF without changing the GFR. Prostaglandins increase RBF by dampening the vasoconstrictor effects of sympathetic nerves and angiotensin II. This effect is important because it prevents severe and potentially harmful vasoconstriction and renal ischemia. Prostaglandin synthesis is stimulated by dehydration and stress (e.g., surgery and anesthesia), angiotensin II, and sympathetic nerves.

Nonsteroidal antiinflammatory drugs (NSAIDs), such as aspirin and ibuprofen, inhibit the synthesis of prostaglandins. Thus administration of these drugs during renal ischemia and hemorrhagic shock is contraindicated because, by blocking the production of prostaglandins, they decrease RBF and increase renal ischemia. Prostaglandins play an increasingly important role in maintaining RBF and GFR as people age. Accordingly, NSAIDs can significantly reduce RBF and GFR in the elderly.

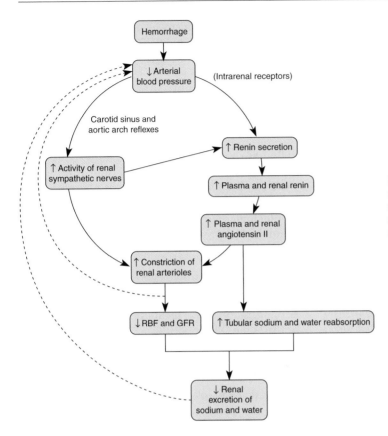

FIGURE 3-10 ■ Pathway by which hemorrhage activates renal sympathetic nerve activity and stimulates the production of angiotensin II. *GFR*, Glomerular filtration rate; *RBF*, renal blood flow. *(Modified from Vander AJ: Renal physiology, ed 2, New York, 1980, McGraw-Hill.)*

IN THE CLINIC

Hemorrhage decreases arterial blood pressure and therefore activates the sympathetic nerves to the kidneys by the baroreceptor reflex (Figure 3-10). Norepinephrine causes intense vasoconstriction of the afferent and efferent arterioles and thereby decreases GFR and RBF. The rise in sympathetic activity also increases the release of epinephrine and renin (renin in turn generates angiotensin II), which causes further vasoconstriction and a fall in RBF. The rise in the vascular resistance of the kidneys and other vascular beds increases the total peripheral resistance. The resulting tendency for blood pressure to increase (Blood pressure = Cardiac output × Total peripheral resistance) offsets the tendency of blood pressure to decrease in response to hemorrhage. Hence this system works to preserve the arterial pressure at the expense of maintaining a normal GFR and RBF.

Nitric Oxide

NO, an endothelium-derived relaxing factor, is an important vasodilator under basal conditions, and it counteracts the vasoconstriction produced by angiotensin II and catecholamines. When blood flow increases, a greater shear force acts on the endothelial cells in the arterioles and increases the production of NO. In addition, a number of vasoactive hormones, including acetylcholine, histamine, bradykinin, and ATP, cause the release of NO from endothelial cells. Increased production of NO causes dilation of the afferent and efferent arterioles in the kidneys. Whereas increased levels of NO decrease the total peripheral resistance, inhibition of NO production increases the total peripheral resistance.

Endothelin

Endothelin is a potent vasoconstrictor secreted by endothelial cells of the renal vessels, mesangial cells,

---

IN THE CLINIC

Abnormal production of nitric oxide (NO) is observed in persons with **diabetes mellitus** and **hypertension**. Excess renal NO production in persons with diabetes may be responsible for glomerular hyperfiltration (i.e., increased GFR) and damage of the glomerulus, which are problems characteristic of this disease. Elevated NO levels increase the glomerular capillary hydrostatic pressure as a result of a decrease in the resistance of the afferent arteriole. The ensuing hyperfiltration is thought to cause glomerular damage. The normal response to an increase in dietary salt intake includes the stimulation of renal NO production, which prevents an increase in blood pressure. In some persons, however, NO production may not increase appropriately in response to an elevation in salt intake, and blood pressure rises.

---

and tubular epithelial cells in response to angiotensin II, bradykinin, epinephrine, and endothelial shear stress. Endothelin causes profound vasoconstriction of the afferent and efferent arterioles and decreases the GFR and RBF. Although this potent vasoconstrictor may not influence the GFR and RBF in resting subjects, endothelin production is elevated in a number of glomerular disease states (e.g., renal disease associated with diabetes mellitus).

Bradykinin

Kallikrein is a proteolytic enzyme produced in the kidneys. Kallikrein cleaves circulating kininogen to bradykinin, which is a vasodilator that acts by stimulating the release of NO and prostaglandins. Bradykinin increases the GFR and RBF.

Adenosine

Adenosine is produced within the kidneys and causes vasoconstriction of the afferent arteriole, thereby reducing the GFR and RBF. As previously mentioned, adenosine plays a role in tubuloglomerular feedback.

Natriuretic Peptides

Secretion of atrial natriuretic peptide (ANP) by the cardiac atria and brain natriuretic peptide (BNP) from the cardiac ventricle increases when the ECF volume is expanded. Both ANP and BNP dilate the afferent arteriole and constrict the efferent arteriole. Therefore ANP and BNP produce a modest increase in the GFR with little change in RBF.

Adenosine Triphosphate

Cells release ATP into the renal interstitial fluid. ATP has dual effects on the GFR and RBF. Under some conditions, ATP constricts the afferent arteriole, reduces RBF and GFR, and may play a role in tubuloglomerular feedback. In contrast, ATP may stimulate NO production and increase the GFR and RBF.

Glucocorticoids

Administration of therapeutic doses of glucocorticoids increases the GFR and RBF.

Histamine

The local release of histamine modulates RBF in the resting state and during inflammation and injury. Histamine decreases the resistance of the afferent and efferent arterioles and thereby increases RBF without elevating the GFR.

Dopamine

The vasodilator dopamine is produced by the proximal tubule. Dopamine has several actions within the kidney, such as increasing RBF and inhibiting renin secretion.

Finally, as illustrated in Figure 3-11, vascular endothelial cells play an important role in regulating the resistance of the renal afferent and efferent arterioles by producing a number of paracrine hormones, including NO, prostacyclin (PGI_2), endothelin, and angiotensin II. These hormones regulate contraction or relaxation of vascular smooth muscle cells in afferent and efferent arterioles and mesangial cells. Shear stress, acetylcholine, histamine, bradykinin, and ATP stimulate the production of NO, which increases the GFR and RBF. **Angiotensin-converting enzyme**, located on the surface of

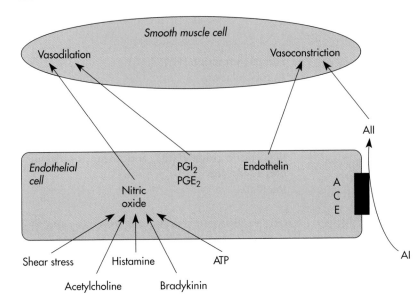

FIGURE 3-11 ■ Examples of the interactions of endothelial cells with smooth muscle and mesangial cells. *ACE,* Angiotensin-converting enzyme; *AI,* angiotensin I; *AII,* angiotensin II; *ATP,* adenosine triphosphate; *PGE₂,* prostaglandin E₂; *PGI₂,* prostacyclin. *(Modified from Navar LG, Inscho EW, Majid SA et al: Paracrine regulation of the renal microcirculation, Physiol Rev 76:425, 1996.)*

endothelial cells lining the afferent arteriole and glomerular capillaries, converts angiotensin I to angiotensin II, which decreases the GFR and RBF. Angiotensin II also is produced locally in the granular cells in the afferent arteriole and proximal tubular cells. PGI_2 and PGE_2 secretion by endothelial cells, stimulated by sympathetic nerve activity and angiotensin II, increases the GFR and RBF. Finally, the release of endothelin from endothelial cells decreases the GFR and RBF.

IN THE CLINIC

Angiotensin-converting enzyme (ACE) degrades and thereby inactivates bradykinin. It also converts angiotensin I, an inactive hormone, to angiotensin II, an active hormone. Thus ACE increases angiotensin II levels and decreases bradykinin levels. Drugs called **ACE inhibitors** (e.g., enalapril and captopril), which reduce systemic blood pressure in patients with hypertension, decrease angiotensin II levels and elevate bradykinin levels. Both effects lower systemic vascular resistance, reduce blood pressure, and decrease renal vascular resistance, thereby increasing GFR and RBF. **Angiotensin II receptor antagonists** (e.g., losartan) also are used to treat high blood pressure. As their name suggests, they block the binding of angiotensin II to the angiotensin II receptor (AT1). These antagonists block the vasoconstrictor effects of angiotensin II on the afferent arteriole; thus they increase GFR and RBF. In contrast to ACE inhibitors, AT1 antagonists do not inhibit kinin metabolism (e.g., bradykinin).

S U M M A R Y

1. Creatinine and inulin clearance can be used to measure the GFR.
2. Clinically, the GFR is evaluated by measuring plasma creatinine concentration.
3. Starling forces across the glomerular capillaries provide the driving force for the ultrafiltration of plasma from the glomerular capillaries into Bowman's space.
4. The glomerular ultrafiltrate is devoid of cellular elements, including red and white blood cells and platelets, and contains very little protein but otherwise is identical to plasma.
5. RBF (1.25 L/min) is about 25% of the cardiac output. RBF determines the GFR; modifies solute and water reabsorption by the proximal tubule; participates in the concentration and dilution of the urine; delivers oxygen, nutrients, and hormones to the cells of the nephron; returns carbon dioxide and reabsorbed fluid and solutes to the general circulation; and delivers substrates for excretion in the urine.
6. Autoregulation allows the GFR and RBF to remain constant despite fluctuations in arterial blood pressure between 90 and 180 mm Hg.
7. Hemorrhage activates renal sympathetic nerves and stimulates angiotensin II production and thereby reduces renal perfusion and urinary excretion of NaCl and water.
8. Sympathetic nerves and angiotensin II are the major hormones that regulate GFR and RBF; however, prostaglandins, NO, endothelin, natriuretic peptides, prostaglandins, bradykinin, and adenosine also affect GFR and RBF.

KEY WORDS AND CONCEPTS

- Clearance
- Mass balance
- Renal plasma flow (RPF)
- Inulin
- Glomerular filtration rate (GFR)
- Creatinine
- Creatinine clearance
- Filtration fraction (FF)
- Autoregulation
- Myogenic mechanism
- Tubuloglomerular feedback
- Juxtaglomerular apparatus (JGA)
- Sympathetic nerves, angiotensin II, prostaglandins, nitric oxide (NO), endothelin, bradykinin, and adenosine
- Renalase

SELF-STUDY PROBLEMS

1. Phlorhizin is a drug that completely inhibits the reabsorption of glucose by the kidneys. The following data are obtained to assess the effect of phlorhizin on the clearance of glucose. Fill in the missing data.

   Before phlorhizin administration

Plasma (inulin):	1 mg/mL
Plasma (glucose):	1 mg/mL
Inulin excretion rate:	100 mg/min
Glucose excretion rate:	0 mg/min
Inulin clearance:	_____ mL/min
Glucose clearance:	_____ mL/min

   After phlorhizin administration

Plasma (inulin):	1 mg/mL
Plasma (glucose):	1 mg/mL
Inulin excretion rate:	100 mg/min
Glucose excretion rate:	_____ mg/min
Inulin clearance:	_____ mL/min
Glucose clearance:	_____ mL/min

   How do you explain the change in glucose excretion and clearance seen with phlorhizin?

2. Finding which of the following substances in the urine would indicate damage to the glomerular ultrafiltration barrier?
   a. Red blood cells
   b. Glucose
   c. Sodium
   d. Proteins

3. Explain how hormones (e.g., sympathetic agonists, angiotensin II, and prostaglandins) change RBF.

4. Explain why the use of NSAIDs (e.g., indomethacin for arthritis) does not affect GFR or RBF in patients with normal renal function and why administration of NSAIDs is not recommended for patients with severe reductions in GFR and RBF.

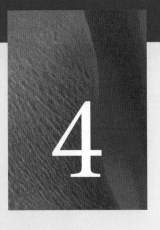

4

RENAL TRANSPORT MECHANISMS: NaCl AND WATER REABSORPTION ALONG THE NEPHRON

■ ■ ■ ■ ■ ■ ■ ■ ■ ■ ■ ■ ■ ■ ■ ■

OBJECTIVES

Upon completion of this chapter, the student should be able to answer the following questions:

1. What three processes are involved in the production of urine?

2. What is the composition of "normal" urine?

3. What transport mechanisms are responsible for sodium chloride (NaCl) reabsorption by the nephron? Where are they located along the nephron?

4. How is water reabsorption "coupled" to NaCl reabsorption in the proximal tubule?

5. Why are solutes, but not water, reabsorbed by the thick ascending limb of Henle's loop?

6. What transport mechanisms are involved in the secretion of organic anions and cations? What is the physiologic relevance of these transport processes?

7. What is glomerulotubular balance, and what is its physiologic importance?

8. What are the major hormones that regulate NaCl and water reabsorption by the kidneys? What is the nephron site of action of each hormone?

9. What is the aldosterone paradox?

The formation of urine involves three basic processes: (1) **ultrafiltration** of plasma by the glomerulus, (2) **reabsorption** of water and solutes from the ultrafiltrate, and (3) **secretion** of select solutes into the tubular fluid. Although an average of 115 to 180 L of fluid for women and 130 to 200 L of fluid for men is filtered by the human glomeruli each day,* less than 1% of

---

*The normal glomerular filtration rate averages 115 to 180 L/day in women and 130 to 200 L/day in men. Thus the volume of the ultrafiltrate represents a volume that is approximately 10 times the extracellular fluid volume. For simplicity, this book assumes that glomerular filtration rate is 180 L/day.

the filtered water and sodium chloride (NaCl) and variable amounts of other solutes are excreted in the urine (Table 4-1). By the processes of reabsorption and secretion, the renal tubules regulate the volume and composition of urine (Table 4-2). Consequently, the tubules precisely control the volume, osmolality, composition, and pH of the intracellular and extracellular fluid compartments. Transport proteins in cell membranes of the nephron mediate the reabsorption and secretion of solutes and water in the kidneys. Approximately 5% to 10% of all human genes code for transport proteins, and genetic and acquired defects in transport proteins are

TABLE 4-1

Filtration, Excretion, and Reabsorption of Water, Electrolytes, and Solutes by the Kidneys

SUBSTANCE	MEASURE	FILTERED*	EXCRETED	REABSORBED	% FILTERED LOAD REABSORBED
Water	L/day	180	1.5	178.5	99.2
Na^+	mEq/day	25,200	150	25,050	99.4
K^+	mEq/day	720	100	620	86.1
Ca^{++}	mEq/day	540	10	530	98.2
HCO_3^-	mEq/day	4320	2	4318	99.9+
Cl^-	mEq/day	18,000	150	17,850	99.2
Glucose	mmol/day	800	0	800	100.0
Urea	g/day	56	28	25	50.0

*The filtered amount of any substance is calculated by multiplying the concentration of that substance in the ultrafiltrate by the glomerular filtration rate (GFR); for example, the filtered load of Na^+ is calculated as $[Na^+]_{ultrafiltrate}$ (140 mEq/L) × GFR (180 L/day) = 25,200 mEq/day.

TABLE 4-2

Composition of Urine*

SUBSTANCE	CONCENTRATION
Na^+	50-130 mEq/L
K^+	20-70 mEq/L
Ammonium	30-50 mEq/L
Ca^{++}	5-12 mEq/L
Mg^{++}	2-18 mEq/L
Cl^-	50-130 mEq/L
Inorganic phosphate	20-40 mEq/L
Urea	200-400 mmol/L
Creatinine	6-20 mmol/L
pH	5.0-7.0
Osmolality	500-800 mOsm/kg H_2O
Glucose	0
Amino acids	0
Protein	0
Blood	0
Ketones	0
Leukocytes	0
Bilirubin	0

*The composition and volume of the urine can vary widely in the healthy state. These values represent average ranges. Water excretion ranges between 0.5 and 1.5 L/day.
Modified from Valtin HV: Renal physiology, ed 2, Boston, 1983, Little Brown.

the cause of many kidney diseases (Table 4-3). In addition, numerous transport proteins are important drug targets. This chapter discusses NaCl and water reabsorption, organic anion and cation transport, the transport proteins involved in solute and water transport, and some of the factors and hormones that regulate NaCl transport. Details on acid-base transport and on K^+, Ca^{++}, and inorganic phosphate (P_i) transport and their regulation are provided in Chapters 7 to 9.

GENERAL PRINCIPLES OF MEMBRANE TRANSPORT

Solutes may be transported across cell membranes by passive mechanisms, active transport mechanisms, or endocytosis. In mammals, solute movement occurs by both passive and active mechanisms, whereas all water movement is passive. The movement of a solute across a membrane is passive if it develops spontaneously and does not require direct expenditure of metabolic energy. **Passive transport** (diffusion) of uncharged solutes occurs from an area of higher concentration to one of lower concentration (i.e., down its chemical concentration gradient). In addition to concentration gradients, the passive diffusion of ions (but not uncharged solutes, such as glucose and urea) is affected by the electrical potential difference (i.e., electrical gradient) across cell membranes and the renal tubules. Cations (e.g., Na^+ and K^+) move to the negative side of

TABLE 4-3

Some Monogenic Renal Diseases Involving Transport Proteins

DISEASES	MODE OF INHERITANCE	GENE(S)	TRANSPORT PROTEIN	NEPHRON SEGMENT	PHENOTYPE
Cystinuria, type I	AR	SLC3A1, SLC7A9	Amino acid symporters	Proximal tubule	Increased excretion of basic amino acids, nephrolithiasis (kidney stones)
Proximal renal tubular acidosis	AR	SLC4A4	Na^+-HCO_3^- symporter	Proximal tubule	Hyperchloremic metabolic acidosis
X-linked nephrolithiasis (Dent disease)	XLR	CLCN, OCRL1	Chloride channel	Distal tubule	Hypercalciuria, nephrolithiasis
Bartter syndrome	AR type I	SLC12A1	Na^+/K^+/$2Cl^-$ symporter	TAL	Hypokalemia, metabolic alkalosis, hyperaldosteronism
	AR type II	KCNJ1	ROMK potassium channel	TAL	Hypokalemia, metabolic alkalosis, hyperaldosteronism
	AR type III	CLCNKB	Chloride channel (basolateral membrane)	TAL	Hypokalemia, metabolic alkalosis, hyperaldosteronism
	AR type IV	BSND, CLCNKA, CLCNKB	Subunit of chloride channel, chloride channels	TAL	Hypokalemia, metabolic alkalosis, hyperaldosteronism
Hypomagnesemia-hypercalciuria syndrome	AR	CLDN16	Claudin-16, also known as paracellin 1	TAL	Hypomagnesemia-hypercalciuria, nephrolithiasis
Gitelman syndrome	AR	SLC12A3	Thiazide-sensitive symporter	Distal tubule	Hypomagnesemia, hypokalemic metabolic alkalosis, hypocalciuria, hypotension
Pseudohypoaldosteronism type I	AR	SCNN1A, SCNN1B, SCNN1G	α, β, and γ subunits of ENaC	Collecting duct	Increased excretion of Na^+, hyperkalemia, hypotension
Pseudohypoaldosteronism type I	AD	MLR	Mineralocorticoid receptor	Collecting duct	Increased excretion of Na^+, hyperkalemia, hypotension
Liddle syndrome	AD	SCNN1B, SCNN1G	β and γ subunits of ENaC	Collecting duct	Decreased excretion of Na^+, hypertension
Nephrogenic diabetes insipidus type 2	AR/AD	AQP2	Aquaporin 2 water channel	Collecting duct	Polyuria, polydipsia, plasma hyperosmolality
Distal renal tubular acidosis	AD/AR	SLC4A1	Cl^-/HCO_3^- antiporter	Collecting duct	Metabolic acidosis, hypokalemia, hypercalciuria, nephrolithiasis
Distal renal tubular acidosis	AR	ATP6N1B	Subunit of H^+ ATPase	Collecting duct	Metabolic acidosis, hypokalemia, hypercalciuria, nephrolithiasis

AD, autosomal dominant; *AR*, autosomal recessive; *ATPase*, adenosine triphosphatase; *ENaC*, epithelial sodium channel; *HCO$_3^-$*, bicarbonate; *ROMK*, renal outer medullary K^+; *TAL*, thick ascending limb of Henle's loop. There are approximately 300 different solute transporter genes that form the so-called SLC (solute carrier) family of genes.
Modified from Nachman RH, Glassock RJ: Glomerular, vascular, and tubulointerstitial diseases. NephSAP (J Am Soc Nephrol Suppl) *9(3):119-211, 2010.*

the membrane, whereas anions⁻ (e.g., Cl^- and bicarbonate [HCO_3^-]) move to the positive side of the membrane. Diffusion of water (**osmosis**) occurs through aquaporin (AQP) water channels in the cell membrane and is driven by osmotic pressure gradients. When water is reabsorbed across tubule segments, the solutes dissolved in the water also are carried along with the water. This process is called **solvent drag** and can account for a substantial amount of solute reabsorption across the proximal tubule. Traditionally, it was thought that the biologically important gases O_2, carbon dioxide (CO_2), and ammonia (NH_3) diffused across the lipid bilayer of plasma membranes. It is now known that these gases also move across the membrane via specific membrane transport proteins (e.g., CO_2 and NH_3 have been shown to cross the membrane via the AQP1 water channel).

In **facilitated diffusion**, transport depends on the interaction of the solute with a specific protein in the membrane that facilitates its movement across the membrane. If defined broadly, the term "facilitated diffusion" can be used to describe several different types of membrane transporters. For example, one form of facilitated diffusion is the diffusion of ions, such as Na^+ and K^+, through aqueous-filled channels created by proteins that span the plasma membrane. Also, the movement of a single molecule across the membrane by a transport protein (**uniport**), such as occurs with urea and glucose, is a form of facilitated diffusion.*

Another form of facilitated diffusion is coupled transport, in which the movement of two or more solutes across a membrane depends on their interaction with a specific transport protein. Coupled transport of two or more solutes in the same direction is mediated by a **symport** mechanism. Examples of symport mechanisms in the kidneys include Na^+-glucose, Na^+–amino acid, and Na^+-P_i symporters in the proximal tubule and the Na^+-K^+-$2Cl^-$ symporter in the thick ascending limb of Henle's loop. Coupled transport of two or more solutes in opposite directions is mediated by an **antiport** mechanism. An Na^+-H^+ antiporter in the proximal tubule mediates Na^+ reabsorption and H^+ secretion. With coupled transporters, at least one of the solutes

usually is transported against its electrochemical gradient. The energy for this uphill movement is derived from the passive downhill movement of at least one of the other solutes into the cell. For example, in the proximal tubule, operation of the Na^+-H^+ antiporter in the apical membrane of the cell results in the movement of H^+ against its electrochemical gradient out of the cell into the tubular lumen. The movement of Na^+ from the tubular lumen into the cell, down its electrochemical gradient, drives the uphill movement of H^+. The uphill movement of H^+ is termed **secondary active transport** to reflect the fact that the movement of H^+ is not directly coupled to the hydrolysis of adenosine triphosphate (ATP) (see below). Instead, the energy is derived from the gradient of the other coupled ion (in this example, Na^+).

Transport is **active** if it is coupled directly to energy derived from metabolic processes (i.e., it consumes ATP). Active transport of solutes usually takes place from an area of lower concentration to an area of higher concentration. In the kidneys, the most prevalent active transport mechanism is sodium-potassium adenosine triphosphatase (Na^+-K^+-ATPase) (or the sodium pump), which is located in the basolateral membrane. The Na^+-K^+-ATPase mechanism is made up of several proteins that together actively move Na^+ out of the cell and K^+ into the cell. Other active transport mechanisms in the kidneys include the H^+-ATPase and H^+-K^+-ATPase mechanisms, which are responsible for H^+ secretion in the collecting duct (see Chapter 8), and the Ca^{++}-ATPase mechanism, which is responsible for Ca^{++} movement from the cell cytoplasm into the blood (see Chapter 9). In addition to these transport ATPases, another large group of ATP-dependent transporters exists that is called **ATP-binding cassette**, or **ABC transporters**. To date, seven groups and more than 40 specific ABC transporters have been identified in humans. They transport a diverse group of solutes, including Cl^-, cholesterol, bile acids, drugs, iron, and organic anions and cations.

Endocytosis is the movement of a substance across the plasma membrane by a process involving the invagination of a piece of membrane until it completely pinches off and forms a vesicle in the cytoplasm. This mechanism is important for the reabsorption of small proteins and macromolecules by the proximal tubule. Because endocytosis requires ATP, it is a form of active transport.

---

*Some authors restrict the term *facilitated diffusion* to this type of transport and use as the classic example the glucose uniporter that brings glucose into many cells (e.g., skeletal muscle).

GENERAL PRINCIPLES OF TRANSEPITHELIAL SOLUTE AND WATER TRANSPORT

As illustrated in Figure 4-1, tight junctions hold renal cells together. Below the tight junctions, the cells are separated by **lateral intercellular spaces**. The tight junctions separate the apical membranes from the basolateral membranes. An epithelium can be compared with a six-pack of soda, in which the cans are the cells and the plastic holder represents the tight junctions.

In the nephron, a substance can be reabsorbed or secreted through cells, the so-called **transcellular pathway**, or between cells, the so-called **paracellular pathway** (see Figure 4-1). Na^+ reabsorption by the proximal tubule is a good example of transport by the transcellular pathway. Na^+ reabsorption in this nephron segment depends on the operation of the Na^+-K^+-ATPase pump (see Figure 4-1). The Na^+-K^+-ATPase pump, which is located exclusively in the basolateral membrane, moves Na^+ out of the cell into the blood and K^+ into the cell. Thus the operation of the Na^+-K^+-ATPase pump lowers intracellular $[Na^+]$ and increases intracellular $[K^+]$. Because intracellular $[Na^+]$ is low (12 mEq/L) and the $[Na^+]$ in tubular fluid is high (140 mEq/L), Na^+ moves across the apical cell membrane, down a chemical concentration gradient from the tubular lumen into the cell. Because the interior of

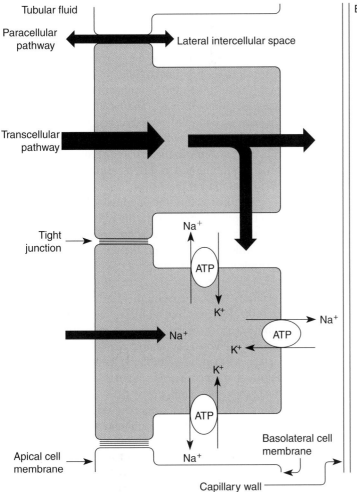

FIGURE 4-1 ■ Paracellular and transcellular transport pathways in the proximal tubule. *ATP,* Adenosine triphosphate.

the cell is electrically negative with respect to the tubular lumen, and depending on the Na^+ transporter, the energy in this electrical gradient also can drive Na^+ into the cell across the apical membrane. The Na^+-K^+-ATPase pump senses the addition of Na^+ to the cell and is stimulated to increase its rate of Na^+ extrusion into the blood, thereby returning intracellular Na^+ to normal levels. Thus transcellular Na^+ reabsorption by the proximal tubule is a two-step process:

1. Movement across the apical membrane into the cell, down a chemical concentration gradient and/or an electrochemical gradient established by the Na^+-K^+-ATPase pump
2. Movement across the basolateral membrane against an electrochemical gradient through the Na^+-K^+-ATPase pump

The reabsorption of Ca^{++} and K^+ across the proximal tubule is a good example of paracellular transport. Some of the water reabsorbed across the proximal tubule traverses the paracellular pathway. Some solutes dissolved in this water, particularly Ca^{++} and K^+, are entrained in the reabsorbed fluid and thereby reabsorbed by the process of solvent drag.

AT THE CELLULAR LEVEL

The tight junction in renal epithelial cells is a specialized membrane domain that creates a barrier that regulates the paracellular diffusion of solutes across the epithelia. Tight junctions are composed of linear arrays of several integral membrane proteins, including occludins, claudins, and several members of the immunoglobulin superfamily. The tight junction complex of proteins has biophysical properties of ion channels, including the ability to allow ions to diffuse selectively across the complex based on size and charge.

NaCl, SOLUTE, AND WATER REABSORPTION ALONG THE NEPHRON

Quantitatively, the reabsorption of NaCl and water represents the major function of nephrons. Approximately 25,000 mEq/day of Na^+ and 179 L/day of water are reabsorbed by the renal tubules (see Table 4-1). In addition, renal transport of many other important solutes is linked either directly or indirectly to Na^+ reabsorption. In the following sections the NaCl and water transport processes of each nephron segment and its regulation by hormones, along with other factors, are presented.

Proximal Tubule

The proximal tubule reabsorbs approximately 67% of filtered water, Na^+, Cl^-, K^+, and other solutes. In addition, the proximal tubule reabsorbs virtually all the glucose and amino acids filtered by the glomerulus. The key element in proximal tubule reabsorption is the Na^+-K^+-ATPase pump in the basolateral membrane. The reabsorption of every substance, including water, is linked in some manner to the operation of the Na^+-K^+-ATPase pump.

Na^+ Reabsorption

Na^+ is reabsorbed by different mechanisms in the first and the second halves of the proximal tubule. In the first half of the proximal tubule, Na^+ is reabsorbed primarily with HCO_3^- and a number of other solutes (e.g., glucose, amino acids, P_i, and lactate). In contrast, in the second half, Na^+ is reabsorbed mainly with Cl^-. This disparity is mediated by differences in the Na^+ transport systems in the first and second halves of the proximal tubule and by differences in the composition of tubular fluid at these sites.

In the first half of the proximal tubule, Na^+ uptake into the cell is coupled with either H^+ or organic solutes (Figure 4-2). Specific transport proteins mediate Na^+ entry into the cell across the apical membrane. For example, the Na^+-H^+ antiporter (see Figure 4-2, A) couples Na^+ entry with H^+ extrusion from the cell. H^+ secretion results in sodium bicarbonate ($NaHCO_3^-$) reabsorption (see Chapter 8). Na^+ also enters proximal tubule cells by several symporter mechanisms, including Na^+-glucose, Na^+–amino acid, Na^+-P_i, and Na^+-lactate (see Figure 4-2, B). The glucose and other organic solutes that enter the cell with Na^+ leave the cell across the basolateral membrane by passive transport mechanisms. Any Na^+ that enters the cell across the apical membrane leaves the cell and enters the blood by the Na^+-K^+-ATPase mechanism. In brief, the reabsorption of Na^+ in the first half of the proximal tubule is coupled to that of HCO_3^-, P_i, and a number of organic molecules, and this process generates a negative transepithelial

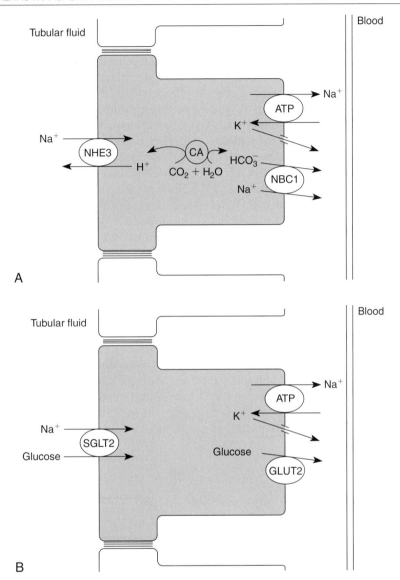

FIGURE 4-2 ■ Na^+ transport processes in the first half of the proximal tubule. These transport mechanisms are present in all cells in the first half of the proximal tubule but are separated into different cells to simplify the discussion. **A,** Operation of the Na^+-H^+ antiporter (*NHE3*) in the apicalmembrane and the Na^+-K^+–adenosine triphosphatase (ATPase) and bicarbonate transporters, including the Cl^--HCO_3^- antiporter (AE2, not shown) and the Na^+- HCO_3^- cotransporter (*NBC1*; see Chapter 8), in the basolateral membrane mediates $NaHCO_3$ reabsorption. Note that a single HCO_3^- transporter (*NBC1*) is illustrated for simplicity. Carbon dioxide (CO_2) and water combine inside the cells to form H^+ and HCO_3^- in a reaction facilitated by the enzyme carbonic anhydrase (*CA*). **B,** Operation of the Na^+-glucose transporter (*SGLT2*) in the apical membrane, in conjunction with the Na^+-K^+-ATPase and glucose transporter (*GLUT2*) in the basolateral membrane, mediates Na^+-glucose reabsorption. Inactivating mutations in the *GLUT2* gene lead to decreased glucose reabsorption in the proximal tubule and glucosuria (i.e., glucose in the urine). Although not shown, Na^+ reabsorption also is coupled with other solutes, including amino acids, P_i, and lactate. Reabsorption of these solutes is mediated by the Na^+–amino acid, Na^+-P_i, and Na^+-lactate symporters located in the apical membrane and the Na^+-K^+-ATPase, amino acid, P_i, and lactate transporters located in the basolateral membrane. Three classes of amino acid transporters have been identified in the proximal tubule: two that transport Na^+ in conjunction with either acidic or basic amino acids and one that does not require Na^+ and transports basic amino acids. *ATP,* Adenosine triphosphate.

voltage across the proximal tubule that provides the driving force for the paracellular reabsorption of Cl^-. The reabsorption of many organic molecules is so avid that they are almost completely removed from the tubular fluid in the first half of the proximal tubule (Figure 4-3). The reabsorption of $NaHCO_3$ Na^+-P_i, and Na^+–organic solutes across the proximal tubule establishes a transtubular osmotic gradient (i.e., the osmolality of the interstitial fluid bathing the basolateral side of the cells is slightly higher than the osmolality of tubule fluid) that provides the driving force for the passive reabsorption of water by osmosis. Because more water than Cl^- is reabsorbed in the first half of the proximal tubule, the Cl^- concentration in tubular fluid rises along the length of the proximal tubule (see Figure 4-3).

In the second half of the proximal tubule, Na^+ is mainly reabsorbed with Cl^- across the transcellular pathway (Figure 4-4). Na^+ is primarily reabsorbed with Cl^- rather than organic solutes or HCO_3^- as the accompanying anion because the Na^+ transport mechanisms in the second half of the proximal tubule differ from those in the first half. Furthermore, the tubular fluid that enters the second half contains very little glucose and amino acids, but the high concentration of Cl^- (140 mEq/L) in tubule fluid exceeds that in the first half (105 mEq/L). The high Cl^- concentration is due to

the preferential reabsorption of Na^+ with HCO_3^- and organic solutes in the first half of the proximal tubule.

The mechanism of transcellular Na^+ reabsorption in the second half of the proximal tubule is shown in Figure 4-4. Na^+ enters the cell across the luminal membrane primarily through the parallel operation of a Na^+-H^+ antiporter and one or more Cl^--base antiporters. Because the secreted H^+ and base combine in the tubular fluid and reenter the cell, the operation of the Na^+-H^+ and Cl^--base antiporters is equivalent to NaCl uptake from tubular fluid into the cell. Na^+ leaves the cell through the Na^+-K^+-ATPase mechanism, and Cl^- leaves the cell and enters the blood through a K^+-Cl^- symporter and a Cl^- channel in the basolateral membrane.

Some NaCl also is reabsorbed across the second half of the proximal tubule by a **paracellular route**. Paracellular NaCl reabsorption occurs because the rise in the Cl^- concentration in the tubule fluid in the first half of the proximal tubule creates a Cl^- concentration gradient (140 mEq/L in the tubule lumen and 105 mEq/L in the interstitium). This concentration gradient favors the diffusion of Cl^- from the tubular lumen across the tight junctions into the lateral intercellular space. Movement of the negatively charged Cl^- causes the tubular fluid to become positively charged relative

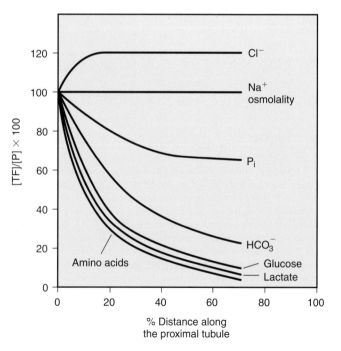

FIGURE 4-3 ■ Concentration of solutes in tubule fluid as a function of length along the proximal tubule. [TF] is the concentration of the substance in tubular fluid; [P] is the concentration of the substance in plasma. Values higher than 100 indicate that relatively less of the solute than water was reabsorbed, and values less than 100 indicate that relatively more of the substance than water was reabsorbed. HCO_3^-, Bicarbonate; P_i, inorganic phosphate. *(Modified from Vander AJ: Renal physiology, ed 4, New York, 1991, McGraw-Hill.)*

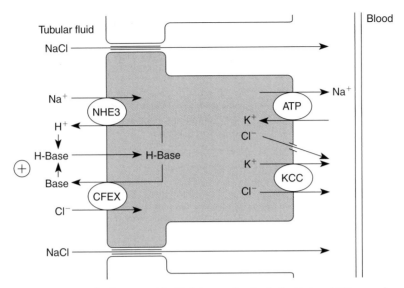

FIGURE 4-4 ■ Na$^+$ transport processes in the second half of the proximal tubule. Na$^+$ and Cl$^-$ enter the cell across the apical membrane through the operation of parallel Na$^+$-H$^+$ and Cl$^-$-base (e.g., formate, oxalate, and bicarbonate) antiporters (*CFEX*). More than one Cl$^-$-base antiporter may be involved in this process, but only one is depicted. The secreted H$^+$ and base combine in the tubular fluid to form an H$^+$-base complex that can recycle across the plasma membrane. Accumulation of the H$^+$-base complex in tubular fluid establishes an H$^+$-base concentration gradient that favors H$^+$-base recycling across the apical plasma membrane into the cell. Inside the cell, H$^+$ and the base dissociate and recycle back across the apical plasma membrane. The net result is sodium chloride (NaCl) uptake across the apical membrane. The base may be hydroxide ions (OH$^-$), formate (HCO$_2^-$), oxalate$^-$, HCO$_3^-$, or sulfate. The lumen-positive transepithelial voltage, indicated by the plus sign inside the circle in the tubular lumen, is generated by the diffusion of Cl$^-$ (lumen to blood) across the tight junction. The high Cl$^-$ concentration of tubular fluid provides the driving force for Cl$^-$ diffusion. Some glucose also is reabsorbed in the second half of the proximal tubule by a mechanism similar to that described in the first half of the proximal tubule, except that the Na$^+$-glucose symporter (*SGLT1* gene) transports 2Na$^+$ with one glucose and has a higher affinity and lower capacity than the Na$^+$-glucose symporter in the first part of the proximal tubule (i.e., SGLT2; not shown). Also, glucose exits the cell across the basolateral membrane through GLUT1 rather than GLUT2, as in the first part of the proximal tubule (not shown). *ATP,* Adenosine triphosphate; *KCC,* KCl cotransporter; *NHE3,* sodium hydrogen exchanger 3.

to the blood. This positive transepithelial voltage causes the diffusion of positively charged Na$^+$ out of the tubular fluid across the tight junction into the blood. Thus in the second half of the proximal tubule, some Na$^+$ and Cl$^-$ are reabsorbed across the tight junctions (the paracellular pathway) by passive diffusion. The reabsorption of NaCl establishes a transtubular osmotic gradient that provides the driving force for the passive reabsorption of water by osmosis.

In summary, the reabsorption of Na$^+$ and Cl$^-$ in the proximal tubule occurs across paracellular and transcellular pathways. Approximately 67% of the NaCl filtered each day is reabsorbed in the proximal tubule. Of this amount, two thirds moves across the transcellular pathway, and the remaining one third moves across the paracellular pathway (Table 4-4).

IN THE CLINIC

Fanconi syndrome is a renal disease that is either hereditary, as a result of an autosomal recessive mutation in *SLC2A2* (the gene that encodes *GLUT2*), or acquired. It often is associated with glucosuria, osteomalacia, acidosis, and hypokalemia. The syndrome results from an impaired ability of the proximal tubule to reabsorb HCO$_3^-$, amino acids, glucose, and low-molecular-weight proteins. Because other segments of the nephron cannot reabsorb these solutes and protein, Fanconi syndrome results in increased urinary excretion of HCO$_3^-$, amino acids, glucose, inorganic phosphate, and low-molecular-weight proteins.

TABLE 4-4			
NaCl Transport Along the Nephron			
SEGMENT	PERCENTAGE OF FILTERED NaCl REABSORBED	MECHANISM OF Na⁺ ENTRY ACROSS APICAL MEMBRANE	MAJOR REGULATORY HORMONES
Proximal tubule	67	Na^+-H^+ antiporter, Na^+ symporter with amino acids and organic solutes, Na^+/H^+-Cl^-/anion antiporter, paracellular	Angiotensin II, norepinephrine, epinephrine, dopamine
Loop of Henle	25	Na^+-K^+-$2Cl^-$ symporter	Aldosterone, angiotensin II
Distal tubule	~5	NaCl symporter	Aldosterone, angiotensin II
Late distal tubule and collecting duct	~3	ENaC Na^+ channels	Aldosterone, ANP, BNP, urodilatin, uroguanylin, guanylin, angiotensin II

ANP, atrial natriuretic peptide; *BNP*, brain natriuretic peptide; *ENaC*, epithelial sodium channel.

Water Reabsorption

The proximal tubule reabsorbs 67% of the filtered water (Table 4-5). The driving force for water reabsorption is a transtubular osmotic gradient established by solute reabsorption (e.g., NaCl and Na^+-glucose). The reabsorption of Na^+ along with organic solutes, HCO_3^-, P_i, and Cl^- from the tubular fluid into the lateral intercellular spaces reduces the osmolality of the tubular fluid and increases the osmolality of the lateral intercellular space (Figure 4-5). Because the proximal tubule is highly permeable to water, primarily because of the expression of aquaporin water channels (AQP1) in the apical and basolateral membranes, water is reabsorbed across cells by osmosis. However, because the tight junctions in the proximal tubule also are permeable to water, some water is reabsorbed across the paracellular pathway between proximal tubular cells. The accumulation of fluid and solutes within the lateral intercellular space increases the hydrostatic pressure in this compartment. This increased hydrostatic pressure forces fluid and solutes into the capillaries.* Thus water reabsorption follows solute reabsorption in the proximal tubule. The reabsorbed fluid is slightly hyperosmotic to plasma. However, this difference in osmolality is so small that it is commonly said that proximal tubule reabsorption is isosmotic (i.e., ~67% of the both the filtered solute and water are reabsorbed). Indeed, little difference is seen in the osmolality of tubular fluid at the start and end of the proximal tubule. An important consequence of osmotic water flow across the proximal tubule is that some solutes, especially K^+ and Ca^{++}, are entrained in the reabsorbed fluid and thereby are reabsorbed by the process of solvent drag (see Figure 4-5). The reabsorption of virtually all organic solutes, HCO_3^-, Cl^-, P_i, and other ions, and water is coupled to Na^+ reabsorption. **Therefore changes in Na^+ reabsorption influence the reabsorption of water and other solutes by the proximal tubule.** This point will be discussed later, notably in Chapter 6, and is especially relevant during volume depletion when increased Na^+ reabsorption by the proximal tubule is accompanied by a parallel increase in HCO_3^- reabsorption, which can lead to metabolic alkalosis (i.e., volume contraction alkalosis).

Protein Reabsorption

Proteins filtered across the glomerulus are reabsorbed in the proximal tubule. As mentioned previously, peptide hormones, small proteins, and small amounts of large proteins such as albumin are filtered by the glomerulus. Overall, only a small percentage of proteins cross the glomerulus and enter Bowman's space (i.e., the concentration of proteins in the glomerular ultrafiltrate is ~40 mg/L). However, the amount of protein filtered per day is significant because the glomerular filtration rate (GFR) is so high:

$$\text{Filtered protein} = GFR \times [\text{Protein}] \text{ in the ultrafiltrate}$$
$$\text{Filtered protein} = 180 \text{ L/day} \times 40 \text{ mg/L} \tag{4-1}$$
$$= 7200 \text{ mg/day, or } 7.2 \text{ g/day}$$

---

*In addition, the protein oncotic pressure in the peritubular capillaries is elevated because of the process of glomerular filtration (see Chapter 3). This elevated pressure also facilitates fluid and solute uptake into the capillary.

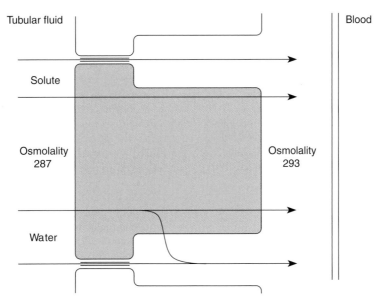

FIGURE 4-5 ■ Routes of water and solute reabsorption across the proximal tubule. The transport of solutes, including Na$^+$, Cl$^-$, and organic solutes, into the lateral intercellular space increases the osmolality of this compartment, which establishes the driving force for osmotic water reabsorption across the proximal tubule. This phenomenon occurs because some Na$^+$-K$^+$-adenosine triphosphatase and some transporters of organic solutes, HCO$_3^-$ and Cl$^-$, are located on the lateral cell membranes and deposit these solutes between cells. Furthermore, some sodium chloride also enters the lateral intercellular space by diffusion across the tight junction (i.e., paracellular pathway). An important consequence of osmotic water flow across the transcellular and paracellular pathways in the proximal tubule is that some solutes, especially K$^+$ and Ca^{++}, are entrained in the reabsorbed fluid and are thereby reabsorbed by the process of solvent drag.

AT THE CELLULAR LEVEL

Water channels called **aquaporins** (AQPs) mediate the transcellular reabsorption of water across many nephron segments. In 2003, Dr. Peter Agre received the Nobel Prize in Chemistry for his discovery that AQPs regulate and facilitate water transport across cell membranes, a process essential to all living organisms. To date, 14 aquaporins have been identified. The AQP family is divided into two groups on the basis of their permeability characteristics. One group (AQPs) is permeable to water (AQP0, AQP1, AQP2, AQP4, AQP5, AQP6, AQP8, AQP11, and AQP12). The other group (aquaglyceroporins) is permeable to water and small solutes, especially glycerol (AQP3, AQP5, AQP7, AQP9, and AQP10). AQPs form tetramers in the plasma membrane of cells, with each subunit forming a water channel. In the kidneys, AQP1 is expressed in the apical and basolateral membranes of the proximal tubule and portions of the descending thin limb of the loop of Henle (see Chapter 5). The importance of AQP1 in renal water reabsorption is underscored by studies in which the *AQP1* gene was "knocked out" in mice. These mice have increased urine output (polyuria) and a reduced ability to concentrate the urine. In addition, the osmotic water permeability of the proximal tubule is fivefold less in mice lacking APQ1 than in normal mice. AQP7 and AQP8 also are expressed in the proximal tubule. AQP2 is expressed in the apical plasma membrane of principal cells in the collecting duct, and its expression in the membrane is regulated by AVP. AQP3 and AQP4 are expressed in the basolateral membrane of principal cells in the collecting duct. Mice deficient in AQP3 or AQP4 (i.e., knockout mice) have defects in the ability to concentrate urine. AQPs also are expressed in many other organs in the body, including the lung, eye, skin, secretory glands, and brain, where they play key physiological roles. For example, AQP4 is expressed in cells that form the blood-brain barrier. Knockout of AQP4 in mice affects the water permeability of the blood-brain barrier such that brain edema is reduced after acute water loading and hyponatremia.

AT THE CELLULAR LEVEL

The endocytosis of protein by the proximal tubule is mediated by apical membrane receptors that specifically bind luminal proteins and peptides. These receptors, called **multiligand endocytic receptors**, can bind a wide range of peptides and proteins and thereby mediate their endocytosis. **Megalin** and **cubilin** mediate protein and peptide endocytosis in the proximal tubule. Both are glycoproteins, with megalin being a member of the low-density lipoprotein receptor gene family.

IN THE CLINIC

Urinalysis is an important and routine tool in disease detection. A thorough analysis of the urine includes macroscopic and microscopic assessments. These assessments are performed by visual assessment of the urine, microscopic examination, and chemical evaluation, which is conducted with use of dipstick reagents strips. The dipstick test is inexpensive and fast (i.e., it can be performed in less than 5 minutes). Dipstick reagent strips test the urine for the presence of many substances, including bilirubin, blood, glucose, ketones, pH, and protein. It is normal to find trace amounts of protein in the urine. Trace amounts of protein in the urine can be derived from two sources: (1) filtration and incomplete reabsorption by the proximal tubule and (2) synthesis by the thick ascending limb of the loop of Henle. Cells in the thick ascending limb produce **Tamm-Horsfall glycoprotein** and secrete it into the tubular fluid. Because the mechanism for protein reabsorption is "upstream" of the thick ascending limb (i.e., proximal tubule), the secreted Tamm-Horsfall glycoprotein appears in the urine. However, more than trace amounts of protein in the urine is indicative of renal disease.

Filtered proteins are either endocytosed intact or are endocytosed after being partially degraded by enzymes on the surface of the proximal tubule cells. Once the proteins and peptides are inside the cell, enzymes digest them into their constituent amino acids, which then leave the cell across the basolateral membrane by transport proteins and are returned to the blood. Normally this mechanism reabsorbs virtually all of the proteins filtered, and hence the urine is essentially protein free. However, because the mechanism is easily saturated, an increase in filtered proteins causes **proteinuria** (i.e., appearance of protein in the urine). Disruption of the glomerular filtration barrier to proteins increases the filtration of proteins and results in proteinuria, which is frequently found in persons with kidney disease.

Organic Anion and Organic Cation Secretion

Cells of the proximal tubule also secrete organic anions and organic cations into the tubule fluid. Secretion of organic anions and cations by the proximal tubule plays a key role in regulating the plasma levels of xenobiotics (e.g., a variety of antibiotics, diuretics, statins, antivirals, antineoplastics, immunosuppressants, neurotransmitters, and nonsteroidal antiinflammatory agents) and toxic compounds derived from endogenous and exogenous sources. Many of the organic anions and cations (see Boxes 4-1 and 4-2) secreted by the proximal tubule are end products of metabolism that circulate in the plasma. Many of these organic compounds are bound to plasma proteins and are not readily filtered. Therefore only a small portion of these potentially toxic substances are eliminated from the body by excretion resulting from filtration alone. Such substances also are secreted from the peritubular capillary into the tubular fluid. These secretory mechanisms are very powerful and can remove virtually all organic anions and cations from the plasma that enters the kidneys. Hence these substances are removed from the plasma by both filtration and secretion. Thus it is important to note that when kidney function is reduced by disease, the urinary excretion of organic anions and cations is severely reduced, which can lead to increased plasma levels of xenobiotics and metabolites.

Figure 4-6 illustrates the mechanisms of organic anion (OA^-) transport across the proximal tubule. These secretory pathways have a maximum transport rate and a low specificity (i.e., they transport many organic anions) and are responsible for the secretion of all organic anions listed in Box 4-1. OA^-s are taken up into the cell, across the basolateral membrane, and against their chemical gradient in exchange for α-ketoglutarate (α-KG) by several OA^-–α-KG antiport mechanisms, including OAT1, OAT2, and OAT3.

BOX 4-1

SOME ORGANIC ANIONS SECRETED BY THE PROXIMAL TUBULE

ENDOGENOUS ANIONS
Cyclic adenosine monophosphate
Cyclic guanosine monophosphate
Bile salts
Hippurate
Oxalate
Prostaglandins: PGE_2, $PGF_{2\alpha}$
Urate
Vitamins: ascorbate, folate

DRUGS
Acetazolamide
Acyclovir

Amoxicillin
Captopril
Chlorothiazide
Furosemide
Losartan
Penicillin
Probenecid
Salicylate (aspirin)
Simvastatin
Bumetanide
Nonsteroidal antiinflammatory drus (e.g., indomethacin)

BOX 4-2

SOME ORGANIC CATIONS SECRETED BY THE PROXIMAL TUBULE

ENDOGENOUS	DRUGS
Creatinine	Atropine
Dopamine	Isoproterenol
Epinephrine	Cimetidine
Norepinephrine	Morphine
	Quinine
	Amiloride
	Procainamide

α-KG accumulates inside the cells by metabolism of glutamate and by an Na^+–α-KG symporter (i.e., the Na^+-dicarboxylate transporter [NaDC3]) also present in the basolateral membrane. Thus OA^- uptake into the cell against an electrochemical gradient is coupled to the exit of α-KG out of the cell, down its chemical gradient generated by the Na^+–α-KG antiport mechanism. The exit of OA^- across the luminal membrane into the tubular fluid is mediated by the multidrug resistance proteins 2 and 4 (MRP2/4) and breast cancer resistance protein 1 (BCRP), which require ATP for their operation (i.e., they are ABC transporters). Recent studies reveal that OAT4 mediates the reabsorption of urate, the end product of purine catabolism, and the secretion of several drugs (see Figure 4-6).

IN THE CLINIC

Because many organic anions compete for the same secretory pathways, elevated plasma levels of one anion often inhibit the secretion of the others. For example, infusing para-amino hippurate (PAH) can reduce penicillin secretion by the proximal tubule. Because the kidneys are responsible for eliminating penicillin, the infusion of PAH into persons who receive penicillin reduces penicillin excretion and thereby extends the biologic half-life of the drug. In World War II, when penicillin was in short supply, hippurates were given with the penicillin to extend the drug's therapeutic effect. Similar competition for secretion by the proximal tubule occurs for organic cations. For example, elevated plasma levels of one cation often inhibit the secretion of the others. The H_2 antagonist cimetidine is used to treat gastric ulcers, and organic cation transport mechanisms in the proximal tubule secrete cimetidine. When cimetidine is given to patients who also receive procainamide (a drug used to treat cardiac arrhythmias), cimetidine reduces the urinary excretion of procainamide (also an organic cation) by competing with this antiarrhythmic drug for the secretory pathway. Thus the coadministration of organic cations can increase the plasma concentrations of both drugs to levels much higher than those seen when the drugs are given alone. This effect can lead to drug toxicity.

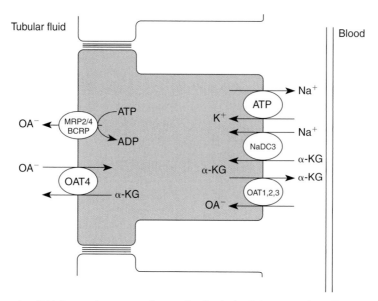

FIGURE 4-6 ■ Organic anion (*OA*⁻) secretion across the proximal tubule. OA⁻s enter the cell across the basolateral membrane by one of three OA⁻–α-ketoglutarate (*α-KG*) antiport mechanisms (organic anion transporter, OAT1, OAT2, OAT3). The uptake of α-KG into the cell, against its chemical concentration gradient, is driven by the movement of Na⁺ into the cell by the Na⁺-dicarboxylate transporter (*NaDC3*). The [Na⁺] inside the cell is low because of the Na⁺-K⁺-adenosine triphosphatase pump itn the basolateral membrane, which transports Na⁺ out the cell in exchange for K⁺. The α-KG recycles across the basolateratl membrane on the OATs in exchange for OA⁻. OA⁻s leave the cell across the apical membrane by multidrug resistance proteins (*MRP2/4*) and breast cancer resistance protein (*BCRP*), which require adenosine triphosphate (*ATP*). OAT4 in the apical membrane also transports OA⁻. OAT4 can reabsorb urate into the cell in exchange for α-KG, or secrete a number of drugs into the tubule lumen in exchange for α-KG. *ADP*, adenosine diphosphate.

Figure 4-7 illustrates the mechanism of organic cation (OC⁺) transport across the proximal tubule. OC⁺s, including xenobiotics such as the antidiabetic agent metformin, the antiviral agent lamivudine, and the anticancer drug oxiliplatin, along with many important monoamine neurotransporters, including dopamine, epinephrine, histamine, and norepinephrine, are secreted by the proximal tubule. OC⁺s are taken up into the cell, across the basolateral membrane, primarily by the OC⁺ transporter 2 (OCT2). Uptake of organic cations is driven by the magnitude of the cell-negative potential difference across the basolateral membrane. Organic cation transport across the luminal membrane into the tubular fluid, which is the rate-limiting step in secretion, is mediated primarily by the electrically neutral multidrug and toxin extrusion transporters (MATEs) and the ABC transporter MDR1 (also known as *P-glycoprotein*). These transport mechanisms mediating OC⁺ secretion are nonspecific; several OC⁺s usually compete for each transport pathway.

Henle's Loop

Henle's loop reabsorbs approximately 25% of the filtered NaCl and 15% of the filtered water. The reabsorption of NaCl in the loop of Henle occurs in both the thin ascending and thick ascending limbs. The descending thin limb does not reabsorb NaCl. Water reabsorption occurs exclusively in some portions of the descending thin limb through AQP1 water channels (see Chapter 5). The ascending limb is impermeable to water. In addition, Ca⁺⁺ and HCO₃⁻ are reabsorbed in the loop of Henle (see Chapters 8 and 9 for more details).

The thin ascending limb reabsorbs NaCl by a passive mechanism. The reabsorption of water but not NaCl in the descending thin limb increases the [NaCl] in tubule fluid entering the ascending thin limb. As the NaCl-rich fluid moves toward the cortex, NaCl diffuses out of tubule fluid across the ascending thin limb into the medullary interstitial fluid, down a concentration gradient directed from tubule fluid to interstitium.

Tubular fluid

Blood

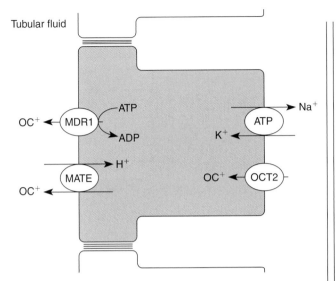

FIGURE 4-7 ■ Organic cation (OC^+) secretion across the proximal tubule. OC^+s enter the cell across the basolateral membrane primarily by OCT2. The uptake of OC^+s into the cell, against their chemical concentration gradient, is driven by the cell-negative potential difference. OC^+s leave the cell across the apical membrane in exchange with H^+ by electrically neutral multidrug and toxin extrusion transporters (*MATE1* and MATE2-K), by multidrug resistance protein (*MDR1*) and, possibly, by two OC^+-H^+ antiporters (OCTN1/2, not shown). *ADP*, Adenosine diphosphate; *ATP*, adenosine triphosphate.

The key element in solute reabsorption by the thick ascending limb is the Na^+-K^+-ATPase pump in the basolateral membrane (Figure 4-8). As with reabsorption in the proximal tubule, the reabsorption of every solute by the thick ascending limb is linked to Na^+-K^+-ATPase. This transporter maintains a low intracellular $[Na^+]$, which provides a favorable chemical gradient for the movement of Na^+ from the tubular fluid into the cell. The movement of Na^+ across the apical membrane into the cell is mediated by the Na^+-K^+-$2Cl^-$ symporter (NKCC2), which couples the movement of Na^+ with K^+ and $2Cl^-$. Using the potential energy released by the downhill movement of Na^+ and Cl^-, this symporter drives the uphill movement of K^+ into the cell. The K^+ channel in the apical plasma membrane plays an important role in NaCl reabsorption by the thick ascending limb. This K^+ channel allows the K^+ transported into the cell by NKCC2 to recycle back into tubule fluid. Because the $[K^+]$ in tubule fluid is relatively low, K^+ recycling is required for the continued operation of NKCC2. An Na^+-H^+ antiporter in the apical cell membrane also mediates Na^+ reabsorption as well as H^+ secretion (HCO_3^- reabsorption) in the thick ascending limb (see Chapter 8). Na^+ leaves the cell across the basolateral membrane through the Na^+-K^+-ATPase pump, whereas K^+, Cl^-, and HCO_3^- leave the cell across the basolateral membrane by separate pathways.

The voltage across the thick ascending limb is important for the reabsorption of several cations. The tubular fluid is positively charged relative to blood because of the unique location of transport proteins in the apical and basolateral membranes. Two points are important: (1) increased NaCl transport by the thick ascending limb increases the magnitude of the positive voltage in the lumen, and (2) this voltage is an important driving force for the reabsorption of several cations, including Na^+, K^+, Mg^{++}, and Ca^{++} across the paracellular pathway (see Figure 4-8). The importance of the paracellular pathway to solute reabsorption is underscored by the observation that inactivating mutations of the tight junction protein claudin-16 reduces Mg^{++} and Ca^{++} reabsorption by the ascending thick limb even when the lumen-positive transepithelial voltage is positive.

In summary, salt reabsorption across the thick ascending limb occurs by the transcellular and paracellular pathways. A total of 50% of NaCl reabsorption is transcellular, and 50% is paracellular. The thick ascending limb does not reabsorb **water** because it does not express water channels (i.e., AQPs), and thus the reabsorption of NaCl and other solutes reduces the osmolality of tubular fluid to less than 150 mOsm/kg H_2O. Thus because the thick ascending limb produces a fluid that is dilute relative to plasma, the ascending limb of the Henle loop is called the **diluting segment**.

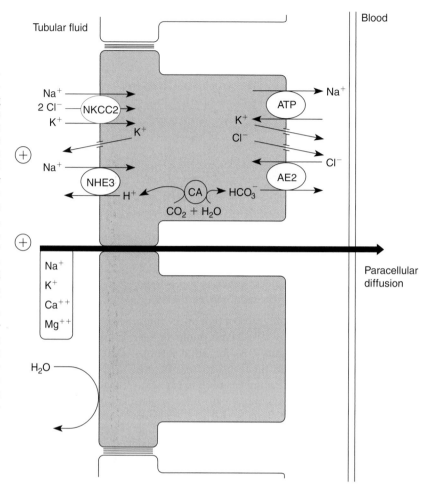

FIGURE 4-8 ■ Transport mechanisms for sodium chloride reabsorption in the thick ascending limb of the loop of Henle. The positive voltage in the lumen plays a major role in driving the passive paracellular reabsorption of cations. Because the apical membrane is conductive primarily to K^+, the apical membrane voltage is more negative than the basolateral membrane voltage, which is conductive to K^+ and Cl^-, thereby resulting in a lumen-positive transepithelial potential. Mutations in the gene encoding the apical membrane K^+ channel, the apical membrane Na^+-K^+-$2Cl^-$ symporter (*NKCC2*), or the basolateral Cl^- channel cause Bartter syndrome (see the clinical box on Bartter syndrome). *AE2*, anion exchanger 2; *ATP*, adenosine triphosphate; *CA*, carbonic anhydrase; CO_2, carbon dioxide; HCO_3^-, bicarbonate; *NHE3*, Na^+-H^+ antiporter 3.

AT THE CELLULAR LEVEL

As previously described in this chapter and in Chapter 2, epithelial cells are joined at their apical surfaces by tight junctions (also knows as **zonula occludens**). A number of proteins now have been identified as components of the tight junction. These proteins include those that span the membrane of one cell and link to the extracellular portion of the same molecule in the adjacent cell (e.g., occludins and claudins), as well as cytoplasmic linker proteins (e.g., ZO-1, ZO-2, and ZO-3) that link the membrane-spanning proteins to the cytoskeleton of the cell. Of these junctional proteins, claudins appear to be important in determining the permeability characteristics of the tight junction. Claudin-16 and

claudin-19 are critical for determining divalent cation permeability of the tight junctions in the thick ascending limb of the Henle loop. Mutations in human claudin-16 and claudin-19 cause familial hypomagnesemia with hypercalciuria and nephrolithiasis. Claudin-2 is permeable to water and may allow paracellular water reabsorption across the proximal tubule. In cultured kidney cells, claudin-4 has been shown to control the Na^+ permeability of the tight junction, and claudin-15 determines whether a tight junction is permeable to cations or anions. Thus the permeability characteristics of the tight junctions in different nephron segments are determined, at least in part, by the specific claudins expressed by the cells in that segment.

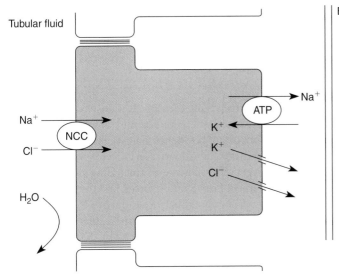

Tubular fluid

Blood

FIGURE 4-9 ■ Transport mechanism for Na^+ and Cl^- reabsorption in the early segment of the distal tubule. This segment is impermeable to water. Mutations in the apical membrane sodium chloride cotransporter gene cause Gitelman syndrome. *ATP*, Adenosine triphosphate; *NCC*, sodium-chloride cotransporter.

IN THE CLINIC

Bartter syndrome is a set of autosomal recessive genetic diseases characterized by hypokalemia, metabolic alkalosis, and hyperaldosteronism (see Table 4-3). Inactivating mutations in the gene coding for the Na^+-K^+-$2Cl^-$ symporter (*SLC12A1*), the apical K^+ channel (*KCNJ1*), or the basolateral Cl^- channel (*ClCNKB*) decrease both sodium chloride (NaCl) and K^+ reabsorption by the ascending thick limb, which in turn causes hypokalemia (i.e., a low plasma $[K^+]$) and a decrease in the extracellular fluid (ECF) volume. The decrease in ECF volume stimulates aldosterone secretion, which in turn stimulates NaCl reabsorption and H^+ secretion by the distal tubule and collecting duct (discussed later in this chapter).

AT THE CELLULAR LEVEL

Gitelman syndrome is an autosomal recessive disorder characterized by metabolic alkalosis, hypokalemia, and hypocalciuria (hypomagnesemia also is seen often). It results from an inactivating mutation of the Na^+-Cl^- symporter gene (*SLC12A3*) that is expressed in the early portion of the distal tubule. The fluid and electrolyte disturbances seen in patients with Gitelman syndrome can be mimicked by administration of thiazide diuretics, which act by inhibiting the sodium chloride transporter.

Cl^- leaves the cell by diffusion through Cl^- channels. NaCl reabsorption is reduced by thiazide diuretics, which inhibit NCC. Thus dilution of the tubular fluid begins in the thick ascending limb and continues in the early segment of the distal tubule.

The last segment of the distal tubule (late distal tubule) and the collecting duct are composed of two cell types: **principal cells** and **intercalated cells**. As illustrated in Figure 4-10, *A*, principal cells reabsorb Na^+ and water and secrete K^+. The α-intercalated cell secretes H^+ and reabsorbs HCO_3^- and K^+ and thus is important in regulating acid-base balance (see Chapter 8) and K^+ balance (see Chapter 7). β-Intercalated cells secrete HCO_3^- and reabsorb H^+ and Cl^- (Figure 4-10, *C*). α-Intercalated cells also reabsorb K^+ by the

Distal Tubule and Collecting Duct

The distal tubule and collecting duct reabsorb approximately 8% of the filtered NaCl, secrete variable amounts of K^+ and H^+, and reabsorb a variable amount of water (~8% to 17%). The initial segment of the distal tubule (the early distal tubule) reabsorbs Na^+, Cl^-, and Ca^{++} and is impermeable to water (Figure 4-9). NaCl entry into the cell across the apical membrane is mediated by a Na^+-Cl^- symporter (NCC). Na^+ leaves the cell through the action of Na^+-K^+-ATPase, and operation of an H^+-K^+-ATPase mechanism located in the apical plasma membrane (Figure 4-10, *B*). Both Na^+ reabsorption and K^+ secretion by principal cells depend on the activity of Na^+-K^+-ATPase in the basolateral membrane (see Figure 4-10, *A*). By maintaining a low intracellular $[Na^+]$, this transporter provides a favorable chemical gradient for the movement of Na^+ from the tubular fluid into the cell. Because Na^+ enters the cell across the apical membrane by diffusion through Na^+-selective channels in the apical membrane, the negative voltage inside the cell facilitates Na^+ entry. Na^+ leaves the cell across the basolateral membrane and enters the blood through the action of Na^+-K^+-ATPase. Na^+ reabsorption generates a lumen-negative voltage across the late distal tubule and collecting duct, which provides the driving force for Cl^- reabsorption across the paracellular pathway. As previously noted, Cl^- also is reabsorbed by β-intercalated cells (Figure 4-10, *C*). Chloride enters the β-intercalated cell across the apical membrane via a Cl^-/HCO_3^- antiporter (Pendrin) and leaves the cell across the basolateral membrane via a Cl^- channel. A variable amount of water is reabsorbed across principal cells in the late distal tubule and collecting duct. Water reabsorption is mediated by the AQP2 water channel located in the apical plasma membrane and AQP3 and AQP4 water channels located in the basolateral membrane of principal cells. In the presence of arginine vasopressin (AVP), water is reabsorbed. By contrast, in the absence of AVP, the distal tubule and collecting duct reabsorb little water (see Chapter 5).

K^+ is secreted from the blood into the tubular fluid by principal cells in two steps (see Figure 4-10, *A*). First, K^+ uptake across the basolateral membrane is mediated by the action of the Na^+-K^+-ATPase pump. Second, K^+ leaves the cell by passive diffusion. Because the K^+ concentration inside the cells is high (~150 mEq/L) and the K^+ concentration in tubular fluid is low (~10 mEq/L), K^+ diffuses down its concentration gradient through apical cell membrane K^+ channels into the tubular fluid. Although the negative potential inside the cells tends to retain K^+ within the cell, the electrochemical gradient across the apical membrane favors K^+ secretion from the cell into the tubular fluid (see Chapter 7). K^+ reabsorption by α-intercalated cells is mediated by

an H^+-K^+-ATPase pump located in the apical cell membrane (Figure 4-10, *B*).

REGULATION OF NaCl AND WATER REABSORPTION

Quantitatively, angiotensin II, aldosterone, catecholamines, natriuretic peptides, and uroguanylin are the most important hormones that regulate NaCl reabsorption and thereby urinary NaCl excretion (Table 4-6). However, other hormones (including dopamine and adrenomedullin), Starling forces, and the phenomenon of glomerulotubular balance influence NaCl reabsorption. AVP is the only major hormone that directly regulates the amount of water excreted by the kidneys.

Angiotensin II has a potent stimulatory effect on NaCl and water reabsorption in the proximal tubule. It also has been shown to stimulate Na^+ reabsorption in the thick ascending limb of the Henle loop, as well as the distal tubule and collecting duct. Angiotensin II is one of the most potent hormones that stimulates NaCl and water reabsorption in the proximal tubule. A decrease in the extracellular fluid (ECF) volume activates the renin-angiotensin-aldosterone system (see Chapter 6 for more details), thereby increasing the plasma concentration of angiotensin II.

Aldosterone, which is synthesized by the glomerulosa cells of the adrenal cortex, stimulates NaCl reabsorption. It acts on the thick ascending limb of the loop of Henle, the late segment of the distal tubule, and the collecting duct. As described in Chapter 6, the late distal tubule and collecting duct are collectively termed the **aldosterone-sensitive distal nephron (ASDN)**. Aldosterone also stimulates K^+ secretion by the late segment of the distal tubule and collecting duct (see Chapter 7). Aldosterone enhances NaCl reabsorption across principal cells in the ASDN by four mechanisms: (1) increasing the amount of Na^+-K^+-ATPase in the basolateral membrane; (2) increasing the expression of the epithelial sodium channel (ENaC) in the apical cell membrane; (3) elevating serum glucocorticoid–stimulated kinase (Sgk) levels, which also increases the expression of ENaC in the apical cell membrane; and (4) stimulating channel-activating protease (CAP1, also called prostatin), a serine protease, which directly activates ENaC channels by proteolysis. Taken together, these actions increase

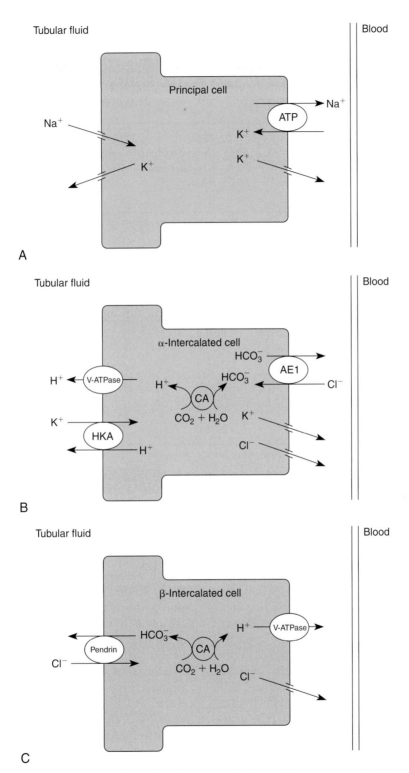

FIGURE 4-10 ■ Transport pathways in principal cells, α-intercalated cells and β-intercalated cells of the late segment of the distal tubule and collecting duct. Principal cells reabsorb Na^+ and secrete K^+. α-intercalated cells secrete H^+ and reabsorb bicarbonate (HCO_3^-) and K^+, and β-intercalated cells secrete HCO_3^- and reabsorb H^+ and Cl^-. *AE1,* anion exchanger 1; *ATP,* adenosine triphosphate; *CA,* carbonic anhydrase; *CO_2,* carbon dioxide; *HKA,* H^+-K^+–adenosine triphosphatase; *V-ATPase,* vacuolar adenosine triphosphatase.

		TABLE 4-5		
		Water Transport Along the Nephron		
SEGMENT	PERCENTAGE OF FILTERED REABSORBED	MECHANISM OF WATER REABSORPTION	HORMONES THAT REGULATE WATER PERMEABILITY
Proximal tubule	67	Passive	None
Loop of Henle	15	Descending thin limb only; passive	None
Distal tubule	0	No water reabsorption	None
Late distal tubule and collecting duct	~8-17	Passive	AVP, ANP,* BNP*

*Atrial natriuretic peptide (ANP) and brain natriuretic peptide (BNP) inhibit arginine vasopressin (AVP)-stimulated water permeability.

		TABLE 4-6	
		Hormones that Regulate NaCl and Water Reabsorption	
HORMONE*	MAJOR STIMULUS	NEPHRON SITE OF ACTION	EFFECT ON TRANSPORT
Angiotensin II	↑ Renin	PT, TAL, DT/CD	↑ NaCl and H_2O reabsorption
Aldosterone	↑ Angiotensin II, ↑ $[K^+]_p$	TAL, DT/CD	↑ NaCl and H_2O reabsorption†
ANP, BNP, urodilatin	↑ ECFV	CD	↓ H_2O and NaCl reabsorption
Uroguanylin, guanylin	Oral ingestion of NaCl	PT, CD	↓ H_2O and NaCl reabsorption
Sympathetic nerves	↓ ECFV	PT, TAL, DT/CD	↑ NaCl and H_2O reabsorption
Dopamine	↑ ECFV	PT	↓ H_2O and NaCl reabsorption
AVP	↑ P_{osm}, ↓ECFV	DT/CD	↑ H_2O reabsorption

*All these hormones act within minutes except aldosterone, which exerts its action on NaCl reabsorption with a delay of 1 hour. Aldosterone achieves its maximal effect after a few days.
†The effect on H_2O reabsorption does not include the thick ascending limb or the early portion of the distal tubule.
ANP, atrial natriuretic peptide; AVP, arginine vasopressin; BNP, brain natriuretic peptide, CD, collecting duct; DT, distal tubule; ECFV, extracellular fluid volume; $[K^+]_p$, plasma K^+ concentration; NaCl, sodium chloride; P_{osm}, plasma osmolality; PT, proximal tubule; TAL, thick ascending limb.

the uptake of Na^+ across the apical cell membrane and facilitate the exit of Na^+ from the cell interior into the blood. The increase in the reabsorption of Na^+ generates a lumen-negative transepithelial voltage across the late segment of the distal tubule and collecting duct. This lumen-negative voltage provides the electrochemical driving force for Cl^- reabsorption across the tight junctions (i.e., paracellular pathway) in the ASDN. Aldosterone secretion is enhanced by hyperkalemia and by volume contraction (i.e., reduced ECF volume) via increased angiotensin II (after activation of the renin-angiotensin system). Aldosterone secretion is decreased by hypokalemia and natriuretic peptides (discussed later in this chapter). Through its stimulation of NaCl reabsorption in the collecting duct, aldosterone also indirectly increases water reabsorption by this nephron segment.

Atrial natriuretic peptide (ANP) and **brain natriuretic peptide** (BNP) inhibit NaCl and water reabsorption. Secretion of ANP by the cardiac atria and BNP by the cardiac ventricles is stimulated by a rise in blood pressure and an increase in the ECF volume. ANP and BNP reduce the blood pressure by decreasing the total peripheral resistance and by enhancing urinary NaCl and water excretion, primarily by increasing GFR and renal blood flow (RBF). These natriuretic peptides vasodilate the afferent and efferent arterioles, which increases GFR and thus the filtration of NaCl, thereby increasing NaCl excretion (see the discussion on glomerulotubular balance later in this chapter for the mechanism). In addition, the increase in RBF decreases the concentration of NaCl in the medullary interstitium, which in turn reduces passive NaCl reabsorption by the thin ascending limb of

AT THE CELLULAR LEVEL

As previously noted, aldosterone stimulates both sodium chloride (NaCl) reabsorption and K$^+$ secretion by the collecting duct. Although both a reduction in the extracellular fluid (ECF) volume (i.e., volume contraction; see Chapter 6) and hyperkalemia (see Chapter 7) increase aldosterone levels, the physiologic response of the kidneys with regard to NaCl and K$^+$ excretion differs in these two conditions. During reduction in the ECF volume, NaCl excretion by the kidneys is reduced, to restore ECF volume, without a change in K$^+$ excretion. By contrast, during hyperkalemia, K$^+$ excretion by the kidneys is increased, to return plasma [K$^+$] to normal, without a change in NaCl excretion. This phenomenon, the apparent independent effects of aldosterone on net urinary Na$^+$ and K$^+$ excretion, is called the **aldosterone paradox**. The paradox can be explained by the observation that although aldosterone increases in both conditions, angiotensin II levels increase only during ECF volume contraction and not during hyperkalemia, and the fact that aldosterone and angiotensin II differentially regulate a number of transport proteins in several nephron segments. The integrated physiological response to a reduction in the ECF volume is depicted in Figure 4-11, *A*. During volume contraction, angiotensin II stimulates NaCl reabsorption by the proximal tubule (not shown in Figure 4-11) and by the distal tubule (early segment) by activating **w**ith **n**o lysine (**K**) kinase (WNK), which enhances NaCl reabsorption by activating NCC. Aldosterone stimulates Na$^+$ reabsorption in principal cells of the collecting duct by activating *SGK1*, which increases the abundance of epithelial sodium channel (ENaC) channels in the apical plasma membrane. Both effects stimulate NaCl reabsorption. Moreover, angiotensin II activates WNK in principal cells, which inhibits K$^+$ secretion via the **r**enal **o**uter **m**edullary **K**$^+$ (**ROMK**) channel, thereby preventing an increase in K$^+$ excretion even though aldosterone levels are elevated. The integrated physiological response to hyperkalemia is depicted in Figure 4-11, *B*. During hyperkalemia, aldosterone stimulates ROMK-mediated K$^+$ secretion by principal cells in the collecting duct by activating WNK (a different WNK than the one that inhibits ROMK), thereby increasing K$^+$ excretion by the kidneys. Because the distal tubule (early segment) is not responsive to aldosterone, this hormone does not stimulate NaCl reabsorption in this nephron segment. In fact, because

angiotensin II levels are not elevated during hyperkalemia, the basal activity of WNK is low, resulting in reduced NaCl reabsorption via NCC (Figure 4-11, *B*). The lack of effect of WNK on NaCl reabsorption in the distal tubule offsets the stimulatory effect of aldosterone on NaCl reabsorption in principal cells of the collecting duct, resulting in no net change in urinary NaCl excretion during hyperkalemia.

AT THE CELLULAR LEVEL

Serum **g**lucocorticoid-stimulated **k**inase (**Sgk**), a serine/threonine kinase, plays an important role in maintaining sodium chloride (NaCl) and K$^+$ homeostasis by regulating NaCl and K$^+$ excretion by the kidneys. Studies in Sgk1 knockout mice reveal that this kinase is required for animals to survive severe NaCl restriction and K$^+$ loading. NaCl restriction and K$^+$ loading enhance plasma (aldosterone), which rapidly (in minutes) increases Sgk1 protein expression and phosphorylation. Phosphorylated Sgk1 enhances epithelial sodium channel (ENaC)-mediated sodium reabsorption in the collecting duct, primarily by increasing the number of ENaC channels in the apical plasma membrane of principal cells and also by increasing the number of Na$^+$-K$^+$ ATPase pumps in the basolateral membrane. Phosphorylated Sgk1 inhibits Nedd4-2, a ubiquitin ligase, which monoubiquitinylates ENaC subunits, targeting them for endocytic removal from the plasma membrane and subsequent destruction in lysosomes. Inhibition of Nedd4-2 by Sgk1 reduces the monoubiquitinylation of ENaC, thereby reducing endocytosis and increasing the number of channels in the membrane. Sgk1 induces a translocation of ROMK from an intracellular pool to the plasma membrane and thereby enhances ROMK-mediated K$^+$ secretion by principal cells. These effects of Sgk1 precede the aldosterone-stimulated increase in ENaC, ROMK, and Na$^+$-K$^+$ ATPase abundance, which leads to a delayed (>4 hours) secondary increase in NaCl and K$^+$ transport by the collecting duct. Activating polymorphisms in Sgk1 cause an increase in blood pressure, presumably by enhanced NaCl reabsorption by the collecting duct, which increases the extracellular fluid volume and thereby blood pressure.

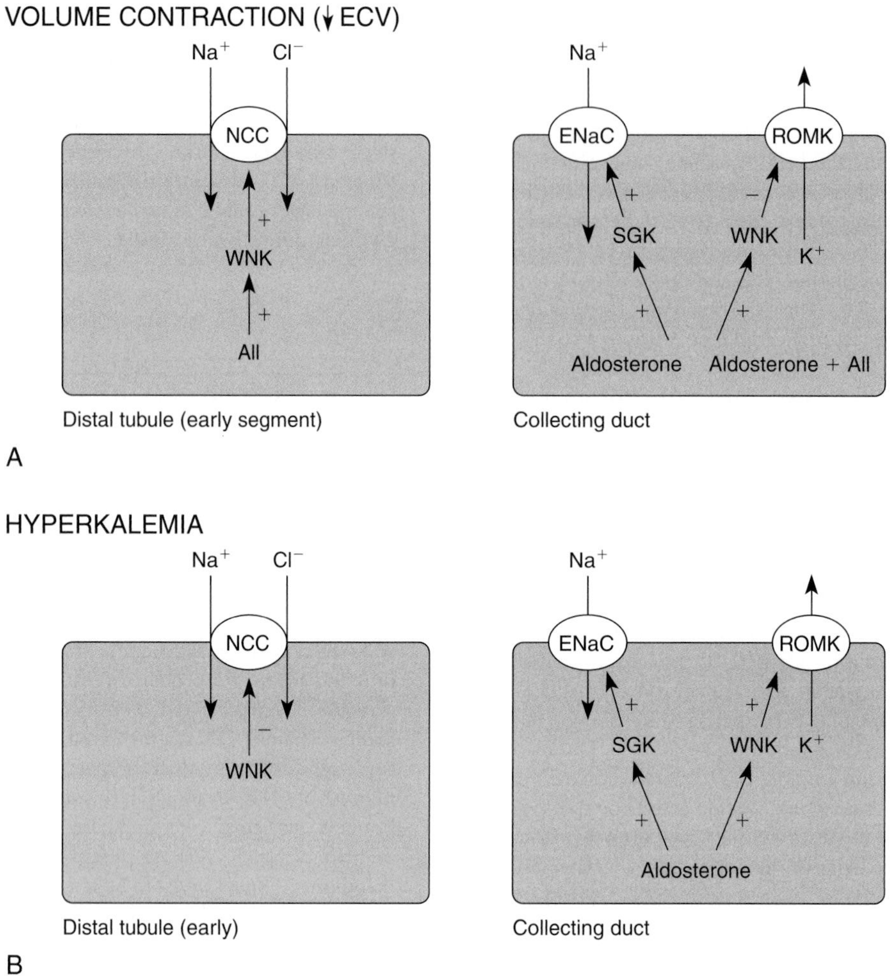

FIGURE 4-11 ■ Volume contraction enhances net sodium chloride (NaCl) reabsorption but has no effect on net K⁺ excretion by the mechanism depicted in (**A**). Hyperkalemia enhances net K⁺ excretion but has no effect on net NaCl excretion by the mechanism depicted in (**B**). *AII*, angiotensin II; *ECV*, effective circulating volume; *ENaC*, epithelial sodium channel; *NCC*, NaCl cotransporter; *ROMK*, K+ channel; *SGK*, serum glucocorticoid kinase; *WNK4*, with no lysine; *(K)*, potassium; +, stimulate; −, inhibit.

the loop of Henle (see Chapter 5 for details on NaCl reabsorption by the thin ascending limb of the loop of Henle). ANP and BNP also inhibit NaCl reabsorption by the medullary portion of the collecting duct and inhibit AVP-stimulated water reabsorption across the collecting duct. Moreover, ANP and BNP also reduce the secretion of AVP from the posterior pituitary. These actions of ANP and BNP are mediated by activation of membrane-bound guanylyl cyclase receptors,

which increase intracellular levels of the second messenger cyclic guanosine monophosphate (cGMP). ANP induces a more profound natriuresis and diuresis than does BNP.

Urodilatin and ANP are encoded by the same gene and have similar amino acid sequences. Urodilatin is a 32-amino-acid hormone that differs from ANP by the addition of four amino acids to the amino terminus. Urodilatin is secreted by the distal

Liddle syndrome is a rare genetic disorder characterized by an increase in the extracellular fluid (ECF) volume that causes an increase in blood pressure (i.e., hypertension). Liddle syndrome is caused by activating mutations in either the β or γ subunit of the epithelial Na^+ channel gene (*ENaC*), which is composed of three subunits, α, β, and γ. These mutations increase the number of Na^+ channels in the apical cell membrane of principal cells and thereby the amount of Na^+ reabsorbed by each channel. In persons with Liddle syndrome, the rate of renal Na^+ reabsorption is inappropriately high, which leads to an increase in the ECF volume and hypertension.

Two different forms of **pseudohypoaldosteronism type 1** (PHA1) exist (i.e., the kidneys waste sodium chloride [NaCl] as they do when aldosterone levels are reduced; however, in PHA1, aldosterone levels are elevated). The autosomal recessive form is caused by inactivating mutations in the α, β, or γ subunit of *ENaC*. The etiology of the autosomal dominant form is an inactivating mutation in the mineralocorticoid receptor. PHA is characterized by an increase in Na^+ excretion, a reduction in the ECF volume, hyperkalemia, and hypotension. Some persons with expanded ECF volume and elevated blood pressure are treated with drugs that inhibit **angiotensin-converting enzyme** (ACE) inhibitors (e.g., captopril, enalapril, and lisinopril) and thereby lower fluid volume and blood pressure. The inhibition of ACE blocks the degradation of angiotensin I to angiotensin II and thereby lowers plasma angiotensin II levels (see Chapter 6 for details). The decline in plasma angiotensin II concentration has three effects. First, NaCl and water reabsorption by the nephron (especially the proximal tubule) decreases. Second, aldosterone secretion decreases, thus reducing NaCl reabsorption in the thick ascending limb, distal tubule, and collecting duct. Third, because angiotensin is a potent vasoconstrictor, a reduction in its concentration permits the systemic arterioles to dilate and thereby lower arterial blood pressure. ACE also degrades the vasodilator hormone bradykinin; thus ACE inhibitors increase the concentration of bradykinin, a vasodilatory hormone. ACE inhibitors decrease the extracellular fluid volume and the arterial blood pressure by promoting renal NaCl and water excretion and by reducing total peripheral vascular resistance.

tubule and collecting duct and is not present in the systemic circulation; thus urodilatin influences only the function of the kidneys. Urodilatin secretion is stimulated by a rise in the blood pressure and an increase in the ECF volume. It inhibits NaCl and water reabsorption across the medullary portion of the collecting duct. Urodilatin is a more potent natriuretic and diuretic hormone than ANP because some of the ANP that enters the kidneys in the blood is degraded by a neutral endopeptidase that has no effect on urodilatin.

Uroguanylin and **guanylin** are produced by neuroendocrine cells in the intestine in response to the oral ingestion of NaCl. These hormones enter the circulation and inhibit NaCl and water reabsorption by the kidneys by activation of membrane-bound guanylyl cyclase receptors, which increases intracellular levels of cGMP. The natriuretic response of the kidneys to a salt load is more pronounced when given orally than when delivered intravenously because oral administration of salt causes the intestinal secretion of uroguanylin and guanylin.

Catecholamines stimulate NaCl reabsorption. Catecholamines released from the sympathetic nerves (norepinephrine) and the adrenal medulla (epinephrine) stimulate NaCl and water reabsorption by the proximal tubule, the thick ascending limb of the loop of Henle, the distal tubule, and the collecting duct. Although sympathetic nerves are not very active when the ECF volume is normal, when ECF volume declines (e.g., after hemorrhage), sympathetic nerve activity rises dramatically and stimulates NaCl and water reabsorption by these four nephron segments.

Dopamine, a catecholamine, is synthesized by cells of the proximal tubule. The action of dopamine is opposite to that of norepinephrine and epinephrine. Dopamine secretion is stimulated by an increase in ECF volume, and its secretion directly inhibits NaCl and water reabsorption in the proximal tubule.

Adrenomedullin is a 52-amino-acid peptide hormone that is produced by a variety of organs including the kidneys. Adrenomedullin induces a marked diuresis and natriuresis, and its secretion is stimulated by congestive heart failure and hypertension. The major effect of adrenomedullin on the kidneys is to increase GFR and RBF and thereby to stimulate indirectly the excretion of NaCl and water (see the previous discussion regarding ANP/BNP).

AVP regulates water reabsorption and is the most important hormone that regulates water reabsorption in the kidneys (see Chapter 5). This hormone is secreted by the posterior pituitary gland in response to an increase in plasma osmolality (1% or more) or a decrease in the ECF volume (>5% to 10% of normal). AVP increases the permeability of the collecting duct to water and thereby increases osmotic water reabsorption across the collecting duct because of the osmotic gradient that exists between tubular fluid and the interstitium (see Chapter 5). AVP has little effect on urinary NaCl excretion.

Starling forces regulate NaCl and water reabsorption across the proximal tubule. As previously described, Na^+, Cl^-, HCO_3^-, amino acids, glucose, and water are transported into the intercellular space of the proximal tubule. Starling forces between this space and the peritubular capillaries facilitate the movement of the reabsorbed fluid into the capillaries. Starling forces across the wall of the peritubular capillaries are the hydrostatic pressures in the peritubular capillary (P_{pc}) and lateral intercellular space (P_i) and the oncotic pressures in the peritubular capillary (π_{pc}) and lateral intercellular space (π_i). Thus the reabsorption of water resulting from Na^+ transport from tubular fluid into the lateral intercellular space is modified by the Starling forces. Thus:

$$Q = K_f[(P_{pc} - P_i) + \sigma(\pi_{pc} - \pi_i)] \tag{4-2}$$

where Q is flow (positive numbers indicate flow from the intercellular space into blood). Starling forces that favor movement from the interstitium into the peritubular capillaries are π_{pc} and P_i (Figure 4-12). The opposing Starling forces are π_i and P_{pc}. Normally the sum of the Starling forces favors the movement of solute and water from the interstitial space into the capillary. However, some of the solutes and fluid that enter the lateral intercellular space leak back into the proximal tubular fluid. Starling forces do not affect transport by the loop of Henle, distal tubule, and collecting duct because these segments are less permeable to water than the proximal tubule.

A number of factors can alter the Starling forces across the peritubular capillaries surrounding the proximal tubule. For example, dilation of the efferent arteriole increases P_{pc}, whereas constriction of the efferent arteriole decreases it. An increase in P_{pc} inhibits solute and water reabsorption by increasing the back-leak of NaCl and **water** across the tight junction, whereas a decrease stimulates reabsorption by decreasing back-leak across the tight junction.

The π_{pc} is partially determined by the rate of formation of the glomerular ultrafiltrate. For example, if one assumes a constant plasma flow in the afferent arteriole, the plasma proteins become less concentrated in the plasma that enters the efferent arteriole and peritubular capillary because less ultrafiltrate is formed (i.e., as GFR decreases). Hence the π_{pc} decreases. The π_{pc} is directly related to the **filtration fraction** (FF) (FF = GFR/RPF). A decrease in the FF resulting from a decrease in GFR, at constant RPF, decreases the π_{pc}. This phenomenon in turn increases the backflow of NaCl and water from the lateral intercellular space into the tubular fluid and thereby decreases net solute and water reabsorption across the proximal tubule. An increase in the FF has the opposite effect.

The importance of Starling forces in regulating solute and water reabsorption by the proximal tubule is underscored by the phenomenon of **glomerulotubular (G-T) balance**. Spontaneous changes in GFR markedly alter the filtered load of Na^+ (filtered load = GFR × [Na^+]). Without rapid adjustments in Na^+ reabsorption to counter the changes in the filtration of Na^+, urine Na^+ excretion would fluctuate widely, disturb the Na^+ balance of the body, and thus alter ECF volume and blood pressure (see Chapter 6 for more details). However, spontaneous changes in GFR do not alter Na^+ excretion in the urine or Na^+ balance when ECF volume is normal because of the phenomenon of G-T balance. When body Na^+ balance is normal (i.e., ECF volume is normal), G-T balance refers to the fact that Na^+ and water reabsorption increases in proportion to the increase in GFR and filtered load of Na^+. Thus a constant fraction of the filtered Na^+ and water is reabsorbed from the proximal tubule despite variations in GFR. The net result of G-T balance is to reduce the impact of GFR changes on the amount of Na^+ and water excreted in the urine.

Two mechanisms are responsible for G-T balance. One is related to the oncotic and hydrostatic pressure

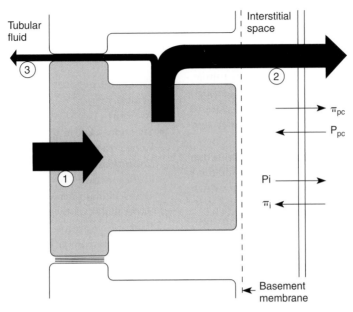

FIGURE 4-12 ■ Routes of solute and water transport across the proximal tubule and the Starling forces that modify reabsorption. The arrow labeled *1* represents solute and water being reabsorbed across the apical membrane. This solute and water then cross the lateral cell membrane. Some solute and water reenter the tubule fluid (indicated by arrow labeled *3*), and the remainder enters the interstitial space and then flows into the capillary (indicated by arrow labeled *2*). The width of the arrows is directly proportional to the amount of solute and water moving by the pathways labeled *1* to *3*. Starling forces across the capillary wall determine the amount of fluid flowing through pathway 2 versus 3. Transport mechanisms in the apical cell membranes determine the amount of solute and water entering the cell (pathway 1). π_i, Interstitial fluid oncotic pressure; π_{pc}, peritubular capillary oncotic pressure; Pi, interstitial hydrostatic pressure; P_{pc}, peritubular capillary hydrostatic pressure. *Thin arrows* across the capillary wall indicate direction of water movement in response to each force.

differences between the peritubular capillaries and the lateral intercellular space (i.e., Starling forces). For example, an increase in the GFR (at constant renal blood flow) raises the protein concentration in the glomerular capillary plasma above normal. This protein-rich plasma leaves the glomerular capillaries, flows through the efferent arterioles, and enters the peritubular capillaries. The increased π_{pc} augments the movement of solute and fluid from the lateral intercellular space into the peritubular capillaries. This action increases net solute and water reabsorption by the proximal tubule.

The second mechanism responsible for G-T balance is initiated by an increase in the filtered load of glucose and amino acids. As discussed earlier, the reabsorption of Na^+ in the first half of the proximal tubule is coupled to that of glucose and amino acids. The rate of Na^+ reabsorption therefore partially depends on the filtered load of glucose and amino acids. As the GFR and filtered load of glucose and amino acids increase, Na^+ and water reabsorption also rises.

In addition to G-T balance, another mechanism minimizes changes in the filtered load of Na^+. As discussed in Chapter 3, an increase in the GFR (and thus in the amount of Na^+ filtered by the glomerulus) activates the tubuloglomerular feedback mechanism. This action returns the GFR and filtration of Na^+ to normal values. Thus spontaneous changes in the GFR (e.g., caused by changes in posture and blood pressure) increase the amount of Na^+ filtered for only a few minutes. The mechanisms that underlie G-T balance maintain urinary Na^+ excretion constant and thereby maintain Na^+ homeostasis (and ECF volume and blood pressure) until the GFR returns to normal.

SUMMARY

1. The four major segments of the nephron (the proximal tubule, the loop of Henle, the distal tubule, and the collecting duct) determine the composition and volume of the urine by the processes of selective reabsorption of solutes and water and secretion of solutes.

2. Tubular reabsorption allows the kidneys to retain the substances that are essential and regulate their levels in the plasma by altering the degree to which they are reabsorbed. The reabsorption of Na^+, Cl^-, other anions, and organic anions and cations together with water constitutes the major function of the nephron. Approximately 25200 mEq of Na^+ and 179 L of water are reabsorbed each day. The proximal tubule cells reabsorb 67% of the glomerular ultrafiltrate, and cells of the Henle loop reabsorb about 25% of the NaCl that was filtered and about 15% of the water that was filtered. The distal segments of the nephron (distal tubule and collecting duct system) have a more limited reabsorptive capacity. However, the final adjustments in the composition and volume of the urine and most of the regulation by hormones and other factors occur in distal segments.

3. Secretion of substances into tubular fluid is a means for excreting various byproducts of metabolism, and it also serves to eliminate exogenous organic anions and cations (e.g., drugs) and toxins from the body. Many organic anions and cations are bound to plasma proteins and therefore are unavailable for ultrafiltration. Thus secretion is their major route of excretion in the urine.

4. Various hormones (including angiotensin II, aldosterone, AVP, natriuretic peptides [ANP and BNP], dopamine, urodilatin, uroguanylin, and guanylin), sympathetic nerves, and Starling forces regulate NaCl reabsorption by the kidneys. AVP is the major hormone that regulates water reabsorption.

KEY WORDS AND CONCEPTS

- Passive transport (diffusion)
- Solvent drag
- Facilitated diffusion
- Uniport
- Coupled transport
- Symport
- Antiport
- Secondary active transport
- Active transport
- Endocytosis
- Tight junctions
- Transcellular pathway
- Paracellular pathway
- Fanconi syndrome
- Glomerulotubular balance (G-T balance)
- Angiotensin II
- Aldosterone
- Aldosterone paradox
- Sympathetic nerves
- Catecholamines
- Vasopressin (AVP)
- Atrial natriuretic peptide (ANP)
- Brain natriuretic peptide (BNP)
- Urodilatin
- Uroguanylin
- Guanylin
- Adrenomedullin
- Peritubular Starling forces
- Bartter syndrome
- Gitelman syndrome
- Liddle syndrome
- Pseudohypoaldosteronism type 1

SELF-STUDY PROBLEMS

1. Consider the amount of water and sodium chloride (NaCl) filtered and reabsorbed by the kidneys each day. What does this tell you about the amount of energy (ATP) expended by the kidneys? Could this explain why the blood flow is so high relative to the size of the kidneys?

2. What are the composition and volume of normal urine produced in a 24-hour period?

3. Compare and contrast passive and active transport.

4. If it were possible to inhibit the Na^+-K^+-ATPase pump in the kidney completely, what would

happen to transcellular and paracellular NaCl reabsorption across the proximal tubule? If GFR was unchanged, how much water and NaCl would appear in the urine every day?

5. Describe the mechanisms and pathways of Na^+, glucose, amino acid, Cl^-, and water reabsorption by the proximal tubule. Which pathways occur in the first phase of reabsorption, and which occur in the second phase? How do Starling forces affect solute and water reabsorption in the proximal tubule?

6. Describe how Na^+ and Cl^- are reabsorbed by the thick ascending limb of the Henle loop. If a diuretic that inhibits NaCl reabsorption (e.g., furosemide) in the thick ascending limb was given to an individual, what would happen to water reabsorption by this segment?

7. What is glomerulotubular balance, and what is the physiological importance of this phenomenon? If the GFR increased without a change in the extracellular fluid volume, what would happen to Na^+ balance if glomerulotubular balance did not exist?

8. What is the aldosterone paradox?

9. List the hormones and factors that regulate NaCl and water reabsorption by the kidneys.

5

REGULATION OF BODY FLUID OSMOLALITY: REGULATION OF WATER BALANCE

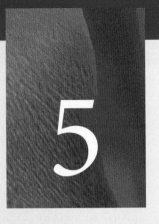

OBJECTIVES

Upon completion of this chapter, the student should be able to answer the following questions:

1. Why do changes in water balance result in alterations in the [Na$^+$] of the extracellular fluid?

2. How is the secretion of arginine vasopressin controlled by changes in the osmolality of the body fluids and in blood volume and pressure?

3. What are the cellular events associated with the action of arginine vasopressin on the collecting duct, and how do they lead to an increase in the water permeability of this segment?

4. What is the role of Henle's loop in the production of both dilute and concentrated urine?

5. What is the composition of the medullary interstitial fluid, and how does it participate in the process of producing concentrated urine?

6. What are the roles of the vasa recta in the process of diluting and concentrating the urine?

7. How is the diluting and concentrating ability of the kidneys quantitated?

As described in Chapter 1, water constitutes approximately 60% of the healthy adult human body. Body water is divided into two compartments (i.e., intracellular fluid and extracellular fluid [ECF]), which are in osmotic equilibrium. Water intake into the body generally occurs orally, and the water ingested is absorbed into the ECF by the gastrointestinal tract via a mechanism similar to that which mediates water absorption by the proximal tubule. However, in clinical situations, intravenous infusion is an important route of water entry. Regardless of the route of entry (oral versus intravenous), water first enters the ECF and then equilibrates with the intracellular fluid. The kidneys are responsible for regulating water balance and under most conditions are the major route for elimination of water from the body (Table 5-1). Other routes of water loss from the body include evaporation from the cells of the skin and respiratory passages. Collectively, water loss by these routes is termed **insensible water loss** because people are unaware of its occurrence. The production of sweat accounts for the loss of additional water. Water loss by this mechanism can increase dramatically in a hot environment, with exercise, or in the presence of fever (Table 5-2). Finally, water can be lost from the gastrointestinal tract. Fecal water loss is normally small (~100 mL/day) but can increase dramatically with diarrhea (e.g., 20 L/day in persons with cholera). Vomiting also can cause gastrointestinal water loss.

TABLE 5-1

Normal Routes of Water Gain and Loss in Adults at Room Temperature (23° C)

ROUTE	mL/DAY
Water Intake	
Fluid*	1200
In food	1000
Metabolically produced from food	300
Total	**2500**
Water Output	
Insensible	700
Sweat	100
Feces	200
Urine	1500
Total	**2500**

*Fluid intake varies widely for both social and cultural reasons.

TABLE 5-2

Effect of Environmental Temperature and Exercise on Water Loss and Intake in Adults

SOURCE OF WATER LOSS	NORMAL TEMPERATURE (mL/DAY)	HOT WEATHER* (mL/DAY)	PRO-LONGED HEAVY EXERCISE* (mL/DAY)
Insensible Loss			
Skin	350	350	350
Lungs	350	250	650
Sweat	100	1400	5000
Feces	200	200	200
Urine*	1500	1200	500
Total loss	2500	3400	6700

*In hot weather and during prolonged heavy exercise, water balance is maintained by increased water ingestion. Decreased excretion of water by the kidneys alone is insufficient to maintain water balance.

Although water loss from sweating, defecation, and evaporation from the lungs and skin can vary depending on the environmental conditions or during pathologic conditions, the loss of water by these routes cannot be regulated. In contrast, the renal excretion of water is tightly regulated to maintain whole-body water balance. The maintenance of water balance requires that water intake and loss from the body are precisely matched. If intake exceeds losses, **positive water balance** exists. Conversely, when intake is less than losses, **negative water balance** exists.

When water intake is low or water losses increase, the kidneys conserve water by producing a small volume of urine that is hyperosmotic with respect to plasma. When water intake is high, a large volume of hypoosmotic urine is produced. In a healthy person, the urine osmolality (U_{osm}) can vary from approximately 50 to 1200 mOsm/kg H_2O, and the corresponding urine volume can vary from approximately 18 to 0.5 L/day.

It is important to recognize that disorders of water balance are manifested by alterations in the body fluid osmolality, which usually are measured by changes in

IN THE CLINIC

When plasma osmolality (P_{osm}) is reduced (i.e., hypoosmolality), water moves from the extracellular fluid into cells, causing them to swell. Symptoms associated with hypoosmolality are related primarily to swelling of brain cells. For example, a rapid decrease in P_{osm} can alter neurologic function and thereby cause nausea, malaise, headache, confusion, lethargy, seizures, and coma. When P_{osm} is increased (i.e., hyperosmolality), water is lost from cells, causing them to shrink. The symptoms of an increase in P_{osm} also are primarily neurologic and include lethargy, weakness, seizures, coma, and even death.

The symptoms associated with changes in body fluid osmolality vary depending on how quickly osmolality is changed. Rapid changes in osmolality (i.e., over hours) are less well tolerated than changes that occur more gradually (i.e., over days to weeks). Indeed, when alterations in body fluid osmolality have developed over an extended period, such persons may be entirely asymptomatic. This situation reflects the ability of cells over time either to eliminate intracellular osmoles, as occurs with hypoosmolality, or to generate new intracellular osmoles in response to hyperosmolality and thus minimize changes in cell volume of the neurons. This ability has important clinical implications when treating a patient with an abnormal plasma osmolality. For example, rapid correction of the osmolality of a person who has had long-standing hypoosmolality of the body fluids can lead to the development of osmotic demyelination syndrome. The syndrome can result in paralysis of multiple muscle groups and can be fatal.

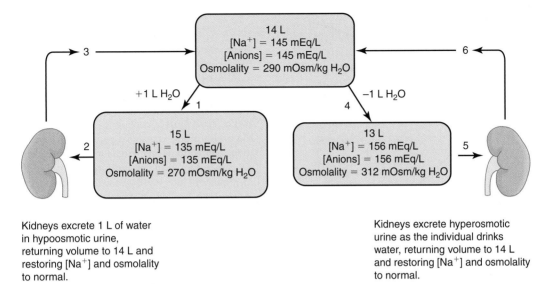

FIGURE 5-1 ▪ Response to changes in water balance. Illustrated are the effects of adding or removing 1 L of water from the extracellular fluid (ECF) of a person weighing 70 kg. *Positive water balance*: (1) Addition of 1 L of water increases the ECF volume and reduces its osmolality. [Na^+] also is decreased (hyponatremia). (2) The normal renal response is to excrete 1 L of water as hypoosmotic urine. (3) As a result of the renal excretion of water, the ECF volume, osmolality, and [Na^+] are returned to normal. *Negative water balance*: (4) The loss of 1 L of water from the ECF decreases its volume and increases its osmolality. The [Na^+] also is increased (hypernatremia). (5) The renal response is to conserve water by excreting a small volume of hyperosmotic urine. (6) With ingestion of water, stimulated by thirst, and the conservation of water by the kidneys, the ECF volume, osmolality, and [Na^+] are returned to normal. The size of the boxes indicates the relative volume of ECF.

plasma osmolality (P_{osm}). Because the major determinant of plasma osmolality is Na^+ (with its anions Cl^- and HCO_3^-), these disorders also result in alterations in the plasma [Na^+] (see Figure 5-1). When an abnormal plasma [Na^+] is observed in an individual, it is tempting to suspect a problem in Na^+ balance. However, the problem usually is related to water balance, not Na^+ balance. As described in Chapter 6, changes in Na^+ balance result in alterations in the volume of the ECF, not its osmolality.

Under steady-state conditions, the kidneys control water excretion independently of their ability to control the excretion of various other physiologically important substances such as Na^+, K^+, and urea (Figure 5-2). Indeed, this ability is necessary for survival because it allows water balance to be achieved without upsetting the other homeostatic functions of the kidneys.

This chapter discusses the mechanisms by which the kidneys maintain water balance by excreting either hypoosmotic (dilute) or hyperosmotic (concentrated) urine (see Figure 5-2). The control of **arginine vasopressin (AVP)** secretion and its important role in regulating the excretion of water by the kidneys also are explained.

ARGININE VASOPRESSIN

AVP, also known as **antidiuretic hormone**, acts on the kidneys to regulate the volume and osmolality of the urine. When plasma AVP levels are low, a large volume of urine is excreted (diuresis), and the urine is dilute.* When plasma levels are high, a small volume of urine is excreted (antidiuresis), and the urine is concentrated. Figure 5-2 illustrates the effect of AVP on the urine flow rate and osmolality. The excretion of

---

*Diuresis is simply a large urine output. When the urine contains primarily water, it is referred to as a *water diuresis,* which is in contrast to the diuresis seen with diuretic agents (see Chapter 10). In the latter case, urine output is large, but the urine contains solute plus water, which sometimes is termed a *solute diuresis.*

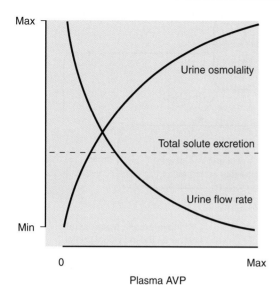

FIGURE 5-2 ■ Relationships between plasma arginine vasopressin (AVP) levels and urine osmolality, urine flow rate, and total solute excretion. *Max,* Maximum; *Min,* minimum.

AT THE CELLULAR LEVEL

The gene for arginine vasopressin (AVP) is found on chromosome 20. It contains approximately 2000 base pairs with three exons and two introns. The gene codes for a 145 amino acid prohormone that consists of a signal peptide, the AVP molecule, neurophysin, and a glycopeptide (copeptin). As the cell processes the prohormone, the signal peptide is cleaved off in the rough endoplasmic reticulum. Once packaged in neurosecretory granules, the preprohormone is further cleaved into AVP, neurophysin, and copeptin molecules. The neurosecretory granules are then transported down the axon to the posterior pituitary and stored in the nerve endings until released. When the neurons are stimulated to secrete AVP, the action potential opens Ca^{++} channels in the nerve terminal, which raises the intracellular $[Ca^{++}]$ and causes exocytosis of the neurosecretory granules. All three peptides are secreted in this process. Neurophysin and copeptin do not have an identified physiologic function.

total solute (e.g., Na^+, K^+, and urea) by the kidneys also is shown. As already noted, AVP does not appreciably alter the excretion of solute, which underscores the fact that AVP controls water excretion and maintains water balance without altering the excretion and homeostatic control of other substances.

AVP is a small peptide that is nine amino acids in length. It is synthesized in neuroendocrine cells located within the supraoptic and paraventricular nuclei of the hypothalamus.* The synthesized hormone is packaged in granules that are transported down the axon of the cell and stored in the nerve terminals located in the neurohypophysis (posterior pituitary). The anatomy of the hypothalamus and pituitary gland is shown in Figure 5-3.

The secretion of AVP by the posterior pituitary can be influenced by several factors. The two primary physiologic regulators of AVP secretion are the osmolality of the body fluids (osmotic) and volume and pressure of the vascular system (hemodynamic). Other factors that can alter AVP secretion include nausea

(stimulates), atrial natriuretic peptide (inhibits), and angiotensin II (stimulates). A number of drugs, prescription and nonprescription, also affect AVP secretion. For example, nicotine stimulates secretion, whereas ethanol inhibits secretion.

Osmotic Control of Arginine Vasopressin Secretion

Changes in the osmolality of body fluids play the most important role in regulating AVP secretion; changes as minor as 1% are sufficient to alter it significantly. Although the neurons in the supraoptic and paraventricular nuclei respond to changes in body fluid osmolality by altering their secretion of AVP, it is clear that separate cells exist in the anterior hypothalamus that sense changes in body fluid osmolality and regulate the activity of the AVP-secreting neurons.† These cells, termed *osmoreceptors*, appear to sense changes in body

---

*Neurons within the supraoptic and paraventricular nuclei synthesize either AVP or the related peptide oxytocin. AVP-secreting cells predominate in the supraoptic nucleus, and the oxytocin-secreting neurons are found primarily in the paraventricular nucleus.

†Osmoreceptors have been identified in the anterior hypothalamus; one of these sites is the organum vasculosum of the lamina terminalis, which is located outside the blood-brain barrier. In addition, the subfornical organ, which is also located in the anterior hypothalamus outside the blood-brain barrier, responds to circulating levels of angiotensin II, which is an important stimulator of AVP secretion.

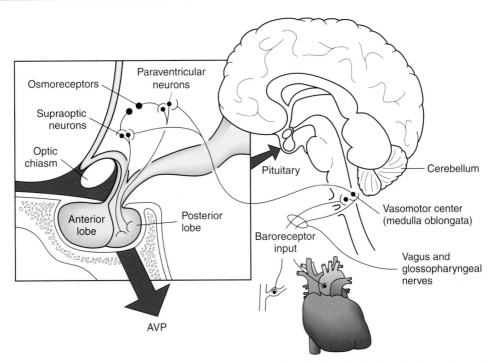

FIGURE 5-3 ▪ Anatomy of the hypothalamus and pituitary gland (midsagittal section) depicting the pathways for arginine vasopressin (*AVP*) secretion. Also shown are pathways involved in regulating AVP secretion. Afferent fibers from the baroreceptors are carried in the vagus and glossopharyngeal nerves. *Inset,* An expanded view of the hypothalamus and pituitary gland.

fluid osmolality by either shrinking or swelling. The osmoreceptors respond only to solutes in plasma that are effective osmoles (see Chapter 1). For example, urea is an ineffective osmole when the function of osmoreceptors is considered. Thus elevation of the plasma urea concentration alone has little or no effect on AVP secretion.

When the effective osmolality of the plasma increases, the osmoreceptors send signals to the AVP synthesizing/secreting cells located in the supraoptic and paraventricular nuclei of the hypothalamus, and AVP synthesis and secretion are stimulated. Conversely, when the effective osmolality of the plasma is reduced, secretion is inhibited. Because AVP is rapidly degraded in the plasma, circulating levels can be reduced to zero within minutes after secretion is inhibited. As a result, the AVP system can respond rapidly to fluctuations in body fluid osmolality.

Figure 5-4, *A*, illustrates the effect of changes in plasma osmolality on circulating AVP levels. The set point of the system is the plasma osmolality value at which AVP secretion begins to increase. Below this set point, virtually no AVP is released. Above this set point, the slope of the relationship is quite steep and accounts for the sensitivity of this system. The set point varies among individuals and is genetically determined. In healthy adults, it varies from 275 to 290 mOsm/kg H_2O (average ~280 to 285 mOsm/kg H_2O). As described later in this chapter, the set point shifts in response to changes in blood volume and pressure. It also shifts during pregnancy, with the osmolality of the mother's body fluids decreasing during the third trimester. The reasons for the shift of the set point during pregnancy are not completely known but likely involve hormones (e.g., relaxin) whose circulating levels are elevated at this stage of pregnancy.

Hemodynamic Control of Arginine Vasopressin Secretion

A decrease in blood volume or pressure also stimulates AVP secretion. The receptors responsible for this response are located in both the low-pressure (left

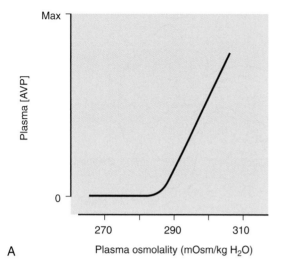

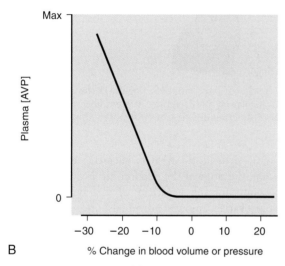

FIGURE 5-4 ■ Osmotic and hemodynamic control of arginine vasopressin (*AVP*) secretion. Depicted are the relationships between plasma AVP levels and plasma osmolality (**A**) and blood volume and pressure (**B**). *Max,* Maximum.

overall vascular volume. The high-pressure receptors respond to arterial pressure. Both groups of receptors are sensitive to stretch of the wall of the structure in which they are located (e.g., the cardiac atrial wall and the wall of the aortic arch) and are termed **baroreceptors**. Signals from these receptors are carried in afferent fibers of the vagus and glossopharyngeal nerves to the brainstem (solitary tract nucleus of the medulla oblongata), which is part of the center that regulates heart rate and blood pressure. Signals then are relayed from the brainstem to the AVP secretory cells of the supraoptic and paraventricular hypothalamic nuclei. The sensitivity of the baroreceptor system is less than that of the osmoreceptors, and a 5% to 10% decrease in blood volume or pressure is required before AVP secretion is stimulated. This phenomenon is illustrated in Figure 5-4, *B.* A number of substances have been shown to alter the secretion of AVP through their effects on blood pressure. These substances include bradykinin and histamine, which lower pressure and thus stimulate AVP secretion, and norepinephrine, which increases blood pressure and inhibits AVP secretion.

Alterations in blood volume and pressure also affect the response to changes in body fluid osmolality (Figure 5-5). With a decrease in blood volume or pressure, the set point is shifted to lower osmolality values and the slope of the relationship is steeper. In terms of survival of the individual, this means that when faced with circulatory collapse, the kidneys continue to conserve water, even though by doing so they reduce the osmolality of the body fluids. With an increase in blood volume or pressure, the opposite occurs. The set point is shifted to higher osmolality values, and the slope is decreased.

Arginine Vasopressin Actions on the Kidneys

The primary action of AVP on the kidneys is to increase the permeability of the collecting duct to water. In addition, and notably, AVP increases the permeability of the medullary portion of the collecting duct to urea. Lastly, AVP stimulates sodium chloride (NaCl) reabsorption by the thick ascending limb of Henle's loop, the distal tubule, and the cortical portion of the collecting duct.

atrium and large pulmonary vessels) and the high-pressure (aortic arch and carotid sinus) sides of the circulatory system. Because the low-pressure receptors are located in the high-compliance side of the circulatory system (i.e., venous) and the majority of blood is in the venous side of the circulatory system, these low-pressure receptors can be viewed as responding to

IN THE CLINIC

Inadequate release of arginine vasopressin (AVP) from the posterior pituitary results in excretion of large volumes of dilute urine (polyuria). To compensate for this loss of water, the individual must ingest large volumes of water (polydipsia) to maintain constant body fluid osmolality. If the individual is deprived of water, the body fluids become hyperosmotic. This condition is called *central diabetes insipidus* or *pituitary diabetes insipidus*. Central diabetes insipidus can be inherited, although this situation is rare. It occurs more commonly after head trauma and with brain neoplasms or infections. Persons with central diabetes insipidus have a urine-concentrating defect that can be corrected by the administration of exogenous AVP.

The inherited (autosomal dominant) form of central diabetes insipidus is caused by a variety of mutations in the AVP gene. In patients with this form of central diabetes insipidus, mutations have been identified in all regions of the AVP gene (i.e., AVP, copeptin, and neurophysin). The most common mutation is found in the neurophysin portion of the gene. In each of these situations, defective trafficking of the peptide occurs, with abnormal accumulation in the endoplasmic reticulum. It is believed that this abnormal accumulation in the endoplasmic reticulum results in death of the AVP secretory cells of the supraoptic and paraventricular nuclei.

The syndrome of inappropriate antidiuretic hormone (ADH) secretion (**SIADH**) is a common clinical problem characterized by plasma AVP levels that are elevated above what would be expected on the basis of body fluid osmolality and blood volume and pressure—hence the term *inappropriate* ADH secretion. In addition, the collecting duct overexpresses water channels, thus augmenting the effect of AVP on the kidney. Persons with SIADH retain water, and their body fluids become progressively hypoosmotic. In addition, their urine is more hyperosmotic than expected on the basis of the low body fluid osmolality. SIADH can be caused by infections and neoplasms of the brain, drugs (e.g., antitumor drugs), pulmonary diseases, and carcinoma of the lung. Many of these conditions stimulate AVP secretion by altering neural input to the AVP secretory cells. However, small cell carcinoma of the lung produces and secretes a number of peptides, including AVP.

Recently, nonpeptide vasopressin receptor antagonists (e.g., conivaptan and tolvaptan) have been developed that can be used to treat SIADH and other conditions in which AVP-dependent water retention by the kidneys occurs (e.g., congestive heart failure and hepatic cirrhosis).

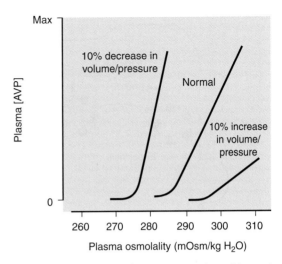

FIGURE 5-5 ■ Interaction between osmotic and hemodynamic stimuli for arginine vasopressin (*AVP*) secretion. With decreased blood volume and pressure, the osmotic set point is shifted to lower plasma osmolality values and the slope is increased. An increase in blood volume and pressure has the opposite effects. *Max,* Maximum.

The actions of AVP on water permeability of the collecting duct have been studied extensively (Figure 5-6). AVP binds to a receptor on the basolateral membrane of the cell. This receptor is termed the V_2 *receptor* (i.e., vasopressin 2 receptor).* Binding to this receptor, which is coupled to adenylyl cyclase through a stimulatory G protein (Gs), increases the intracellular levels of cyclic adenosine monophosphate (cAMP). The rise in intracellular cAMP activates protein kinase A, which ultimately results in an increase in the number of aquaporin (AQP)-2 water channels in the apical membrane of the cell and the synthesis of more AQP-2. With the removal of AVP, the number of AQP-2 water channels in the apical membrane is reduced, thereby rendering the membrane impermeable to water. Because the basolateral

---

*A different AVP receptor (V_1 receptor) is present on vascular smooth muscle. This receptor mediates the vasoconstrictor response to AVP. It is this action that accounts for the term *vasopressin*.

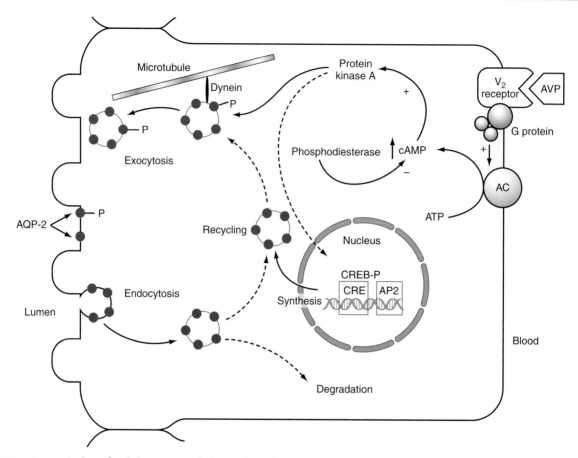

FIGURE 5-6 ■ Action of arginine vasopressin (*AVP*) through the vasopressin 2 (*V₂*) receptor on the principal cell of the late distal tubule and collecting duct. *AC,* Adenylyl cyclase; *AP2,* aquaporin-2 gene; *AQP-2,* aquaporin-2; *ATP,* adenosine triphosphate; *cAMP,* cyclic adenosine monophosphate; *CRE,* cAMP response element; *CREB-P,* phosphorylated cAMP response element binding protein; *P,* phosphorylated proteins. *(Modified from Brown D, Nielsen S: The cell biology of vasopressin action. In Brenner BM, editor:* The kidney, *ed 7, Philadelphia, 2004, WB Saunders.)*

membrane is freely permeable to water because of the presence of AQP-3 and AQP-4 water channels, any water that enters the cell through apical membrane water channels exits across the basolateral membrane, resulting in net absorption of water from the tubule lumen.

AVP also increases the permeability of the terminal portion of the inner medullary collecting duct to urea. This increase in permeability results in an increase in urea reabsorption and an increase in the osmolality of the medullary interstitial fluid. The inner medullary collecting duct expresses two different urea transporters (UTs: UT-A1 and UT-A3. UT-A1 is found in the apical membrane and UT-A3 is found in the basolateral membrane. AVP, acting through adenylyl cyclase

and the cAMP/protein kinase A cascade, increases the permeability of the apical membrane to urea. This increase in permeability is associated with phosphorylation of UT-A1 and UT-A3. Increasing the osmolality of the interstitial fluid of the renal medulla also increases the permeability of the collecting duct to urea. This effect is mediated by the phospholipase C pathway and involves protein kinase C phosphorylation. Thus this effect is separate from and additive to that of AVP.

AVP also stimulates the reabsorption of NaCl by the thick ascending limb of Henle's loop and by the distal tubule and cortical segment of the collecting duct. It is thought that stimulation of thick ascending limb NaCl transport, in particular, may help maintain

AT THE CELLULAR LEVEL

The gene for the **V₂ receptor** is located on the X chromosome. It codes for a 371-amino-acid protein that is in the family of receptors that have seven membrane-spanning domains and are coupled to heterotrimeric G proteins. As shown in Figure 5-6, binding of AVP to its receptor on the basolateral membrane activates adenylyl cyclase. The increase in intracellular cyclic adenosine monophosphate (cAMP) then activates protein kinase A, which results in phosphorylation of aquaporin (AQP)-2 water channels, which reduces the endocytic removal of AQP-2 from the apical membrane and also results in increased transcription of the AQP-2 gene through activation of a cAMP response element. AVP also increases the rate of insertion of vesicles containing AQP-2 into the apical membrane by facilitating their movement along microtubules driven by the molecular motor dynein. Once near the apical membrane, proteins called SNAREs interact with vesicles containing AQP-2 and facilitate the fusion of these vesicles with the membrane. The net addition of AQP-2 to the apical membrane, resulting from reduced endocytosis and increased insertion, allows more water to enter the cell driven by the osmotic gradient (lumen osmolality < cell osmolality). The water then exits the cell across the basolateral membrane through AQP-3 and AQP-4 water channels, which are constitutively present in the basolateral membrane. When the V₂ receptor is not occupied by AVP, clathrin-mediated endocytosis of AQP-2 is enhanced and the exocytic insertion of AQP-2 is reduced, which decreases the total number of AQP-2 channels in the apical membrane, rendering the apical membrane once again impermeable to water.

Recently, persons have been found who have activating (gain-of-function) mutations in the V₂ receptor gene. Thus the receptor is constitutively activated even in the absence of AVP. These persons have laboratory findings similar to those seen in the syndrome of inappropriate antidiuretic hormone secretion (SIADH), including reduced plasma osmolality, hyponatremia (reduced plasma [Na⁺]), and urine more concentrated than would be expected from the reduced body fluid osmolality. However, unlike persons with SIADH, in whom circulating levels of AVP are elevated and thus responsible for water retention by the kidneys, these persons have undetectable levels of AVP in their plasma. This new clinical entity has been termed "nephrogenic syndrome of inappropriate antidiuresis."

AT THE CELLULAR LEVEL

The collecting ducts of some persons do not respond normally to arginine vasopressin (AVP). These persons cannot maximally concentrate their urine and consequently have polyuria and polydipsia. This clinical entity is termed **nephrogenic diabetes insipidus** to distinguish it from central diabetes insipidus. Nephrogenic diabetes insipidus can result from a number of systemic disorders and, more rarely, occurs as a result of inherited disorders. Many of the acquired forms of nephrogenic diabetes insipidus are the result of decreased expression of aquaporin-2 (AQP-2) in the collecting duct. Decreased expression of AQP-2 has been documented in the urine-concentrating defects associated with hypokalemia, lithium ingestion (some degree of nephrogenic diabetes insipidus develops in 35% of persons who take lithium for bipolar disorder), ureteral obstruction, a low-protein diet, and hypercalcemia. The inherited forms of nephrogenic diabetes insipidus reflect mutations in the AVP receptor (V₂ receptor) gene or the AQP-2 gene. Approximately 90% of hereditary forms of nephrogenic diabetes insipidus are the result of mutations in the V₂ receptor gene, with the other 10% being the result of mutations in the AQP-2 gene. Because the gene for the V₂ receptor is located on the X chromosome, these inherited forms are X-linked. Most of these mutations result in trapping of the receptor in the endoplasmic reticulum of the cell; only a few cases result in the surface expression of a V₂ receptor that does not bind AVP. The gene coding for AQP-2 is located on chromosome 12 and is inherited as both an autosomal recessive and an autosomal dominant defect. As noted in Chapters 1 and 4, aquaporins exist as homotetramers. This homotetramer formation explains the difference between the two forms of nephrogenic diabetes insipidus. In the recessive form, heterozygotes produce both normal AQP-2 and defective AQP-2 molecules. The defective AQP-2 monomer is not delivered to the plasma membrane, and thus the homotetramers that do form contain only normal AQP-2 molecules. Accordingly, mutations in both alleles would be required to produce nephrogenic diabetes insipidus. In the autosomal dominant form, the defective monomers can form tetramers with normal monomers, as well as defective monomers. However, these tetramers cannot be delivered to the plasma membrane.

the hyperosmotic medullary interstitium that is necessary for absorption of water from the medullary portion of the collecting duct (discussed later in this chapter).

THIRST

In addition to affecting the secretion of AVP, changes in plasma osmolality and blood volume or pressure lead to alterations in the perception of thirst. When body fluid osmolality is increased or the blood volume or pressure is reduced, a person perceives thirst. Of these stimuli, hypertonicity is the more potent. An increase in plasma osmolality of only 2% to 3% produces a strong desire to drink, whereas decreases in blood volume and pressure in the range of 10% to 15% are required to produce the same response.

As already discussed, people have a genetically determined threshold for AVP secretion (i.e., a body fluid osmolality above which AVP secretion increases). Similarly, people have a genetically determined threshold for triggering the sensation of thirst. However, the thirst threshold is higher than the threshold for AVP secretion. On average, the threshold for AVP secretion is approximately 285 mOsm/kg H_2O, whereas the thirst threshold is approximately 295 mOsm/kg H_2O. Because of this difference, thirst is stimulated at a body fluid osmolality at which AVP secretion is already stimulated.

The neural centers involved in regulating water intake (the thirst center) are located in the same region of the hypothalamus involved with regulating AVP secretion. However, it is not certain if the same cells serve both functions. Indeed, the thirst response, like the regulation of AVP secretion, occurs only in response to effective osmoles (e.g., NaCl). Even less is known about the pathways involved in the thirst response to decreased blood volume or pressure, but it is believed that the pathways are the same as those involved in the volume- and pressure-related regulation of AVP secretion. Angiotensin II, acting on cells of the thirst center (subfornical organ), also evokes the sensation of thirst. Because angiotensin II levels are increased when blood volume and pressure are reduced, this effect of angiotensin II contributes to the homeostatic response that restores and maintains the body fluids at their normal volumes.

The sensation of thirst is satisfied by the act of drinking even before sufficient water is absorbed from the gastrointestinal tract to correct the plasma osmolality. Oropharyngeal and upper gastrointestinal receptors appear to be involved in this response. However, relief of the thirst sensation by these receptors is short lived, and thirst is completely satisfied only when the plasma osmolality or blood volume or pressure is corrected.

It should be apparent that the AVP and thirst systems work in concert to maintain water balance. An increase in the plasma osmolality evokes drinking and, through AVP action on the kidneys, the conservation of water. Conversely, when the plasma osmolality is decreased, thirst is suppressed and, in the absence of AVP, renal water excretion is enhanced. However, most of the time fluid intake is dictated by cultural factors and social situations, which is especially the case when thirst is not stimulated. In this situation, maintaining a normal body fluid osmolality relies solely on the ability of the kidneys to excrete water. How the kidney accomplishes this task is discussed in detail in the following sections of this chapter.

RENAL MECHANISMS FOR DILUTION AND CONCENTRATION OF THE URINE

Under normal circumstances, the excretion of water is regulated separately from the excretion of solutes (see Figure 5-2). For this separate regulation to occur, the kidneys must be able to excrete urine that is either hypoosmotic or hyperosmotic with respect to the body fluids. This ability to excrete urine of varying osmolality in turn requires that solute be separated from water at some point along the nephron. As discussed in Chapter 4, the reabsorption of solute in the proximal tubule results in the reabsorption of a proportional amount of water. Hence solute and water are not separated in this portion of the nephron. Moreover, this proportionality between proximal tubule water and solute reabsorption occurs regardless of whether the kidneys excrete dilute or concentrated urine. Thus the proximal tubule reabsorbs a large portion of the filtered solute and water but does not produce dilute or concentrated tubular fluid. The loop of Henle, in particular the thick ascending limb, is the major site where solute and water are separated. Thus the excretion of both dilute and concentrated urine requires normal function of the loop of Henle.

IN THE CLINIC

With adequate access to water, the thirst mechanism can prevent the development of hyperosmolality. Indeed, it is this mechanism that is responsible for the polydipsia seen in response to the polyuria of both central and nephrogenic diabetes insipidus. Water intake also is influenced by social and cultural factors. Thus persons ingest water even in the absence of the thirst sensation. Normally the kidneys are able to excrete this excess water because they can excrete up to 18 L/day of urine. However, in some instances, the volume of water ingested exceeds the kidneys' capacity to excrete water, especially over short periods. When this situation occurs, the body fluids become hypoosmotic. An example of how water intake can exceed the capacity of the kidneys to excrete water is found in long-distance runners. A study of participants in the **Boston Marathon** found that hyponatremia developed in 13% of the runners during the course of the race.* This finding reflected the practice of some runners of ingesting water, or other hypotonic drinks, during the race to remain "well hydrated." In addition, water is produced from the metabolism of glycogen and triglycerides used as fuels by the exercising muscle. Because over the course of the race they ingested and generated more water through metabolism than their kidneys were able to excrete, hyponatremia developed. In some racers, the hyponatremia was severe enough to elicit the neurologic symptoms described previously.

Throughout the popular media, one can find articles urging us to drink eight 8-oz glasses of water a day (the **8 × 8 recommendation**). Drinking this volume of water is said to provide innumerable health benefits. As a result, it seems that everyone now has a water bottle as his or her constant companion. Although ingesting this volume of water over the course of a day (approximately 2 L) does not harm most persons, no scientific evidence exists to support the beneficial health claims ascribed to the 8 × 8 recommendation.† Indeed, most persons get adequate amounts of water through the foods they ingest and the fluids taken with those meals.

The maximum amount of water that can be excreted by the kidneys depends on the amount of solute excreted, which in turn depends on food intake. For example, with maximally dilute urine (urine osmolality [U_{osm}] = 50 mOsm/kg H_2O), the maximum urine output of 18 L/day is achieved only if the solute excretion rate is 900 mmol/day.

$$U_{osm} = \text{Solute excretion/Volume excreted}$$
$$50 \text{ mOsm/kg } H_2O = 900 \text{ mmol/18 L} \qquad (5\text{-}1)$$

If solute excretion is reduced, as commonly occurs in elderly people with reduced food intake, the maximum urine output decreases. For example, if solute excretion is only 400 mmol/day, a maximum urine output (at U_{osm} = 50 mOsm/kg H_2O) of only 8 L/day can be achieved. Thus persons with reduced food intake have a reduced capacity to excrete water.

*Almond CS, Shin AY, Fortescue EB et al: Hyponatremia among runners in the Boston Marathon, *N Engl J Med* 352:1150-1556, 2005.
†Valtin H: "Drink at least eight glasses of water a day." Really? Is there scientific evidence for "8 × 8"? *Am J Physiol Reg Integr Comp Physiol* 283:R993, 2002.

The excretion of hypoosmotic urine is relatively easy to understand. The nephron simply must reabsorb solute from the tubular fluid and not allow water reabsorption to occur as well. The reabsorption of solute without concomitant water reabsorption occurs in some portions of the descending limb and along the entire ascending limb of Henle's loop. Under appropriate conditions (i.e., in the absence of AVP), the distal tubule and collecting duct also dilute the tubular fluid. The excretion of hyperosmotic urine is more complex and thus more difficult to understand. This process in essence involves removing water from the tubular fluid without solute. Because water movement is passive, driven by an osmotic gradient, the kidney must generate a hyperosmotic compartment that then reabsorbs water osmotically from the tubular fluid. The compartment in the kidney where this reabsorption occurs is the interstitial space of the renal medulla.

It has long been recognized that Henle's loop is associated with the kidneys' ability to excrete hyperosmotic urine. Indeed, only birds and mammals can excrete hyperosmotic urine, and among vertebrates, only the avian and mammalian kidneys have loops of Henle. Moreover, some animals, such as desert rodents, have extremely long loops of Henle and excrete urine with an osmolality that can exceed 5000 mOsm/kg H_2O. This extraordinary ability to concentrate the urine allows the animals to survive without the need to drink water, because they obtain sufficient water in the food (e.g., seeds) that they ingest.

For more than 50 years our understanding of how the loop of Henle is able to generate a hyperosmotic environment within the renal medulla was focused on the process of **countercurrent multiplication**. By this process, solute (principally NaCl) is reabsorbed without water from the ascending limb of Henle's loop into the surrounding medullary interstitium. This reabsorption decreases the osmolality in the tubular fluid and raises the osmolality of the interstitium at this point. The increased osmolality of the interstitium then causes water to be reabsorbed from the descending limb of Henle's loop, thus increasing the tubular fluid osmolality in this segment. Thus at any point along the loop of Henle, the fluid in the ascending limb has an osmolality less than fluid in the adjacent descending limb. This osmotic difference was termed the **single effect**. Because of the countercurrent flow of tubular fluid in the descending (fluid flowing into the medulla) and ascending (fluid flow out of the medulla) limbs, this single effect could be multiplied. The multiplication of this single effect results in an osmotic gradient within the medullary interstitium, where the tip of the papilla has an osmolality of 1200 mOsm/kg H_2O, compared with 300 mOsm/kg H_2O at the corticomedullary junction. Although it is simple in concept, it is now clear that countercurrent multiplication cannot fully explain the process by which the loop of Henle generates a hyperosmotic medullary interstitium.* Given our evolving understanding, specifically of the urine concentrating mechanism, what follows is a simplified explanation that highlights several key concepts:

1. Urine is concentrated by the AVP-dependent reabsorption of water from the collecting duct.
2. Reabsorption of NaCl from the ascending limb of Henle's loop generates a high [NaCl] in the medullary interstitium (up to 600 mmol/L at the tip of the papilla), which then drives water reabsorption from the collecting duct.
3. Urea accumulates in the medullary interstitium (up to 600 mmol/L), which allows the kidneys to excrete urine with the same high urea concentration. This phenomenon allows large amounts of urea to be excreted with relatively little water.

Figure 5-7 summarizes the essential features of the mechanisms whereby the kidneys excrete either a dilute or a concentrated urine.

First, how the kidneys excrete dilute urine (**water diuresis**) when AVP levels are low or zero is considered. The following numbers refer to those encircled in Figure 5-7, *A*.

1. Fluid entering the descending thin limb of the loop of Henle from the proximal tubule is isosmotic with respect to plasma. This state reflects the essentially isosmotic nature of solute and water reabsorption in the proximal tubule (see Chapter 4). (Note: Water is reabsorbed from the segments of the proximal tubule via AQP-1.)
2. Depending on the nephron type (i.e., short-looped nephrons versus long-looped nephrons [see Figure 2-2]), some water will be reabsorbed by the thin descending limb. Importantly, this water reabsorption is limited to the outer medulla and the outermost portion of the inner medulla. By confining water reabsorption to these outer portions of the medulla, less water is added to the deepest part of the inner medullary interstitial space, thus preserving the hyperosmolality of this region of the medulla. (Note: Water is reabsorbed via AQP-1).
3. In the inner medulla, the terminal portion of the descending thin limb and all of the thin ascending limb is impermeable to water. (Note: AQP-1 is not expressed.) These same nephron segments express the Cl^- transporter ClC-K1, which

---

*Recent anatomic studies have looked at the localization of specific membrane transporters in the nephron segments of the renal medulla and the spatial relationships between these nephron segments and capillaries (i.e., vasa recta), which may create microenvironments that facilitate the concentration of tubular fluid. In addition, it has been proposed that the regular contraction of the renal calyx that surrounds each pyramid (see Chapter 2) also may contribute to the generation of hyperosmotic tubular fluid in water-permeable medullary nephron segments. In this model, compression of glycosaminoglycans in the medullary interstitium during calyx contraction generates a force that upon recoil (i.e., relaxation of the calyx) draws water out of water-permeable nephron segments and thereby concentrates the tubular fluid.

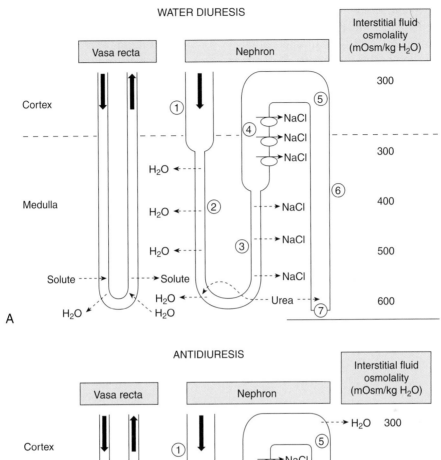

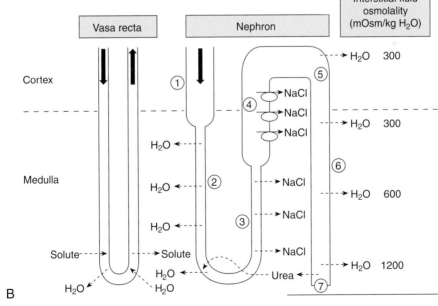

FIGURE 5-7 ■ Schematic of nephron segments involved in dilution and concentration of the urine. Henle's loops of juxtamedullary nephrons are shown. **A,** Mechanism for the excretion of dilute urine (water diuresis). Arginine vasopressin (AVP) is absent, and the collecting duct is essentially impermeable to water. Note also that during a water diuresis, the osmolality of the medullary interstitium is reduced as a result of increased vasa recta blood flow and the entry of some urea into the medullary collecting duct. **B,** Mechanism for the excretion of a concentrated urine (antidiuresis). Plasma AVP levels are maximal, and the collecting duct is highly permeable to water. Under this condition, the medullary interstitial gradient is maximal. See the text for a detailed description of the numbered steps.

mediates Cl⁻ reabsorption with Na⁺ following passively via the paracellular pathway. This passive reabsorption of NaCl without concomitant water reabsorption begins the process of diluting the tubular fluid.

4. The thick ascending limb of the loop of Henle also is impermeable to water and actively reabsorbs NaCl from the tubular fluid and thereby dilutes it further (see Chapter 4). Dilution occurs to such a degree that this segment often is referred to as the **diluting segment** of the kidney. Fluid leaving the thick ascending limb is hypoosmotic with respect to plasma (approximately 150 mOsm/kg H_2O).

5. The distal tubule and cortical portion of the collecting duct actively reabsorb NaCl. In the absence of AVP, these segments are not permeable to water (i.e., AQP-2 is not present in the apical membrane of the cells). Thus when AVP is absent or present at low levels (i.e., decreased plasma osmolality), the osmolality of tubule fluid in these segments is reduced further because NaCl is reabsorbed without water. Under this condition, fluid leaving the cortical portion of the collecting duct is hypoosmotic with respect to plasma (approximately 50-100 mOsm/kg H_2O).

6. The medullary collecting duct actively reabsorbs NaCl. Even in the absence of AVP, this segment is slightly permeable to water, and some water is reabsorbed.

7. The urine has an osmolality as low as approximately 50 mOsm/kg H_2O and contains low concentrations of NaCl. The volume of urine excreted can be as much as 18 L/day, or approximately 10% of the glomerular filtration rate (GFR).

Next, how the kidneys excrete concentrated urine (**antidiuresis**) when plasma osmolality and plasma AVP levels are high is considered. The following numbers refer to those encircled in Figure 5-7, *B*.

1-4. These steps are similar to those for production of dilute urine. An important point in understanding how a concentrated urine is produced is to recognize that while reabsorption of NaCl by the ascending thin and thick limbs of the loop of Henle dilutes the tubular fluid, the reabsorbed NaCl accumulates in the medullary interstitium

and raises the osmolality of this compartment. The accumulation of NaCl in the medullary interstitium is crucial for the production of urine hyperosmotic to plasma because it provides the osmotic driving force for water reabsorption by the medullary collecting duct. As already noted, AVP stimulates NaCl reabsorption by the thick ascending limb of Henle's loop. This action is thought to maintain the medullary interstitial gradient at a time when water is being added to this compartment from the medullary collecting duct, which would tend to dissipate the gradient.

5. Because of NaCl reabsorption by the ascending limb of the loop of Henle, the fluid reaching the collecting duct is hypoosmotic with respect to the surrounding interstitial fluid. Thus an osmotic gradient is established across the collecting duct. In the presence of AVP, which increases the water permeability of the last half of the distal tubule and the collecting duct by increasing the number of AQP-2 water channels in the luminal membrane of the cells, water diffuses out of the tubule lumen, and the tubule fluid osmolality increases. This diffusion of water out of the lumen of the collecting duct begins the process of urine concentration. The maximum osmolality that the fluid in the distal tubule and cortical portion of the collecting duct can attain is approximately 290 mOsm/kg H_2O (i.e., the same as plasma), which is the osmolality of the interstitial fluid and plasma within the cortex of the kidney.

6. As the tubular fluid descends deeper into the medulla, water continues to be reabsorbed from the collecting duct, increasing the tubular fluid osmolality to 1200 mOsm/kg H_2O at the tip of the papilla.

7. The urine produced when AVP levels are elevated has an osmolality of 1200 mOsm/kg H_2O and contains high concentrations of urea and other nonreabsorbed solutes. The urine volume under this condition can be as low as 0.5 L/day.

Under most conditions, a relatively constant volume of tubular fluid is delivered to the AVP-sensitive portions of the nephron (late distal tubule and collecting duct). Plasma AVP levels then determine the amount of water that is reabsorbed by these segments. When AVP levels are low, a relatively small volume of water is reabsorbed by these segments, and a large volume of hypoosmotic urine is excreted (up to 10% of the filtered water). When AVP levels are high, a large volume of water is reabsorbed by these same segments, and a small volume of hyperosmotic urine is excreted (<1% of filtered water). During antidiuresis, most of the water is reabsorbed in the distal tubule and cortical and outer medullary portions of the collecting duct. Thus a relatively small volume of fluid reaches the inner medullary collecting duct, where it is then reabsorbed. This distribution of water reabsorption along the length of the collecting duct (i.e., cortex > outer medulla > inner medulla) allows for the maintenance of a hyperosmotic interstitial environment in the inner medulla by minimizing the amount of water entering this compartment.

AT THE CELLULAR LEVEL

Water movement across the various segments of the nephron occurs through water channels (aquaporins [AQPs]). The proximal tubule and portions of some thin descending limbs of Henle's loop are highly permeable to water, and these segments express high levels of AQP-1 in both the apical and basolateral membranes. The vasa recta also are highly permeable to water and express AQP-1. AQP-7 and AQP-8 also are expressed in the proximal tubule. As already discussed, AQP-2 is responsible for arginine vasopressin (AVP)-regulated water movement across the apical membrane of principal cells of the late distal tubule and collecting duct, and AQP-3 and AQP-4 are responsible for water movement across the basolateral membrane.

Mice lacking the AQP-1 gene have been created. These mice have a urine-concentrating defect with increased urine output. Several persons have been found who also lack the normal AQP-1 gene. Interestingly, these persons do not have polyuria. However, when challenged by water deprivation, they are able to concentrate their urine to only approximately half of what is seen in a healthy person.

Role of Urea

As noted, a hyperosmotic renal medullary interstitium is critically important in concentrating the urine and provides the driving force for reabsorption of water from the collecting duct. The principal solutes within

the renal medullary interstitium are NaCl and urea, but the concentration of these solutes is not uniform throughout the medulla (i.e., a gradient exists from cortex to papilla). Other solutes also accumulate in the medulla (e.g., ammonium [NH_4^+] and K^+), but the most abundant solutes are NaCl and urea. For simplicity, this discussion assumes that NaCl and urea are the only solutes.

At the junction of the medulla with the cortex, the interstitial fluid has an osmolality of approximately 300 mOsm/kg H_2O, with virtually all osmoles attributable to NaCl.* The concentrations of both NaCl and urea increase progressively with increasing depth into the medulla. When maximally concentrated urine is excreted, the medullary interstitial fluid osmolality is approximately 1200 mOsm/kg H_2O at the papilla (Figure 5-6, B). Of this value, approximately 600 mOsm/kg H_2O is attributed to NaCl and 600 mOsm/kg H_2O is attributed to urea. As described later, NaCl is an effective osmole in the inner medulla and thus is responsible for driving water reabsorption from the medullary collecting duct. The high urea concentration of the medullary interstitial fluid allows this solute to be excreted at a high concentration (600 mmol/L) in a small volume of urine, thus limiting the amount of water that otherwise would be needed to excrete the daily load of urea.†

The medullary gradient for NaCl results from the accumulation of NaCl reabsorbed by the segments of Henle's loop (see the previous discussion). Urea accumulation within the medullary interstitium is more complex and occurs most effectively when hyperosmotic urine is excreted (i.e., antidiuresis). When dilute urine is produced, especially over extended periods,

---

*In the presentation that follows, it is assumed that the osmolality of the interstitial fluid of the medulla progressively increases from the corticomedullary junction to the papillary tip. However, based on new anatomic studies, it is likely that more regional variability in interstitial osmolality exists.

†In a person consuming a typical diet, the kidneys must excrete 450 mmol/day of urea. At a maximal urine [urea] of 600 mmol/L, this amount of urea can be excreted in 0.75 L of urine. However, if the maximal urine [urea] is reduced because of a decrease in the medullary interstitial fluid [urea], a larger volume of water would need to be excreted to excrete the 450 mmol/day of urea (e.g., 2.25 L of urine would be required if the maximal urine [urea] was only 200 mmol/L). This would severely restrict the ability of the kidneys to maintain water balance when P_{osm} is elevated.

the osmolality of the medullary interstitium declines (compare Figure 5-7, *A* and *B*). This reduced osmolality is almost entirely caused by a decrease in the concentration of urea. This decrease reflects washout by the vasa recta (discussed in a later section of this chapter) and diffusion of urea from the interstitium into the tubular fluid within the medullary portion of the collecting duct. (Note: The cortical and outer medullary portions of the collecting have a low permeability to urea, whereas the inner medullary portion has a relatively high permeability because of the presence of UT-A1 and UT-A3.)

Urea is not synthesized in the kidney but is generated by the liver as a product of protein metabolism. It enters the tubular fluid via glomerular filtration. Approximately half of this filtered urea is reabsorbed by the proximal tubule. During antidiuresis, water reabsorption by the cortical and outer medullary portions of the collecting duct leads to an increase in the urea concentration of the tubular fluid. When this fluid reaches the portion of the inner medullary collecting duct that express UT-A1 and UT-A3, urea is reabsorbed. The reabsorption of urea is further enhanced by the high levels of AVP, which increase the expression of the UTs. Some of this reabsorbed urea is secreted into thin descending limbs of Henle's loops via UT-A2, and some enters vasa recta via UT-B. The urea that is secreted into the descending thin limbs of Henle's loops is then trapped in the nephron until it again reaches the medullary collecting duct, where it can reenter the medullary interstitium. Thus urea recycles from the interstitium to the nephron and back into the interstitium. This process of recycling facilitates the accumulation of urea in the medullary interstitium, where it can attain a concentration at the tip of the papilla of 600 mmol/L. It is the high concentration of urea in the interstitial fluid that prevents the diffusion of urea out of the lumen of the inner medullary collecting duct into the interstitium, thereby facilitating urea excretion in the urine.

As described, the hyperosmotic medulla is essential for concentrating the tubular fluid within the collecting duct. Because water reabsorption from the collecting duct is driven by the osmotic gradient established in the medullary interstitium, urine can never be more concentrated than that of the interstitial fluid in the papilla. Thus any condition that reduces the medullary

interstitial osmolality impairs the ability of the kidneys to maximally concentrate the urine. However, because the inner medullary collecting duct is highly permeable to urea, especially in the presence of AVP, urea cannot drive water reabsorption across this nephron segment (i.e., urea is an ineffective osmole). Instead, the urea in the tubular fluid and medullary interstitium equilibrate and a small volume of urine with a high concentration of urea is excreted. It is the medullary interstitial NaCl concentration that is responsible for reabsorbing water from the inner medullary collecting duct and thereby concentrating the nonurea solutes (e.g., NH_4^+ salts, K^+ salts, and creatinine) in the urine.

AT THE CELLULAR LEVEL

The expression of the urea transporter (UT-A1) in the inner medullary collecting duct is increased by arginine vasopressin (AVP) via a cyclic adenosine monophosphate–mediated mechanism. UT-A1 expression also is increased by hyperosmolality. This effect is mediated by changes in intracellular Ca^{++} and protein kinase C activity. Thus the effects of AVP and hyperosmolality are separate and additive. The expression of UT-A3 and UT-A2 also is increased by AVP. Knockout mice have been created that lack the UT-A1/UT-A3 collecting duct transporters, the UT-A2 thin descending limb transporter, or the UT-B vasa recta transporter. All of these animals have some degree of impairment of urinary concentration. Humans with genetic loss of UT-B exhibit a similar urinary concentrating defect as the knockout mouse model.

Vasa Recta Function

The **vasa recta**, the capillary networks that supply blood to the medulla, are highly permeable to solute and water. As with the loop of Henle, the vasa recta form a parallel set of hairpin loops within the medulla (see Chapter 2). Not only do the vasa recta bring nutrients and oxygen to the medullary nephron segments but, more importantly, they also remove the water and solute that is continuously added to the medullary interstitium by these nephron segments. The ability of the vasa recta to maintain the medullary interstitial gradient is flow dependent. A substantial increase in vasa recta blood flow dissipates the medullary gradient. Alternatively, decreased blood flow reduces oxygen delivery to the nephron segments within the medulla. Because transport of salt and other solutes requires oxygen and adenosine triphosphate, reduced medullary blood flow decreases salt and solute transport by nephron segments in the medulla. As a result, the medullary interstitial osmotic gradient cannot be maintained, which also reduces the ability to concentrate the urine.

ASSESSMENT OF RENAL DILUTING AND CONCENTRATING ABILITY

Assessment of renal water handling includes measurements of urine osmolality and the volume of urine excreted. The range of urine osmolality is from 50 to 1200 mOsm/kg H_2O. The corresponding range in urine volume is 18 to as little as 0.5 L/day. These ranges are not fixed, but they vary from person to person and, as noted previously, depend on the amount of water ingested and lost from nonrenal routes, as well as the amount of solute excreted.

As emphasized in this chapter, the ability of the kidneys to dilute or concentrate the urine requires the separation of solute and water. This separation of solute and water in essence generates a volume of water that is "free of solute." When the urine is dilute, **solute-free water** is excreted from the body. When the urine is concentrated, solute-free water is returned to the body (i.e., conserved). The concept of **free water clearance** (C_{H_2O}) provides a way to calculate the amount of solute-free water generated by the kidneys, either when dilute urine is excreted or when concentrated urine is formed. As its name denotes, C_{H_2O} is directly derived from the concept of renal clearance discussed in Chapter 3.

To calculate C_{H_2O}, the clearance of total solute by the kidneys must be calculated. This clearance of total solute (i.e., osmoles, whether effective or ineffective) from plasma by the kidneys is termed the **osmolar clearance (C_{osm})** and can be calculated as follows:

$$C_{OSM} = \frac{U_{OSM} \times \dot{V}}{P_{OSM}} \tag{5-2}$$

where U_{osm} is the urine osmolality, $\dot{V}$ is the urine flow rate, and P_{osm} is the osmolality of plasma. C_{osm} has

units of volume/unit time. C_{H_2O} is then calculated as follows:

$$C_{H_2O} = \dot{V} - C_{osm} \tag{5-3}$$

By rearranging equation 5-3; it should be apparent that

$$\dot{V} = C_{H_2O} + C_{osm} \tag{5-4}$$

In other words, it is possible to partition the total urine output ($\dot{V}$) into two hypothetical components. One component contains all the urine solutes and has an osmolality equal to that of plasma (i.e., U_{osm} = P_{osm}). This volume is defined by C_{osm} and represents a volume from which there has been no separation of solute and water. The second component is a volume of solute-free water (i.e., C_{H_2O}).

When dilute urine is produced, the value of C_{H_2O} is positive, indicating that solute-free water is excreted from the body. When concentrated urine is produced, the value of C_{H_2O} is negative, indicating that solute-free water is retained in the body. By convention, negative C_{H_2O} values are expressed as $T^C_{H_2O}$ (**tubular conservation of water**).

Calculating C_{H_2O} and $T^C_{H_2O}$ can provide important information about the function of the portions of the nephron involved in producing dilute and concentrated urine. Whether the kidneys excrete or reabsorb free water depends on the presence of AVP. When AVP is absent or AVP levels are low, solute-free water is excreted. When AVP levels are high, solute-free water is reabsorbed.

The following factors are necessary for the kidneys to excrete a maximal amount of solute-free water (C_{H_2O}):

1. AVP must be absent. Without AVP, the collecting duct does not reabsorb a significant amount of water.
2. The tubular structures that separate solute from water (i.e., dilute the luminal fluid) must function normally. In the absence of AVP, the following nephron segments can dilute the luminal fluid:
   - Thin ascending limb of Henle's loop
   - Thick ascending limb of Henle's loop
   - Distal tubule
   - Collecting duct

Because of its high transport rate, the thick ascending limb is quantitatively the most important of these segments involved in the separation of solute and water.

3. An adequate amount of tubular fluid must be delivered to the aforementioned nephron sites for maximal separation of solute and water. Factors that reduce delivery (e.g., decreased GFR or enhanced proximal tubule reabsorption) impair the kidneys' ability to excrete solute-free water.

Similar requirements also apply to the conservation of water by the kidneys ($T^C_{H_2O}$). For the kidneys to conserve water maximally, the following conditions must exist:

1. An adequate amount of tubular fluid must be delivered to the nephron segments in which separation of solute from water occurs. The important segment in the separation of solute and water is the thick ascending limb of Henle's loop. Delivery of tubular fluid to Henle's loop depends on GFR and proximal tubule reabsorption.

2. Reabsorption of NaCl by the nephron segments must be normal; again, the most important segment is the thick ascending limb of Henle's loop.

3. A hyperosmotic medullary interstitium must be present. The interstitial fluid osmolality is maintained by NaCl reabsorption by Henle's loop (conditions 1 and 2) and by effective accumulation of urea. Urea accumulation in turn depends on adequate dietary protein intake.

4. Maximum levels of AVP must be present and the collecting duct must respond normally to AVP.

IN THE CLINIC

The concept of free-water clearance as just described does not distinguish between effective and ineffective osmoles, either in the plasma or in the urine. However, urea, which can account for half of total urine osmoles, is not an effective osmole when the movement of water between intracellular fluid and extracellular fluid is considered (see Chapter 1). Accordingly, when one wants to understand how the handling of

water by the kidneys contributes to the maintenance of whole-body water balance, it is more appropriate to consider only the solutes that are effective osmoles. For plasma (i.e., extracellular fluid), the effective osmoles are Na^+ and its attendant anions. For urine, they are the nonurea solutes.

The importance of using effective osmoles in determining the impact of renal water handling on whole-body water balance (i.e., body fluid osmolality) is illustrated by the following example. A patient has an elevated plasma [urea], and his plasma [Na^+] also is increased to 150 mEq/L. His total plasma osmolality (including urea) is 320 mOsm/kg H_2O, but his effective plasma osmolality (calculated as 2 × plasma [Na^+]) is only 300 mOsm/kg H_2O. His urine osmolality is 600 mOsm/kg H_2O, with 300 mOsm/kg H_2O related to urea and 300 mOsm/kg H_2O related to nonurea solutes. His urinary flow rate is 3 L/day.

According to equations 5-2 and 5-3, his total osmolar clearance (C_{osm}) and free-water clearance (C_{H_2O}) are as follows:

$$C_{OSM} = \frac{600 \text{ mOsm/kg } H_2O \times 3 \text{ L/day}}{320 \text{ mOsm/kg } H_2O} = 5.6 \text{ L/day}$$

$$(5\text{-}5)$$

$$C_{H_2O} = 3 \text{ L/day} - 5.6 \text{ L/day} = -2.6 \text{ L/day} \ (T^C_{H_2O})$$

$$(5\text{-}6)$$

Thus it appears that the kidneys are conserving 2.6 L/day of solute-free water, which would be an appropriate response to correct the elevated plasma osmolality. However, when C_{osm} and C_{H_2O} are analyzed from the perspective of effective osmoles, the following results are obtained:

$$C_{OSM} = \frac{300 \text{ mOsm/kg } H_2O \times 3 \text{ L/day}}{300 \text{ mOsm/kg } H_2O} = 3 \text{ L/day}$$

$$(5\text{-}7)$$

$$C_{H_2O} = 3 \text{ L/day} - 3 \text{ L/day} = 0 \text{ L/day} \quad (5\text{-}8)$$

When viewed from the more appropriate perspective of effective osmoles, it thus is apparent that the kidneys are not reabsorbing solute-free water and the patient's kidneys are not correcting the hyperosmolality.

SUMMARY

1. The osmolality and volume of the body fluids are maintained within a narrow range despite wide variations in water and solute intake. The kidneys play the central role in this regulatory process by virtue of their ability to vary the excretion of water and solutes.

2. Regulation of body fluid osmolality requires that water intake and loss from the body be equal. This process involves the integrated interaction of the AVP secretory and thirst centers of the hypothalamus and the ability of the kidneys to excrete urine that is either hypoosmotic or hyperosmotic with respect to the body fluids.

3. When body fluid osmolality increases, AVP secretion and thirst are stimulated. AVP acts on the kidneys to increase the permeability of the collecting duct to water. Hence water is reabsorbed from the lumen of the collecting duct, and a small volume of hyperosmotic urine is excreted. This renal conservation of water, together with increased water intake, restores body fluid osmolality to normal.

4. When body fluid osmolality decreases, AVP secretion and thirst are suppressed. In the absence of AVP, the collecting duct is impermeable to water and a large volume of hypoosmotic urine is excreted. With this increased excretion of water and a decreased intake of water caused by suppression of thirst, the osmolality of the body fluids is restored to normal.

5. Central to the process of concentrating and diluting the urine is Henle's loop. The transport of NaCl by Henle's loop allows the separation of solute and water, which is essential for the elaboration of hypoosmotic urine. By the same mechanism, the interstitial fluid in the medullary portion of the kidney is rendered hyperosmotic. This hyperosmotic medullary interstitial fluid in turn provides the osmotic driving force for the reabsorption of water from the lumen of the collecting duct when AVP is present.

6. Disorders of water balance result in alterations in body fluid osmolality. Because Na^+ and its attendant anions (Cl^- and HCO_3^-) are the major osmotically active particles in the ECF, changes in body fluid osmolality are manifested by a change in the plasma $[Na^+]$. Positive water balance (intake > excretion) results in a decrease in the body fluid osmolality and thus hyponatremia. Negative water balance (intake < excretion) results in an increase in body fluid osmolality and thus hypernatremia.

7. The handling of water by the kidneys is quantitated by measuring the amount of solute-free water that is either excreted (C_{H_2O}) or reabsorbed ($T^C_{H_2O}$). Maximal excretion of solute-free water requires normal nephron function (especially the thick ascending limb of Henle's loop), adequate delivery of tubular fluid to the nephrons, and the absence of AVP. Maximal reabsorption of solute-free water requires normal nephron function (especially the thick ascending limb of Henle's loop), adequate delivery of tubular fluid to the nephrons, a hyperosmotic medullary interstitium, the presence of AVP, and responsiveness of the collecting duct to AVP.

KEY WORDS AND CONCEPTS

- Insensible water loss
- Arginine vasopressin (AVP), also known as antidiuretic hormone (ADH)
- Diuresis
- Antidiuresis
- Supraoptic nuclei
- Paraventricular nuclei
- Neurohypophysis (posterior pituitary)
- Osmoreceptors
- Effective osmole
- Ineffective osmole
- Set point (for osmotic control of AVP secretion)
- Baroreceptors
- Polyuria
- Polydipsia
- Central diabetes insipidus
- Pituitary diabetes insipidus
- Syndrome of inappropriate secretion of ADH (SIADH)
- Nephrogenic syndrome of inappropriate antidiuresis
- Nephrogenic diabetes insipidus
- Aquaporin (AQP)

- Thirst
- Diluting segment (thick ascending limb of Henle's loop)
- Concurrent multiplication (by Henle's loop)
- Free-water clearance (C_{H_2O})
- Tubular conservation of water ($T^C_{H_2O}$)

SELF-STUDY PROBLEMS

1. A person's blood is drawn, and the following values are obtained (see Appendix B for normal values):

Plasma [Na^+]	135 mEq/L
Serum [glucose]	100 mg/dL
Serum [blood urea nitrogen]	100 mg/dL
P_{osm}	310 mOsm/kg H_2O

Would plasma AVP levels in this person be elevated or suppressed?

2. In the following table, indicate the expected osmolality of tubular fluid in the absence and presence of AVP (assume that the plasma osmolality is 300 mOsm/kg H_2O and osmolality of the medullary interstitium is 1200 mOsm/kg H_2O at the papilla).

Nephron site	0-AVP	Maximum AVP
Proximal tubule	_____	_____
Beginning of thin descending limb	_____	_____
Beginning of thin ascending limb	_____	_____
End of thick ascending limb	_____	_____
End of cortical collecting duct	_____	_____
Urine	_____	_____

3. The ability of the kidneys to concentrate the urine maximally is impaired under each of the following conditions:
   a. Decreased renal perfusion (i.e., decreased GFR)
   b. Administration of a diuretic that inhibits active NaCl transport by the thick ascending limb of Henle's loop
   c. Nephrogenic diabetes insipidus
   d. Defect in the urea transporter in the vasa recta

What are the mechanisms responsible for the observed impairment in the kidneys' concentrating ability during each of these conditions?

4. A person must excrete 800 mOsm of solute in a 24-hour period. What volume of urine is required if the person can concentrate the urine to only 400 mOsm/kg H_2O? What volume of urine is required if this person can concentrate the urine to 1200 mOsm/kg H_2O?

5. A person excretes 6 L/day of urine having an osmolality of 200 mOsm/kg H_2O. If plasma osmolality is 280 mOsm/kg H_2O, what are the total osmolar clearance and C_{H_2O}?

6

REGULATION OF EXTRACELLULAR FLUID VOLUME AND NaCl BALANCE

OBJECTIVES

Upon completion of this chapter, the student should be able to answer the following questions:

1. Why do changes in Na⁺ balance alter the volume of extracellular fluid?

2. What is the effective circulating volume, how is it influenced by changes in Na⁺ balance, and how does it influence renal Na⁺ excretion?

3. What are the mechanisms by which the body monitors the effective circulating volume?

4. What are the major signals acting on the kidneys to alter their excretion of Na⁺?

5. How do changes in extracellular fluid volume alter Na⁺ transport in the different segments of the nephron, and how do these changes in transport regulate renal Na⁺ excretion?

6. What are the mechanisms involved in the formation of edema, and what role do the kidneys play in this process?

The major solutes of the extracellular fluid (ECF) are the salts of Na^+. Of these, sodium chloride (NaCl) is the most abundant. Because NaCl is also the major determinant of ECF osmolality, alterations in Na^+ balance commonly are assumed to disturb ECF osmolality. However, under normal circumstances, this is not the case because the arginine vasopressin (AVP) and thirst systems maintain body fluid osmolality within a very narrow range. For example, the addition of NaCl to the ECF (without water) increases the Na^+ concentration and osmolality of this compartment (intracellular fluid osmolality also increases because of osmotic equilibration with the ECF) (Figure 6-1). This increase in osmolality in turn stimulates thirst and the release of AVP from the posterior pituitary. The increased ingestion of water in response to thirst, together with the AVP-induced decrease in water excretion by the kidneys (so-called **antidiuresis**), quickly restores ECF osmolality to normal. However, the volume of the ECF increases in proportion to the amount of water ingested, which in turn depends on the amount of NaCl added to the ECF. Thus in the new steady state, the addition of NaCl to the ECF is equivalent to adding an isosmotic solution, and the volume of this compartment increases. Conversely, a decrease in the NaCl content of the ECF lowers the volume of this compartment (see Figure 6-1). The kidneys are the major route for excretion of NaCl from the body. Only about 10% of the Na^+ lost from the body each day is lost by nonrenal routes (e.g., in perspiration and feces).

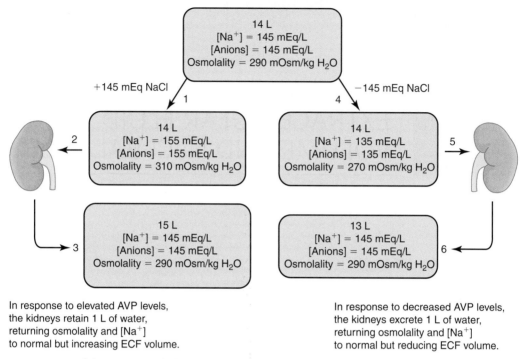

In response to elevated AVP levels, the kidneys retain 1 L of water, returning osmolality and [Na⁺] to normal but increasing ECF volume.

In response to decreased AVP levels, the kidneys excrete 1 L of water, returning osmolality and [Na⁺] to normal but reducing ECF volume.

FIGURE 6-1 ■ Impact of changes in Na⁺ balance on the volume of the extracellular fluid (*ECF*). *1,* Addition of sodium chloride (NaCl) (without water) to the ECF increases [Na⁺] and osmolality. *2,* The increase in ECF osmolality stimulates the secretion of arginine vasopressin (*AVP*) from the posterior pituitary, which then acts on the kidneys to conserve water. *3,* Decreased renal excretion of water together with water ingestion restores plasma osmolality and plasma [Na⁺] to normal. However, the volume of the ECF is now increased by 1 L. *4,* Removal of NaCl (without water) from the ECF decreases the plasma [Na⁺] and plasma osmolality. *5,* The decrease in ECF osmolality inhibits AVP secretion. In response to the decrease in plasma AVP, the kidneys excrete water. *6,* Increased renal excretion of water returns the plasma [Na⁺] and plasma osmolality to normal. However, the volume of the ECF is now decreased by 1 L. As illustrated, changes in Na⁺ balance alter the volume of the ECF because of the efficiency of the AVP system in maintaining a normal body fluid osmolality.

Thus the kidneys are critically important in regulating the volume of the ECF. Under normal conditions, the kidneys keep the volume of the ECF constant by adjusting the excretion of NaCl to match the amount ingested in the diet. If ingestion exceeds excretion, ECF volume increases above normal, whereas the opposite occurs if excretion exceeds ingestion.

IN THE CLINIC

It has been observed that the kidneys excrete sodium chloride (NaCl) more quickly when the NaCl is administered orally versus by an intravenous infusion. This observation has led to the search for factors within the gastrointestinal tract that might modulate the renal excretion of NaCl. Indeed, neuroendocrine cells that produce the peptide hormones **uroguanylin** and **guanylin** in response to NaCl ingestion have been identified in the intestine. These hormones increase NaCl and water excretion by the kidneys (uroguanylin > guanylin) by inhibiting Na⁺ reabsorption in both the proximal tubule and collecting duct. Interestingly, the kidneys also produce uroguanylin and guanylin, suggesting that they also might play a paracrine role in the intrarenal regulation of NaCl excretion. The potential importance of these peptides in regulating renal NaCl excretion is seen in mice lacking the uroguanylin gene. These mice have a blunted natriuretic response to an oral NaCl load, and they also have increased blood pressure.

The typical diet contains approximately 140 mEq/day of Na^+ (8 g of NaCl), and thus daily Na^+ excretion is also about 140 mEq/day. However, the kidneys can vary the excretion of Na^+ over a wide range. Excretion rates as low as 10 mEq/day can be attained when persons are placed on a low-salt diet. Conversely, the kidneys can increase their excretion rate to more than 1000 mEq/day when challenged by the ingestion of a high-salt diet. These changes in Na^+ excretion can occur with only modest changes in the ECF volume and steady-state Na^+ content of the body.

The response of the kidneys to abrupt changes in NaCl intake typically takes several hours to several days, depending on the magnitude of the change. During this transition period, the intake and excretion of Na^+ are not matched as they are in the steady state. Thus the individual experiences either **positive Na^+ balance** (intake > excretion) or **negative Na^+ balance** (intake < excretion). However, by the end of the transition period, a new steady state is established, and intake once again equals excretion. Provided that the AVP and thirst systems are intact and normal, alterations in Na^+ balance change the volume, but not the Na^+ concentration, of the ECF. Changes in ECF volume can be monitored by measuring body weight because 1 L of ECF equals 1 kg of body weight.

In this chapter the physiology of the receptors that monitor ECF volume is reviewed and the various signals that act on the kidneys to regulate NaCl excretion and thereby ECF volume are explained. In addition, the responses of the various portions of the nephron to these signals are considered. Finally, the pathophysiologic mechanisms involved in the formation of edema are presented, with emphasis on the role of NaCl handling by the kidneys.

CONCEPT OF EFFECTIVE CIRCULATING VOLUME

As described in Chapter 1, the ECF is subdivided into two compartments: blood plasma and interstitial fluid. Plasma volume is a determinant of vascular volume and thus blood pressure and cardiac output. The maintenance of Na^+ balance, and thus ECF volume, involves a complex system of sensors and effector signals that act primarily on the kidneys to regulate the excretion of NaCl. As can be appreciated from the

dependence of vascular volume, blood pressure, and cardiac output on ECF volume, this complex system is designed to ensure adequate tissue perfusion. Because the primary sensors of this system are located in the large vessels of the vascular system, changes in vascular volume, blood pressure, and cardiac output are the principal factors regulating renal NaCl excretion (described later in this chapter).

In a healthy person, changes in ECF volume result in parallel changes in vascular volume, blood pressure, and cardiac output. Thus a decrease in ECF volume, a situation termed **volume contraction**, results in reduced vascular volume, blood pressure, and cardiac output. Conversely, an increase in ECF volume, a situation termed **volume expansion**, results in increased vascular volume, blood pressure, and cardiac output. The degree to which these cardiovascular parameters change depends on the degree of volume contraction or expansion and the effectiveness of cardiovascular reflex mechanisms. When a person is in negative Na^+ balance, ECF volume is decreased and renal NaCl excretion is reduced. Conversely, with positive Na^+ balance, an increase in ECF volume occurs, which results in enhanced renal NaCl excretion (i.e., **natriuresis**).

However, in some pathologic conditions (e.g., congestive heart failure and hepatic cirrhosis), the renal excretion of NaCl is not reflective of the ECF volume. In both of these situations, the volume of the ECF is increased. However, instead of increased renal NaCl excretion, as would be expected, a reduction in the renal excretion of NaCl occurs. To explain renal Na^+ handling in these situations, it is necessary to understand the concept of **effective circulating volume (ECV)**. Unlike the ECF, the ECV is not a measurable and distinct body fluid compartment. The ECV refers to the portion of the ECF that is contained within the vascular system and is "effectively" perfusing the tissues (*effective blood volume* is another commonly used term). More specifically, the ECV reflects the perfusion of those portions of the vascular system that contain the volume sensors (described later in this chapter).

In healthy persons, ECV varies directly with the volume of the ECF and, in particular, the volume of the vascular system (arterial and venous), the arterial blood pressure, and cardiac output. However, as noted, this is not the case in certain pathologic conditions. In the remaining sections of this chapter, the

IN THE CLINIC

Patients with congestive heart failure frequently have an increase in the volume of the extracellular fluid (ECF), which is manifested as accumulation of fluid in the lungs (**pulmonary edema**) and peripheral tissues (**peripheral edema**). This excess fluid is the result of sodium chloride (NaCl) and water retention by the kidneys. The kidneys' response (i.e., retention of NaCl and water) appears paradoxical because the ECF volume is increased. However, because of poor cardiac performance, perfusion of the portions of the vascular system that contain the volume sensors is reduced (i.e., decreased effective circulating volume). Therefore the volume sensors misinterpret these signals as indicative of ECF volume contraction and respond by increasing NaCl and water retention by the kidneys, thereby exacerbating a vicious cycle of impaired cardiac function and increased NaCl and water reabsorption.

Large volumes of fluid accumulate in the peritoneal cavity of patients with advanced hepatic cirrhosis. This fluid, called **ascites**, is a component of the ECF and results from NaCl and water retention by the kidneys. Again, the response of the kidneys in this situation seems paradoxical if only ECF volume is considered. With advanced hepatic cirrhosis, blood pools in the splanchnic circulation (i.e., the damaged liver impedes the drainage of blood from the splanchnic circulation by the portal vein). Thus volume and pressure are reduced in the portions of the vascular system where the volume sensors are found and, as in the case of congestive heart failure, the volume sensors interpret reduced effective circulating volume as decreased ECF volume and respond accordingly. Hence the kidneys respond as they normally would to ECF volume contraction, resulting in NaCl and water retention and an increase in ECF volume, which results in the accumulation of ascites fluid.

BOX 6-1
VOLUME AND Na$^+$ SENSORS

I. Vascular
  A. Low-pressure cardiopulmonary circuit
    1. Cardiac atria
    2. Pulmonary vasculature
  B. High-pressure arterial circuit
    1. Cartoid sinus
    2. Aortic arch
    3. Juxtaglomerular apparatus of the kidney
II. Central nervous system
III. Hepatic

---

relationship between ECF volume and renal NaCl excretion in healthy adults, where changes in ECV and ECF volume occur in parallel, is examined.

VOLUME-SENSING SYSTEMS

The ECF volume (or ECV) is monitored by multiple sensors (Box 6-1). A number of the sensors are located in the vascular system, and they monitor its fullness and pressure. These receptors typically are called volume receptors; because they respond to pressure-induced stretch of the walls of the receptor (e.g., blood vessels or cardiac atria), they also are referred to as baroreceptors (see Chapter 5). The sensors within the liver and central nervous system (CNS) are less well understood and do not seem to be as important as the vascular sensors in monitoring the ECF volume.

Volume Sensors in the Low-Pressure Cardiopulmonary Circuit

Volume sensors (i.e., baroreceptors), which are located within the walls of the cardiac atria, right ventricle, and large pulmonary vessels, respond to distention of these structures. Because the low-pressure venous side of the circulatory system has a high compliance, these sensors respond mainly to the "fullness" of the vascular system. These baroreceptors send signals to the brainstem through afferent fibers in the glossopharyngeal and vagus nerves. The activity of these sensors modulates both sympathetic nerve outflow and AVP secretion. For example, a decrease in filling of the pulmonary vessels and cardiac atria increases sympathetic nerve activity and stimulates AVP secretion. Conversely, distention of these structures decreases sympathetic nerve activity. In general, 5% to 10% changes in blood volume and pressure are necessary to evoke a response.

The cardiac atria possess an additional mechanism related to the control of renal NaCl excretion. The myocytes of the atria synthesize and store a peptide hormone. This hormone, termed **atrial natriuretic peptide (ANP)**, is released when the atria are distended, which, by mechanisms outlined later in this chapter, reduces blood pressure and increases the excretion of NaCl and water by the kidneys. The ventricles of the heart also produce a natriuretic peptide termed **brain natriuretic peptide (BNP)**, so named because it was first isolated from the brain. Like ANP, BNP is released from the ventricular myocytes by distention of the ventricles. Its actions are similar to those of ANP.

Volume Sensors in the High-Pressure Arterial Circuit

Baroreceptors also are present in the arterial side of the circulatory system; they are located in the wall of the aortic arch, carotid sinus, and afferent arterioles of the kidneys. The aortic arch and carotid baroreceptors send input to the brainstem through afferent fibers in the glossopharyngeal and vagus nerves. The response to this input alters sympathetic outflow and AVP secretion. Thus a decrease in blood pressure increases sympathetic nerve activity and AVP secretion. An increase in pressure tends to reduce sympathetic nerve activity (and activate parasympathetic nerve activity). The sensitivity of the high-pressure baroreceptors is similar to that in the low-pressure side of the vascular system; 5% to 10% changes in pressure are needed to evoke a response.

The **juxtaglomerular apparatus** of the kidneys (see Chapter 2), particularly the afferent arteriole, responds directly to changes in pressure. If perfusion pressure in the afferent arteriole is reduced, renin is released from the myocytes. Renin secretion is suppressed when perfusion pressure is increased. As described later in this chapter, renin determines blood levels of angiotensin II and aldosterone, both of which play an important role in regulating renal NaCl excretion.

Of the two classes of baroreceptors, those on the high-pressure side of the vascular system appear to be more important in influencing sympathetic tone and AVP secretion. For example, patients with congestive heart failure often have an increased vascular volume with dilation of the atria and ventricles, which would be expected to decrease sympathetic tone and inhibit AVP secretion via the low-pressure baroreceptors.

However, sympathetic tone often is increased and AVP secretion often is stimulated in these patients (the renin-angiotensin-aldosterone system also is activated). This phenomenon reflects the activation of baroreceptors in the high-pressure arterial circuit in response to reduced blood pressure and cardiac output secondary to the failing heart (i.e., the high-pressure baroreceptors detect a reduced ECV and misinterpret this signal as indicative of reduced ECF volume).

Hepatic Sensors

The liver also contains volume sensors that can modulate renal NaCl excretion, although they are not as important as the vascular sensors. One type of hepatic sensor responds to pressure within the hepatic vasculature and therefore functions in a manner similar to the baroreceptors in the low- and high-pressure vascular circuits. A second type of sensor also appears to exist in the liver. This sensor responds to $[Na^+]$ of the portal blood entering the liver. Afferent signals from both types of sensors are sent to the same area of the brainstem where afferent fibers from both the low- and high-pressure circuit baroreceptors converge. Increased pressure within the hepatic vasculature or an increase in portal blood [Na^+] results in a decrease in efferent sympathetic nerve activity.* As described later in this chapter, this decreased sympathetic nerve activity leads to an increase in renal NaCl excretion.

Central Nervous System Na⁺ Sensors

As with the hepatic sensors, the CNS sensors do not appear to be as important as the vascular sensors in monitoring the ECF volume and controlling renal NaCl excretion. Nevertheless, alterations in the [Na^+] of blood carried to the brain in the carotid arteries or the [Na^+] of the cerebrospinal fluid modulate renal NaCl excretion. For example, if the [Na^+] in either the carotid artery blood or the cerebrospinal fluid is increased, a decrease in renal sympathetic nerve activity occurs, which in turn leads to an increase in renal NaCl excretion. The hypothalamus appears to be the site where these sensors are located. Angiotensin II and natriuretic peptides are generated in the hypothalamus. These locally generated signals, together with systemically generated angiotensin II and natriuretic peptides, appear to play a role in modulating the CNS Na^+-sensing system.

Of the volume and Na^+ sensors just described, those located in the vascular system are better understood. Moreover, their function in health and disease explains quite effectively the regulation of renal NaCl excretion. Therefore the remainder of this chapter focuses on the vascular volume sensors (i.e., baroreceptors) and their role in regulating renal NaCl excretion.

Volume Sensor Signals

When the vascular volume sensors have detected a change in ECV, which under normal conditions reflects ECF volume, they send signals to the kidneys, which result in appropriate adjustments in NaCl and

---

*The hepatic sensors also appear to be involved in the regulation of gastrointestinal NaCl absorption. For example, when [Na^+] of the portal vein blood is increased, a reflex reduction in jejunal NaCl absorption occurs.

■ ■ ■ ■ ■ ■ ■ ■ ■ ■ ■ ■
BOX 6-2
SIGNALS INVOLVED IN THE CONTROL OF RENAL NaCl AND WATER EXCRETION

RENAL SYMPATHETIC NERVES (↑ ACTIVITY: ↓ NaCl EXCRETION)
↓ GFR
↑ Renin secretion
↑ Na^+ reabsorption along the nephron

RENIN-ANGIOTENSIN-ALDOSTERONE (↑ SECRETION: ↓ NaCl EXCRETION)
↑ Angiotensin II stimulates Na^+ reabsorption along the nephron
↑ Aldosterone stimulates Na^+ reabsorption in the thick ascending limb of Henle's loop, distal tubule, and collecting duct
↑ Angiotensin II stimulates AVP secretion

NATRIURETIC PEPTIDES: ANP, BNP, AND URODILATIN (↑ SECRETION: ↑ NaCl EXCRETION)
↑ GFR
↓ Renin secretion
↓ Aldosterone secretion (indirect through angiotensin II and direct on adrenal gland)
↓ NaCl and water reabsorption by the collecting duct
↓ AVP secretion and inhibition of AVP action on the distal tubule and collecting duct

AVP (↑ SECRETION: ↓ H_2O EXCRETION)
↑ H_2O reabsorption by the distal tubule and collecting duct

ANP, Atrial natriuretic peptide; *AVP*, arginine vasopressin; *BNP*, brain natriuretic peptide; *GFR*, glomerular filtration rate; *NaCl*, sodium chloride.

---

water excretion. Accordingly, when the ECF volume is expanded, renal NaCl and water excretion are increased. Conversely, when the ECF volume is contracted, renal NaCl and water excretion are reduced. The signals involved in coupling the volume sensors to the kidneys are both neural and hormonal. These signals are summarized in Box 6-2, as are their effects on renal NaCl and water excretion.

Renal Sympathetic Nerves

As described in Chapter 2, sympathetic nerve fibers innervate the afferent and efferent arterioles of the glomerulus, as well as the nephron cells. With negative Na^+ balance (i.e., ECF volume contraction), baroreceptors in both the low- and high-pressure vascular circuits stimulate the sympathetic input to the kidneys. This stimulation has the following effects:

1. The afferent and efferent arterioles constrict in response to α-adrenergic stimulation. This vasoconstriction predominantly affects the afferent arteriole, effectively reducing hydrostatic pressure within the glomerular capillary lumen and decreasing glomerular filtration. The resulting reduction in the glomerular filtration rate (GFR) reduces the filtered load of Na^+ to the nephrons.
2. Renin secretion is stimulated by the cells of the afferent arterioles in response to β-adrenergic receptor stimulation. As described later, renin ultimately increases the circulating levels of angiotensin II and aldosterone.
3. NaCl reabsorption along the nephron is directly stimulated by α-adrenergic stimulation, effectively reducing the fraction of filtered Na^+ that is ultimately excreted. Quantitatively, the most important segment influenced by sympathetic nerve activity is the proximal tubule.

As a result of these combined actions, increased renal sympathetic nerve activity decreases net NaCl excretion, an adaptive response that works to restore ECF volume to normal, which is a state termed **euvolemia**. With positive Na^+ balance (i.e., ECF volume expansion), renal sympathetic nerve activity is reduced, which generally reverses the effects just described.

Renin-Angiotensin-Aldosterone System

Cells in the afferent arterioles (**juxtaglomerular cells**) are the site of synthesis, storage, and release of the proteolytic enzyme renin. Three factors are important in stimulating renin secretion:

1. *Perfusion pressure.* When perfusion pressure to the kidneys is reduced, renin secretion by the afferent arteriole is stimulated. Conversely, an increase in perfusion pressure inhibits renin release by the afferent arteriole.

AT THE CELLULAR LEVEL

A new "renal hormone" has been discovered recently, a flavin adenine dinucleotide–dependent amine oxidase named **renalase**. Renalase is similar in structure to monoamine oxidase and breaks down catecholamines (e.g., epinephrine and norepinephrine). Several tissues (e.g., skeletal muscle, heart, and small intestine) express renalase, but the kidneys secrete the enzyme into the circulation. Because persons with chronic renal failure have very low levels of renalase in their plasma, the kidney is probably the primary source of the circulating enzyme. In experimental animals, infusion of renalase decreases blood pressure and heart contractility. Although the precise role of renalase in cardiovascular function and blood pressure regulation is not known, it may be important in modulating the effects of the sympathetic nervous system and especially the effects of the sympathetic nerves on the kidney.

---

2. *Sympathetic nerve activity.* Activation of the sympathetic nerve fibers that innervate the afferent arterioles increases renin secretion via β-adrenergic receptor stimulation. Renin secretion is decreased as renal sympathetic nerve activity is decreased.
3. *Delivery of NaCl to the macula densa.* Delivery of NaCl to the macula densa regulates the GFR by a process termed **tubuloglomerular feedback** (see Chapter 3). In addition, the macula densa plays a role in renin secretion. When NaCl delivery to the macula densa is decreased, renin secretion is enhanced. Conversely, an increase in NaCl delivery inhibits renin secretion. It is likely that macula densa–mediated renin secretion helps to maintain systemic arterial pressure under conditions of a reduced intravascular volume. For example, when intravascular volume is reduced, perfusion of body tissues (including the kidneys) decreases, which in turn decreases the GFR and the filtered amount of NaCl. The reduced delivery of NaCl to the macula densa then stimulates renin secretion, which acts through angiotensin II (a potent vasoconstrictor) to increase the blood pressure and thereby maintain tissue perfusion.

AT THE CELLULAR LEVEL

Although many tissues express renin (e.g., brain, heart, and adrenal gland tissues), the primary source of circulating renin is the kidneys. Renin is secreted by juxtaglomerular cells located in the afferent arteriole. At the cellular level, renin secretion is mediated by the fusion of renin-containing granules with the luminal membrane of the cell. This process is stimulated by a *decrease* in intracellular [Ca^{++}], a response opposite to that of most secretory cells where secretion is normally stimulated by an *increase* in intracellular [Ca^{++}]. Renin release is also stimulated by an increase in intracellular cyclic adenosine monophosphate levels. Thus anything that increases intracellular [Ca^{++}] inhibits renin secretion, which includes stretch of the afferent arteriole (myogenic control of renin secretion), angiotensin II (feedback inhibition), and endothelin. Conversely, anything that increases intracellular cyclic adenosine monophosphate stimulates renin secretion, which includes norepinephrine acting through β-adrenergic receptors and prostaglandin E$_2$.

Increases in intracellular cyclic guanosine monophosphate have been shown to stimulate renin secretion in some situations and to inhibit secretion in others. Notably, two substances that increase intracellular cyclic guanosine monophosphate are natriuretic peptides and nitric oxide. Nitric oxide stimulates renin secretion, whereas atrial natriuretic peptide and brain natriuretic peptide are inhibitory. The control of renin secretion by the macula densa (see Chapter 3) may involve paracrine factors such as prostaglandin E$_2$ (which stimulates renin secretion when NaCl delivery to the macula densa is decreased) and adenosine (which inhibits renin secretion when NaCl delivery to the macular densa is increased).

Figure 6-2 summarizes the essential components of the renin-angiotensin-aldosterone system. Renin alone does not have a physiological function; it functions as a proteolytic enzyme. Its principal substrate is a circulating protein, **angiotensinogen**, which is

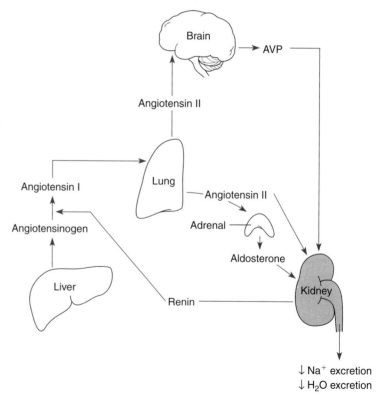

FIGURE 6-2 ■ Schematic representation of the essential components of the renin-angiotensin-aldosterone system. Activation of this system results in a decrease in the excretion of Na$^+$ and water by the kidneys. Note: Angiotensin I is converted to angiotensin II by an angiotensin-converting enzyme, which is present on all vascular endothelial cells. As shown, the endothelial cells within the lungs play a significant role in this conversion process. *AVP,* Arginine vasopressin.

produced by the liver. Angiotensinogen is cleaved by renin to yield a 10-amino-acid peptide, **angiotensin I.** Angiotensin I also has no known physiological function, and it is further cleaved to an 8-amino-acid peptide, **angiotensin II,** by a converting enzyme (**angiotensin-converting enzyme [ACE]**) found on the surface of vascular endothelial cells. Pulmonary and renal endothelial cells are important sites for the bioconversion of angiotensin I to angiotensin II. ACE also degrades bradykinin, a potent vasodilator. Angiotensin II has several important physiologic functions, including:

1. Stimulation of aldosterone secretion by the adrenal cortex
2. Arteriolar vasoconstriction, which increases blood pressure
3. Stimulation of AVP secretion and thirst
4. Enhancement of NaCl reabsorption by the proximal tubule, thick ascending limb of Henle's loop, the distal tubule, and even the collecting duct; of these segments, the effect on the proximal tubule is quantitatively the largest

Angiotensin II is an important secretagogue for **aldosterone.** An increase in the plasma K^+ concentration is the other important stimulus for aldosterone secretion (see Chapter 7). Aldosterone is a steroid hormone produced by the glomerulosa cells of the adrenal cortex. Aldosterone acts in a number of ways on the kidneys (see Chapter 4). With regard to the regulation of the ECF volume, aldosterone reduces NaCl excretion by stimulating its reabsorption by the thick ascending limb of the loop of Henle, portions of the distal tubule, and the collecting duct. (The portions of the distal tubule that functionally respond to aldosterone together with the collecting duct are referred to as the **aldosterone-sensitive distal nephron [ASDN].**) The effect of aldosterone on renal NaCl excretion depends mainly on its ability to stimulate Na^+ reabsorption in the ASDN.

Aldosterone has many cellular actions in cells of the ASDN (see Chapter 4 for details). Notably, it increases the abundance of the apical membrane Na^+-Cl^- symporter in the cells of the distal tubule (DCT2 segment; see previous At the Cellular Level box) and the abundance of the epithelial Na^+ channel in the

---

AT THE CELLULAR LEVEL

The distal tubule can be divided into three distinct segments based on the presence of specific membrane transporters. The first segment after the macula densa (DCT1) expresses a Na^+-Cl^- symporter, which is specifically inhibited by the thiazide class of diuretics (see Chapter 10). The next segment (DCT2) expresses the Na^+-Cl^- symporter and the epithelial Na^+ channel. The last segment of the distal tubule (connecting tubule), like the collecting duct, expresses only the epithelial Na^+ channel.

Aldosterone selectivity and sensitivity are conferred by the presence of mineralocorticoid receptors, as well as the presence of the enzyme **11β-hydroxysteroid dehydrogenase 2** (11β-HSD2). Because the mineralocorticoid receptor also binds glucocorticoids, 11β-HSD2 is required for aldosterone specificity because it metabolizes glucocorticoids and thus prevents them from binding to the mineralocorticoid receptor. The mineralocorticoid receptor is found throughout the distal tubule and collecting duct. However, 11β-HSD2 is only found in the DCT2, the connecting tubule, and collecting duct. Thus the aldosterone-sensitive distal nephron consists of the DCT2 and connecting tubule (collectively termed the late distal tubule) and the collecting duct. Accordingly, the DCT1 segment is referred to as the early distal tubule.

---

apical membrane of principal cells in the late portion of the distal tubule and collecting duct. By this action, Na^+ entry into the cells across the apical membrane is increased. Extrusion of Na^+ from the cell across the basolateral membrane occurs via the Na^+-K^+–adenosine triphosphatase (ATPase) pump, the abundance of which is also increased by aldosterone. Thus aldosterone increases net reabsorption of Na^+ from the tubular fluid by ASDN segments, and reduced levels of aldosterone decrease the amount of Na^+ reabsorbed by these segments.

As noted, aldosterone also enhances Na^+ reabsorption by cells of the thick ascending limb of the loop of Henle. This action probably reflects increased entry of Na^+ into the cell across the apical membrane (probably by the apical membrane Na^+-K^+-$2Cl^-$ symporter) and increased extrusion from the cell by the basolateral membrane Na^+-K^+-ATPase pump.

As summarized in Box 6-2, activation of the renin-angiotensin-aldosterone system, as occurs with ECF volume depletion, decreases the excretion of NaCl by the kidneys. Conversely, this system is suppressed by ECF volume expansion, thereby enhancing renal NaCl excretion.

Natriuretic Peptides

The body produces a number of substances, including ANP and BNP, that act on the kidneys to increase Na$^+$ excretion.* Of these substances, natriuretic peptides produced by the heart and kidneys are best understood and are the focus of the following discussion.

The heart produces two natriuretic peptides. Atrial myocytes primarily produce and store the peptide hormone ANP, and ventricular myocytes primarily produce and store BNP. Both peptides are secreted in response to myocardial wall stretch (i.e., during cardiac dilatation that accompanies volume expansion and/or heart failure), and they act to relax vascular smooth muscle and promote NaCl and water excretion by the kidneys. The kidneys also produce a related natriuretic peptide termed **urodilatin**. Its actions are limited to promoting NaCl excretion by the kidneys. In general, the actions of these natriuretic peptides, as they relate to renal NaCl and water excretion, antagonize those of the renin-angiotensin-aldosterone system. Natriuretic peptide actions include:

1. Afferent arteriolar vasodilation and efferent arteriolar vasoconstriction within the glomerulus, which increases the GFR and the filtered amount of Na$^+$.
2. Inhibition of renin secretion by the juxtaglomerular cells of the afferent arterioles.
3. Inhibition of aldosterone secretion by the glomerulosa cells of the adrenal cortex. This inhibition occurs by two mechanisms: (1) inhibition of renin secretion by the juxtaglomerular cells, thereby reducing angiotensin II–induced aldosterone secretion, and (2) direct inhibition of aldosterone secretion by the glomerulosa cells of the adrenal cortex.
4. Inhibition of NaCl reabsorption by the collecting duct, which also is caused in part by reduced levels of aldosterone. However, the natriuretic peptides also act directly on the collecting duct cells. Through the second messenger, cyclic guanosine monophosphate, natriuretic peptides inhibit Na$^+$ channels in the apical membrane and thereby decrease Na$^+$ reabsorption. This effect occurs predominantly in the medullary portion of the collecting duct.
5. Inhibition of AVP secretion by the posterior pituitary and AVP action on the collecting duct. These effects decrease water reabsorption by the collecting duct and thus increase excretion of water in the urine.

---

*Uroguanylin and adrenomedullin are two additional examples of these substances. Uroguanylin increases renal NaCl excretion and may serve to regulate the renal excretion of ingested NaCl. Adrenomedullin is produced by many tissues, including the heart, kidneys, and the adrenal medulla (from whence its name is derived). It is secreted in response to a number of factors (e.g., cytokines, angiotensin II, endothelin, and increased shear stress on endothelial cells). Although structurally distinct from ANP and BNP, its actions are similar in that it reduces blood pressure, increases GFR, suppresses angiotensin II–induced secretion of aldosterone, and causes increased NaCl excretion.

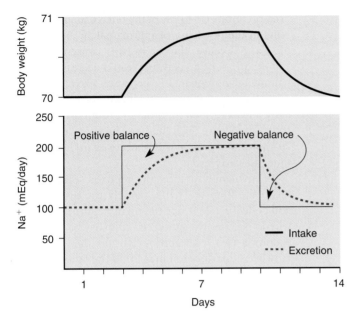

FIGURE 6-3 ■ Response to step increases and decreases in NaCl intake. Na+ excretion by the kidneys (*dashed line*) lags behind abrupt changes in Na+ intake (*lower panel, solid line*). The change in extracellular fluid volume that occurs during the periods of positive and negative Na+ balance is reflected in acute alterations in body weight.

These effects of the natriuretic peptides increase the net excretion of NaCl and water by the kidneys. Hypothetically, a reduction in the circulating levels of these peptides would be expected to decrease NaCl and water excretion, but convincing evidence for this effect has not been reported.

Arginine Vasopressin

As discussed in Chapter 5, a decreased ECF volume stimulates AVP secretion by the posterior pituitary. The elevated levels of AVP decrease water and NaCl excretion by the kidneys, which serve to reestablish euvolemia.

CONTROL OF RENAL NaCl EXCRETION DURING EUVOLEMIA

The maintenance of Na+ balance and therefore euvolemia requires the precise matching of the amount of NaCl ingested and the amount excreted from the body. As already noted, the kidneys are the major route for NaCl excretion. Accordingly, in a euvolemic person, we can equate daily urine NaCl excretion with daily NaCl intake.

The amount of NaCl excreted by the kidneys can vary widely. Under conditions of salt restriction (i.e., a low NaCl diet), virtually no Na+ appears in the urine.

Conversely, in persons who ingest large quantities of NaCl, renal Na+ excretion can exceed 1000 mEq/day. The kidneys require several days to respond maximally to variations in dietary NaCl intake. During the transition period, excretion does not match intake, and the person is in either positive (intake > excretion) or negative (intake < excretion) Na+ balance. This phenomenon is illustrated in Figure 6-3. When Na+ balance is altered during these transition periods, the ECF volume changes in parallel. Water excretion, regulated by AVP, also is adjusted to keep plasma osmolality constant, effectively resulting in isosmotic changes in ECF volume. Thus with positive Na+ balance, the ECF volume expands, whereas with negative Na+ balance, the ECF volume contracts (see Figure 6-1). In both cases no change in plasma [Na+] occurs. These changes in ECF volume can be detected by monitoring changes in body weight. Ultimately, renal excretion reaches a new steady state and NaCl excretion once again is matched to intake. The time course for the adjustment of renal NaCl excretion varies (from hours to days) and depends on the magnitude of the change in NaCl intake. Adaptation to large changes in NaCl intake requires a longer time than adaptation to small changes in intake.

The general features of Na+ handling along the nephron must be understood to comprehend how renal Na+ excretion is regulated. (See Chapter 4 for the

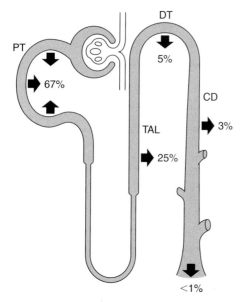

FIGURE 6-4 ■ Segmental Na⁺ reabsorption. The percentage of the filtered amount of Na⁺ reabsorbed by each nephron segment is indicated. *CD,* Collecting duct; *DT,* distal tubule; *PT,* proximal tubule; *TAL,* thick ascending limb.

cellular mechanisms of Na⁺ transport along the nephron.) Most (67%) of the filtered amount of Na⁺ is reabsorbed by the proximal tubule. An additional 25% is reabsorbed by the thick ascending limb of the loop of Henle, and the remainder is largely reabsorbed by the distal tubule and collecting duct (Figure 6-4).

In a normal adult, the filtered amount of Na⁺ is approximately 25,000 mEq/day.

$$\begin{aligned}
\text{Filtered amount of Na}^+ &= (GFR)(\text{plasma }[\text{Na}^+]) \\
&= (180 \text{ L/day})(140 \text{ mEq/L}) \\
&= 25,200 \text{ mEq/day}
\end{aligned} \qquad (6\text{-}1)$$

With a typical diet, less than 1% of this filtered amount is excreted in the urine (approximately 140 mEq/day).* Because of the large amount of filtered Na⁺, small changes in Na⁺ reabsorption by the nephron can profoundly affect Na⁺ balance and thus the volume of the ECF. For example, an increase in Na⁺

---

*The percentage of the filtered amount excreted in the urine is termed fractional excretion (amount excreted/amount filtered). In this example, the fractional excretion of Na⁺ is 140 mEq/day ÷ 25,200 mEq/day = 0.005, or 0.5%.

excretion from 1% to 3% of the filtered amount represents an additional loss of approximately 500 mEq/day of Na⁺. Because the ECF Na⁺ concentration is 140 mEq/L, such an Na⁺ loss would decrease the ECF volume by more than 3 L (i.e., water excretion would parallel the loss of Na⁺ to maintain body fluid osmolality constant: [500 mEq/day]/[140 mEq/L] = 3.6 L/day of fluid loss). Such fluid loss in a person weighing 70 kg would represent a 26% decrease in the ECF volume (see Chapter 1).

In euvolemic subjects, the nephron segments distal to the loop of Henle, namely the distal tubule and collecting duct, are the main nephron segments where Na⁺ reabsorption is adjusted to maintain excretion at a level appropriate for dietary intake. However, this does not mean that the other portions of the nephron are not involved in this process. Because the reabsorptive capacity of the distal tubule and collecting duct is limited, the upstream segments of the nephron (i.e., the proximal tubule and loop of Henle) must reabsorb the bulk of the filtered amount of Na⁺. Thus during euvolemia, Na⁺ handling by the nephron can be explained by two general processes:

1. Na⁺ reabsorption by the proximal tubule and loop of Henle is regulated so that a relatively constant portion of the filtered amount of Na⁺ is delivered to the distal tubule. The combined action of the proximal tubule and loop of Henle reabsorbs approximately 92% of the filtered amount of Na⁺, and thus 8% of the filtered amount is delivered to the distal tubule.
2. Reabsorption of this remaining portion of the filtered amount of Na⁺ by the distal tubule and collecting duct is regulated so that the amount of Na⁺ excreted in the urine closely matches the amount ingested in the diet at steady state. Thus these later nephron segments make final adjustments in Na⁺ excretion to maintain the euvolemic state.

Mechanisms for Maintaining Constant Na⁺ Delivery to the Distal Tubule

A number of mechanisms maintain delivery of a constant fraction of the filtered amount of Na⁺ to the beginning of the distal tubule. These processes are autoregulation of the GFR (a mechanism that keeps the filtered amount of Na^+ constant), glomerulotubular balance, and load dependence of Na^+ reabsorption by the loop of Henle.

Autoregulation of the GFR (see Chapter 3) allows maintenance of a relatively constant filtration rate over a wide range of perfusion pressures. Because the filtration rate is constant, the delivery of filtered Na^+ to the nephrons also is kept constant. Despite the autoregulatory control of the GFR, small variations in GFR occur. If these changes were not compensated for by an appropriate adjustment in Na^+ reabsorption by the nephron, Na^+ excretion would change markedly. Fortunately, Na^+ reabsorption in the euvolemic state, especially by the proximal tubule, changes in parallel with changes in the GFR. This phenomenon is termed **glomerulotubular (G-T) balance** (see Chapter 4). Thus if the GFR increases, the amount of Na^+ reabsorbed by the proximal tubule increases proportionately. The opposite occurs if the GFR decreases.

The final mechanism that helps maintain the constant delivery of Na^+ to the beginning of the collecting duct involves the ability of the loop of Henle to increase its reabsorptive rate in response to increased delivery of Na^+.

Regulation of Distal Tubule and Collecting Duct Na^+ Reabsorption

When delivery of Na^+ is constant, small adjustments in distal tubule and, to a lesser degree, collecting duct Na^+ reabsorption are sufficient to balance excretion with intake. (As already noted, as little as a 2% change in fractional Na^+ excretion produces more than a 3 L change in the volume of the ECF.) Aldosterone is the primary regulator of Na^+ reabsorption by the distal tubule and collecting duct and thus of Na^+ excretion under this condition. When aldosterone levels are elevated, Na^+ reabsorption by these segments is increased (excretion is decreased). When aldosterone levels are decreased, Na^+ reabsorption is decreased (excretion is increased).

In addition to aldosterone, a number of other factors, including natriuretic peptides, prostaglandins, uroguanylin, adrenomedullin, and sympathetic nerves, alter Na^+ reabsorption by the distal tubule

and collecting duct. However, the relative effects of these other factors on the regulation of Na^+ reabsorption by these segments during euvolemia are unclear.

As long as variations in the dietary intake of NaCl are minor, the mechanisms previously described can regulate renal Na^+ excretion appropriately and thereby maintain euvolemia. However, these mechanisms cannot effectively handle significant changes in NaCl intake. When NaCl intake changes significantly, ECF volume expansion or ECF volume contraction occurs. In such cases, additional factors are invoked to act on the kidneys to adjust Na^+ excretion and thereby reestablish the euvolemic state.

The excretion rate of Na^+ by the kidneys can be quantitated in the following way:

$$U_{Na^+} \times \dot{V} = GFR \times P_{Na^+} - R \qquad (6\text{-}2)$$

where $U_{Na^+} \times \dot{V}$ is the excretion rate in mEq/time (U_{Na^+} is the urine $[Na^+]$ and $\dot{V}$ is the urine flow rate), $GFR \times P_{Na^+}$ is the filtered amount of Na^+ (GFR is the glomerular filtration rate and P_{Na^+} is the plasma $[Na^+]$), and R is the amount of Na^+ reabsorbed by the nephron.

CONTROL OF Na^+ EXCRETION WITH VOLUME EXPANSION

During ECF volume expansion, baroreceptors in both the high- and low-pressure vascular circuits send signals to the kidneys. These signals result in increased excretion of NaCl and water. The signals acting on the kidneys include:

1. Decreased activity of the renal sympathetic nerves
2. Increased release of ANP and BNP from the heart and urodilatin by the kidneys
3. Inhibition of AVP secretion from the posterior pituitary and decreased AVP action on the collecting duct
4. Decreased renin secretion and thus decreased production of angiotensin II
5. Decreased aldosterone secretion, which is a consequence of reduced angiotensin II levels, and elevated natriuretic peptide levels

The integrated response of the nephron to these signals is illustrated in Figure 6-5. Three general

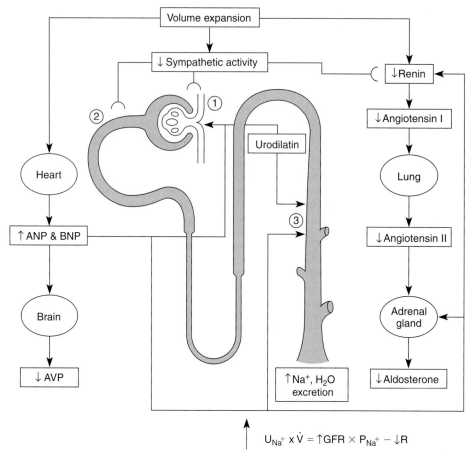

FIGURE 6-5 ▓ Integrated response to extracellular fluid volume expansion. See the text for a detailed description of the numbered response. *ANP,* Atrial natriuretic peptide; *AVP,* arginine vasopressin; *BNP,* brain natriuretic peptide; *GFR,* glomerular filtration rate; P_{Na+}, plasma [Na^+]; *R,* tubular reabsorption of Na^+; $U_{Na+} \times \dot{V}$, Na^+ excretion rate.

responses to ECF volume expansion occur (the numbers correlate with those circled in Figure 6-5):

1. *The GFR increases.* The GFR increases mainly as a result of the decrease in sympathetic nerve activity. Sympathetic fibers innervate the afferent and efferent arterioles of the glomerulus and control their diameter. Decreased sympathetic nerve activity leads to arteriolar dilation. Because afferent arteriolar dilation is greater than efferent dilation, the hydrostatic pressure within the glomerular capillary is increased, thereby increasing the filtration pressure and the GFR. Note that the corresponding filtration fraction decreases

because the renal plasma flow increases to a greater degree than the GFR. Natriuretic peptides, which are increased during ECF volume expansion, also promote an increase in GFR via differential direct effects on the afferent (vasodilation) and efferent (vasoconstriction) arterioles. With the increase in the GFR, the filtered amount of Na^+ increases.

2. *The reabsorption of Na^+ decreases in the proximal tubule and loop of Henle.* Several mechanisms act to reduce Na^+ reabsorption by the proximal tubule, but the precise role of each of these mechanisms remains unresolved. Because activation of the sympathetic nerve fibers that innervate this nephron

segment stimulates Na^+ reabsorption, the decreased sympathetic nerve activity that results from ECF volume expansion decreases Na^+ reabsorption. In addition, angiotensin II directly stimulates Na^+ reabsorption by the proximal tubule. Because angiotensin II levels also are reduced by ECF volume expansion, proximal tubule Na^+ reabsorption decreases accordingly. Increased hydrostatic pressure within the glomerular capillaries also increases the hydrostatic pressure within the peritubular capillaries. In addition, the decrease in filtration fraction reduces the peritubular oncotic pressure. These alterations in the capillary Starling forces reduce the absorption of solute (e.g., NaCl) and water from the lateral intercellular space and thus reduce proximal tubular reabsorption. (See Chapter 4 for a complete description of this mechanism.) Both the increase in the filtered amount of NaCl and the decrease in NaCl reabsorption by the proximal tubule result in the delivery of more NaCl to the loop of Henle. Because activation of the sympathetic nerves and aldosterone stimulate NaCl reabsorption by the loop of Henle, the reduced nerve activity and low aldosterone levels that occur with ECF volume expansion serve to reduce NaCl reabsorption by this nephron segment. Thus the fraction of the filtered amount delivered to the distal tubule is increased.

3. *Na^+ reabsorption decreases in the distal tubule and collecting duct.* As noted, the amount of Na^+ delivered to the distal tubule exceeds that observed in the euvolemic state (the amount of Na^+ delivered to the distal tubule varies in proportion to the degree of ECF volume expansion). This increased amount of delivered Na^+ can overwhelm the reabsorptive capacity of the distal tubule and the collecting duct, an effect heightened by the reduced reabsorptive capacity of these segments associated with increased circulating natriuretic peptides and decreased circulating aldosterone levels.

The final component in the response to ECF volume expansion is the excretion of water. As Na^+ excretion increases, plasma osmolality begins to fall, which decreases the secretion of AVP. AVP secretion also is decreased in response to the elevated levels of natriuretic peptides. In addition, these natriuretic peptides inhibit the action of AVP on the collecting duct. Together, these effects decrease water reabsorption by the collecting duct and thereby increase water excretion by the kidneys. Thus the excretion of Na^+ and water occur in concert; euvolemia is restored, and body fluid osmolality remains constant. The time course of this response (hours to days) depends on the magnitude of the ECF volume expansion. Thus if the degree of ECF volume expansion is small, the mechanisms just described generally restore euvolemia within 24 hours. However, with larger degrees of ECF volume expansion, the response can take several days.

In brief, the renal response to ECF volume expansion involves the integrated action of all parts of the nephron: (1) the filtered amount of Na^+ is increased, (2) the proximal tubule and loop of Henle reabsorption is reduced (the glomerular filtration rate is increased and proximal reabsorption is decreased, and thus G-T balance does not occur under this condition), and (3) the delivery of Na^+ to the distal tubule is increased. This increased delivery, along with the inhibition of distal tubule and collecting duct reabsorption, results in the excretion of a larger fraction of the filtered amount of Na^+ and thus restores euvolemia.

CONTROL OF Na^+ EXCRETION WITH VOLUME CONTRACTION

During ECF volume contraction, volume sensors in both the high- and low-pressure vascular circuits send signals to the kidneys that reduce NaCl and water excretion. The signals that act on the kidneys include:

1. Increased renal sympathetic nerve activity
2. Increased secretion of renin, which results in elevated angiotensin II levels and thus increased secretion of aldosterone by the adrenal cortex
3. Stimulation of AVP secretion by the posterior pituitary

The integrated response of the nephron to these signals is illustrated in Figure 6-6. The general response is as follows (the numbers correlate with those circled in Figure 6-6):

1. *The GFR decreases.* Afferent and efferent arteriolar constriction occurs as a result of increased renal

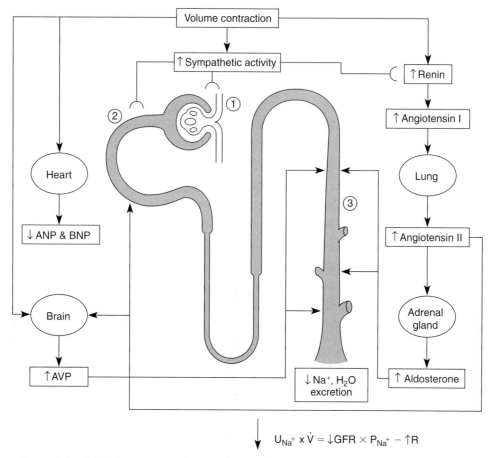

$$U_{Na^+} \times \dot{V} = \downarrow GFR \times P_{Na^+} - \uparrow R$$

FIGURE 6-6 ■ Extracellular fluid volume contraction. See the text for a detailed description of the numbered response. *ANP,* Atrial natriuretic peptide; *AVP,* arginine vasopressin; *BNP,* brain natriuretic peptide; *GFR,* glomerular filtration rate; P_{Na^+}, plasma [Na^+]; *R,* tubular reabsorption of Na^+; $U_{Na^+} \times \dot{V}$, Na^+ excretion rate.

sympathetic nerve activity. The effect is greater on the afferent than on the efferent arteriole. This vasoconstriction causes the hydrostatic pressure in the glomerular capillary to fall and thereby decreases the GFR. The filtration fraction increases because the renal plasma flow decreases more than the GFR, but the absolute decrease in the GFR reduces the filtered load of Na^+.

2. *Na^+ reabsorption by the proximal tubule and loop of Henle is increased.* Several mechanisms augment Na^+ reabsorption in the proximal tubule. For example, increased sympathetic nerve activity and angiotensin II levels directly stimulate Na^+ reabsorption. The decreased hydrostatic

pressure within the glomerular capillaries also leads to a decrease in the hydrostatic pressure within the peritubular capillaries. In addition, the increased filtration fraction results in an increase in the peritubular oncotic pressure. These alterations in the capillary Starling forces facilitate the movement of fluid from the lateral intercellular space into the capillary and thereby stimulate the reabsorption of solute (e.g., NaCl) and water by the proximal tubule. (See Chapter 4 for a complete description of this mechanism). The reduced amount of filtered Na^+ and enhanced proximal tubule reabsorption decrease the delivery of Na^+ to the loop of Henle. Increased sympathetic nerve activity, as well as elevated levels of angiotensin II and aldosterone, stimulate Na$^+$ reabsorption by the thick ascending limb. Because sympathetic nerve activity is increased and angiotensin II and aldosterone levels are elevated during ECF volume contraction, increased Na$^+$ reabsorption by this segment is expected. Thus less Na$^+$ is delivered to the distal tubule.

3. *Na$^+$ reabsorption by the distal tubule and collecting duct is enhanced.* The small amount of Na$^+$ that is delivered to the distal tubule is almost completely reabsorbed because transport in this segment and the collecting duct is enhanced. This stimulation of Na$^+$ reabsorption by the distal tubule and collecting duct is induced by increased angiotensin II and aldosterone levels (increased sympathetic nerve activity also will stimulate Na$^+$ reabsorption).

Finally, water reabsorption by the late portion of the distal tubule and the collecting duct is enhanced by AVP (AVP also stimulates limited Na$^+$ reabsorption in the late distal tubule and collecting duct), the levels of which are elevated through activation of the low- and high-pressure vascular volume sensors and by the elevated levels of angiotensin II. As a result, water excretion is reduced.

Because both water and Na$^+$ are retained by the kidneys in equal proportions, euvolemia is reestablished and body fluid osmolality remains constant. The time course of this expansion of the ECF (hours to days) and the degree to which euvolemia is attained depend on the magnitude of the ECF volume contraction and the dietary intake of Na$^+$. Thus the kidneys reduce Na$^+$ excretion and euvolemia can be restored more quickly if additional NaCl is ingested in the diet.

In brief, the nephron's response to ECF volume contraction involves the integrated action of all its segments: (1) the filtered amount of Na$^+$ is decreased, (2) proximal tubule and loop of Henle reabsorption is enhanced (the GFR is decreased and proximal reabsorption is increased and thus G-T balance does not occur under this condition), and (3) the delivery of Na$^+$ to the distal tubule is reduced. This decreased delivery, together with enhanced Na$^+$ reabsorption by the distal tubule and collecting duct, virtually eliminates Na$^+$ from the urine.

EDEMA

Edema is the accumulation of excess fluid within the interstitial space. As described in Chapter 1, Starling forces across the capillary wall determine the movement of fluid into and out of the vascular compartment in exchange with the extravascular interstitial compartment. Alterations of these forces under pathologic conditions can lead to increased movement of fluid from the vascular space into the interstitium, resulting in edema formation.

The role of the kidneys in the formation of edema can be appreciated by recognizing that the interstitial compartment typically must contain 2 to 3 L of excess fluid before edema is clinically evident (e.g., swelling of the ankles). The source of this fluid is the vascular compartment (i.e., plasma), which has a volume of 3 to 4 L in healthy persons. Alterations in the Starling forces that would accompany a 2 to 3 L fluid shift out of the vascular compartment into the interstitial compartment would be predicted to limit such marked fluid movement and the decline in blood pressure that would attend such a marked fluid shift. However, retention of NaCl and water by the kidneys maintains intravascular compartment volume, thereby maintaining the blood pressure and facilitating interstitial fluid redistribution and edema development.

Alterations in Starling Forces

In Chapter 1, the Starling forces and their effect on fluid movement across the capillary wall were explained. Edema results from changes in the Starling forces that alter these fluid dynamics. Recall that fluid movement across a capillary wall is driven by hydrostatic and oncotic pressure gradients:

$$\text{Filtration rate} = K_f[(P_c - P_i) - \sigma(\pi_c - \pi_i)] \qquad (6\text{-}3)$$

where K_f is the filtration coefficient of the capillary wall (a measure of the intrinsic wall permeability and the surface area available for fluid flow), P_c and P_i are the hydrostatic pressures within the lumen of the capillary and the interstitium, respectively, σ is the reflection coefficient for protein across the capillary wall (approximately 0.9 for skeletal muscle), and π_c and π_i

are the oncotic pressures generated by protein within the capillary lumen and the interstitium, respectively.

Capillary Hydrostatic Pressure (P_c)

Increasing the P_c favors the movement of fluid out of the capillary or retards its movement into the capillary, thereby promoting edema formation. Normally the resistance of the precapillary arteriole is well regulated such that changes in systemic blood pressure do not result in marked alterations in P_c. However, postcapillary resistance is not regulated to the same degree, and thus alterations in the pressure within the venous side of the circulation have significant effects on P_c. Consequently, an increase in the venous pressure elevates P_c, which increases the movement of fluid into the interstitium, resulting in the accumulation of edema fluid. Common causes for increased venous pressure include venous thrombosis and congestive heart failure.

Plasma Oncotic Pressure (π_c)

A decrease in π_c would be expected to favor movement of fluid out of the capillary lumen and inhibit its reabsorption from the interstitium. Because albumin is the most abundant plasma protein, alterations in π_c result primarily from changes in the plasma [albumin]. However, it is important to remember that changes in plasma protein concentration result in parallel changes in the protein concentration of the interstitial fluid. This phenomenon reflects the fact that the reflection coefficient for protein is 0.9 and thus proteins can cross the capillary wall. Because of the parallel changes in capillary and interstitial fluid protein concentration, the oncotic pressure gradient across the capillary wall ($\pi_c - \pi_i$) may not change appreciably.

Lymphatic Obstruction

As noted in Chapter 1, the lymphatic system serves to return interstitial fluid formed by capillary filtration to the vascular system. Obstruction of a lymphatic duct interferes with this process, and as a result interstitial fluid accumulates in the portion of the body drained by the obstructed duct (i.e., edema forms). As this interstitial fluid accumulates, the interstitial hydrostatic pressure increases, and eventually a new steady state is reached where the Starling forces are once again balanced and no additional fluid accumulates. However, unless the obstruction is corrected, the area

IN THE CLINIC

Edema can be classified as localized or generalized. **Localized edema**, as the name denotes, represents the abnormal accumulation of interstitial fluid in a specific area or region of the body. Common causes of localized edema include insect stings and lymphatic obstruction. The venom of many stinging or biting insects contains substances that either directly increase capillary permeability or cause the release of mediators of inflammation that have a similar effect. In addition, the venom or inflammatory mediators may cause vasodilation. Increasing the permeability of the capillary, or in some cases the postcapillary venule, increases the filtration coefficient (K_f) and also can decrease the protein reflection coefficient. Both effects can increase fluid movement out of the capillary, with the latter effect also altering the Starling forces by changing the protein oncotic pressure gradient. Starling forces are further altered in response to the vasodilation (i.e., capillary hydrostatic pressure [P_c] is increased). The net effect of these changes is that more fluid moves out of the capillary into the interstitium and localized swelling occurs. Lymphatic obstruction often accompanies surgical treatment of tumors. For example, in some women with breast cancer, regional lymph nodes that drain the affected breast are surgically removed. When those located in the axilla are removed, the draining of lymph from that arm may be impaired. As a result, edema may develop in the arm.

Generalized edema results when Starling forces across all capillary beds are altered. Edema may be present in the lungs (i.e., **pulmonary edema**) or throughout the systemic circulation (i.e., **peripheral edema**). Peripheral edema is most commonly observed in the feet, ankles, and legs, where the force of gravity magnifies the changes in Starling forces (i.e., further increases P_c) and thereby causes more fluid to leave the capillary and enter the interstitium. One of the most common causes of generalized edema is congestive heart failure. In this condition, blood accumulates in the venous side of the circulation, raising P_c, which in turn causes fluid to move out of the capillary into the interstitium.

Generalized edema is also seen with renal diseases associated with the **nephrotic syndrome**. In the nephrotic syndrome, glomerular capillary permeability is altered, allowing large quantities of albumin to be lost in the urine (**albuminuria**). If the rate of loss exceeds the rate at which albumin is synthesized by the liver, the plasma [albumin] falls. The reduction in plasma protein concentration, and thus π_c, was thought to be the primary cause of edema formation in patients with the nephrotic syndrome. Because the oncotic pressure gradient across the capillary wall may not change appreciably (i.e., interstitial protein oncotic pressure also falls), it is likely that other factors are responsible for, or at least contribute to, the abnormal accumulation of fluid in the interstitial compartment. Supporting this notion is the observation that edema does not spontaneously develop in rats deficient for albumin. It is now known that one of these other factors is primary NaCl retention by the distal tubule and collecting duct. With damage to the glomerular filtration barrier, the serum protein plasminogen enters the renal tubules where it is cleaved to form plasmin by the serine protease urokinase (produced by proximal tubule cells). Plasmin, also a serine protease, then cleaves the γ-subunit of the epithelial Na^+ channels present in the apical membrane of cells in the late distal tubule and collecting duct, thereby increasing the open time of these channels. This phenomenon results in increased Na^+ (and Cl^-) reabsorption. The ensuing retention of NaCl (along with water) increases vascular volume and thereby leads to an increase in P_c, increased movement of fluid into the interstitial compartment, and thus edema formation.

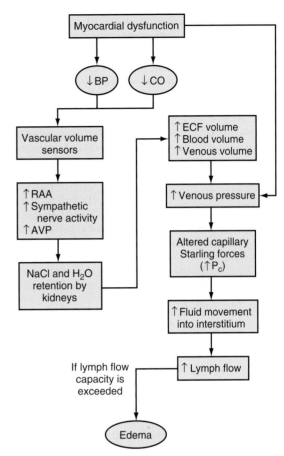

FIGURE 6-7 ■ Mechanisms involved in the formation of generalized edema in a person with congestive heart failure. As indicated, edema forms when the capacity of the lymphatic system to return interstitial fluid to the systemic circulation is exceeded. *AVP,* Arginine vasopressin; *BP,* blood pressure; *CO,* cardiac output; *ECF,* extracellular fluid; *NaCl,* sodium chloride; P_c, capillary hydrostatic pressure; *RAA,* renin-angiotensin-aldosterone.

drained by the obstructed lymphatic duct remains edematous even in this new steady state.

Capillary Permeability

An increase in capillary permeability favors increased movement of fluid across the capillary wall and thus accumulation of excess fluid in the interstitial compartment. The increased permeability also can alter the capillary reflection coefficient for protein(s), allowing more protein across the capillary and thus altering the protein oncotic pressure gradient $(\pi_c - \pi_i)$.

Role of the Kidneys

The role of the kidneys in edema-forming states is best illustrated by considering the situation that exists with heart failure (Figure 6-7). Because of decreased cardiac performance, venous pressure is elevated and

perfusion of the kidneys impaired. The increase in venous pressure alters the Starling forces (i.e., increased P_c) and causes fluid to accumulate in the interstitium. At the same time, decreased cardiac performance (decreased cardiac output and blood pressure) reduces the ECV, which is misinterpreted by the body's vascular volume sensors as a decrease in ECF volume. The fall in ECF volume activates the renal sympathetic nerves and the renin-angiotensin-aldosterone system and causes AVP secretion. In response to these signals, the kidneys retain NaCl and water, as already described. This retention of isotonic fluid expands the ECF volume and thus blood volume, thereby helping perpetuate a vicious cycle of fluid accumulation that can further exacerbate congestive heart failure. Intravascular volume expansion also contributes to the increased P_c, increased interstitial fluid accumulation, and edema formation.

As fluid begins to accumulate in the interstitium, it is taken up by the lymphatics and returned to the systemic circulation. As noted in Chapter 1, thoracic duct and right lymphatic duct flow is approximately 1 to 4 L/day. The lymphatic system can increase this flow up to 20 L/day. Because a significant amount of lymph returns to the circulation at the level of regional lymph nodes, the actual amount of interstitial fluid returned

to the systemic circulation by the lymphatic system can exceed 20 L/day. Nevertheless, the capacity of the lymphatic system has a limit. When this limit is reached, edema fluid begins to accumulate.

The importance of NaCl retention by the kidneys in edema formation provides two approaches for treatment. The first involves dietary manipulation. The ultimate source of NaCl is the diet. Thus if dietary intake of NaCl is restricted, the amount that can be retained by the kidneys is reduced and edema formation is limited. The second approach is to inhibit the kidneys' ability to retain NaCl. This inhibition is accomplished clinically by the use of diuretics, which, as described in Chapter 10, inhibit Na^+ transport mechanisms in the nephron. Thus NaCl excretion is increased and NaCl retention is blunted.

SUMMARY

1. The volume of the ECF is determined by Na^+ balance. When Na^+ intake exceeds excretion, the ECF volume increases (positive Na^+ balance). Conversely, when Na^+ excretion exceeds intake, the ECF volume decreases (negative Na^+ balance). The kidneys are the primary route for Na^+ excretion.

2. The kidneys adjust NaCl excretion in response to changes in ECV. The ECV reflects adequate tissue perfusion and is dependent on the ECF volume, the intravascular volume, arterial blood pressure, and cardiac output. ECF is sensed primarily by the vascular volume sensors. In the absence of disease, ECV, ECF volume, vascular volume, arterial blood pressure, and cardiac output change in parallel (i.e., they increase with positive Na^+ balance and decrease with negative Na^+ balance). In some pathologic conditions (e.g., congestive heart failure), changes in ECV, ECF volume, vascular volume, arterial blood pressure, and cardiac output are uncoupled and do not occur in parallel. The kidneys always adjust Na^+ excretion to changes in the ECV (decreased Na^+ excretion with decreased ECV and increased Na^+ excretion with increased ECV) as detected by the vascular volume sensors.

3. The coordination of Na^+ intake and excretion and thus the maintenance of a normal ECF volume involves neural (renal sympathetic nerves) and

hormonal (renin-angiotensin-aldosterone, uroguanylin, natriuretic peptides, and AVP) regulatory factors and effector mechanisms.

4. Under normal conditions (euvolemia), Na^+ excretion by the kidneys is matched to the amount of Na^+ ingested in the diet. The kidneys accomplish this feat by reabsorbing virtually all of the filtered amount of Na^+ (typically less than 1% of the filtered load is excreted). During euvolemia, the distal tubule and collecting duct are responsible for making small adjustments in urinary Na^+ excretion to maintain Na^+ balance. The major factor regulating distal tubule and collecting duct Na^+ reabsorption is aldosterone, which acts to stimulate Na^+ reabsorption.

5. With ECF volume expansion, volume sensors in both the low- and high-pressure vascular circuits initiate responses that contribute to increased excretion of Na^+ by the kidneys and a return to the euvolemic state. The components of this response include a decrease in sympathetic outflow to the kidney, a suppression of the renin-angiotensin-aldosterone system, and release of natriuretic peptides from the heart (ANP and BNP) and kidneys (urodilatin). The combined actions of these effectors serve to enhance the GFR, increase the filtered amount of Na^+, and reduce Na^+ reabsorption by

the nephron. Together, these changes in renal Na⁺ handling enhance net NaCl excretion.

6. With ECF volume contraction, the aforementioned sequence of events is reversed (increased sympathetic outflow to the kidney, activation of the renin-angiotensin-aldosterone system, and suppression of natriuretic peptide secretion). This reversal decreases the GFR, enhances reabsorption of Na⁺ by the nephron, and thus reduces NaCl excretion.

7. The development of generalized edema requires alterations in the Starling forces across capillary walls favoring the accumulation of fluid in the interstitium and retention of NaCl and water by the kidneys.

KEY WORDS AND CONCEPTS

- Extracellular fluid (ECF)
- Effective circulating volume (ECV)
- Natriuresis
- Fractional Na⁺ excretion
- Positive Na⁺ balance
- Negative Na⁺ balance
- Congestive heart failure
- Euvolemia
- ECF volume expansion
- ECF volume contraction
- Atrial natriuretic peptide (ANP)
- Brain natriuretic peptide (BNP)
- Urodilatin
- Uroguanylin
- Adrenomedullin
- Renalase
- Juxtaglomerular apparatus
- Sympathetic nerve fibers
- Renin-angiotensin-aldosterone system
- Angiotensinogen
- Angiotensin-converting enzyme (ACE)
- Aldosterone
- Hypoaldosteronism
- Hyperaldosteronism
- Pulmonary edema
- Generalized edema
- Localized edema
- Nephrotic syndrome

SELF-STUDY PROBLEMS

1. A person experiences an acute episode of vomiting and diarrhea and loses 3 kg in body weight over a 24-hour period. A blood sample shows that the plasma [Na⁺] is normal at 142 mEq/L. Indicate whether the following parameters would be increased, decreased, or unchanged (i.e., normal values) from what they were before this illness.

   Plasma osmolality   _____
   ECF volume   _____
   ECV   _____
   Plasma AVP levels   _____
   Urine osmolality   _____
   Sensation of thirst   _____

2. A person is euvolemic and ingests a diet containing 100 mEq/day of Na⁺ on average. What would be the estimated Na⁺ excretion rate for this person over a 24-hour period in the steady state?

3. Indicate whether the regulatory signals listed are increased or decreased in response to changes in ECF volume.

	Volume Expansion	Volume Contraction
Renal sympathetic nerve activity	_____	_____
ANP and BNP levels	_____	_____
Angiotensin II levels	_____	_____
Aldosterone levels	_____	_____
AVP levels	_____	_____

4. Pulmonary and peripheral edema have developed in a 65-year-old man with congestive heart failure. During the past 2 weeks, his weight has increased by 4 kg and his plasma [Na⁺] has remained unchanged at 145 mEq/L. Assuming that the entire weight gain is the result of accumulation of edema fluid, calculate the following:

   Volume of accumulated edema fluid   _____ L
   Amount of Na⁺ retained by the kidneys   _____ mEq

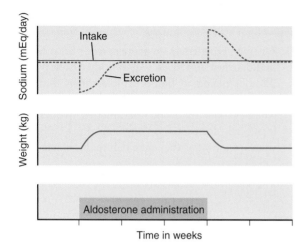

increases (i.e., negative Na⁺ balance) but returns to its initial level over several days. Delineate the mechanisms involved in these transient changes in Na⁺ excretion.

6. A 55-year-old woman has congestive heart failure. On physical examination, she is found to have peripheral and pulmonary edema. Her plasma $[Na^+]$ is normal at 142 mEq/L. For each of the following elements, predict whether the values would be increased, decreased, or unchanged from what would be predicted for a healthy person.

ECF volume   _____
ECV   _____
Plasma osmolality   _____
Fractional Na⁺ excretion _____
Renal sympathetic nerve activity _____
ANP and BNP levels   _____
Angiotensin II levels   _____
Aldosterone levels   _____
AVP levels   _____

5. As shown in the illustration above, administration of high dosages of aldosterone to a healthy person leads to a transient retention of Na⁺ by the kidneys (i.e., positive Na⁺ balance). However, after several days, Na⁺ excretion increases to the level before hormone administration. When the hormone is stopped, Na⁺ excretion transiently

7

REGULATION OF POTASSIUM BALANCE

OBJECTIVES

Upon completion of this chapter, the student should be able to answer the following questions:

1. How does the body maintain K⁺ homeostasis?

2. What is the distribution of K⁺ within the body compartments? Why is this distribution important?

3. What are the hormones and factors that regulate plasma K⁺ levels? Why is this regulation important?

4. How do the various segments of the nephron transport K⁺, and how does the mechanism of K⁺ transport by these segments determine how much K⁺ is excreted in the urine?

5. Why are the distal tubule and collecting duct so important in regulating K⁺ excretion?

6. How do plasma K⁺ levels, aldosterone, vasopressin, tubular fluid flow rate, and acid-base balance influence K⁺ excretion?

Potassium, which is one of the most abundant cations in the body, is critical for many cell functions, including cell volume regulation, intracellular pH regulation, DNA and protein synthesis, growth, enzyme function, resting membrane potential, and cardiac and neuromuscular activity. Despite wide fluctuations in dietary K⁺ intake, [K⁺] in cells and extracellular fluid (ECF) remains remarkably constant. Two sets of regulatory mechanisms safeguard K⁺ homeostasis. First, several mechanisms regulate the [K⁺] in the ECF. Second, other mechanisms maintain the amount of K⁺ in the body constant by adjusting renal K⁺ excretion to match dietary K⁺ intake. The kidneys regulate K⁺ excretion.

OVERVIEW OF K⁺ HOMEOSTASIS

Total body K⁺ is 50 mEq/kg of body weight, or 3500 mEq for a person weighing 70 kg. A total of 98% of the K⁺ in the body is located within cells, where its average [K⁺] is 150 mEq/L. A high intracellular [K⁺] is required for many cell functions, including cell growth and division and volume regulation. Only 2% of total body K⁺ is located in the ECF, where its normal concentration is approximately 4 mEq/L. [K⁺] in the ECF that exceeds 5.0 mEq/L constitutes **hyperkalemia**. Conversely, [K⁺] in the ECF of less than 3.5 mEq/L constitutes **hypokalemia**.

Hypokalemia is one of the most common electrolyte disorders in clinical practice and can be observed in as

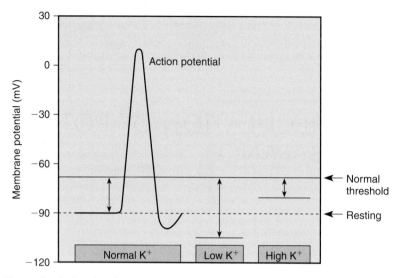

FIGURE 7-1 ■ The effects of variations in plasma K^+ concentration on the resting membrane potential of skeletal muscle. Hyperkalemia causes the membrane potential to become less negative and decreases the excitability by inactivating fast Na^+ channels, which are responsible for the depolarizing phase of the action potential. Hypokalemia hyperpolarizes the membrane potential and thereby reduces excitability because a larger stimulus is required to depolarize the membrane potential to the threshold potential. Resting indicates the "normal" resting membrane potential. Normal threshold indicates the membrane threshold potential.

many as 20% of hospitalized patients. The most common causes of hypokalemia include administration of diuretic drugs (see Chapter 10), surreptitious vomiting (i.e., bulimia), and severe diarrhea. Gitelman syndrome (a genetic defect in the Na^+-Cl^- symporter in the apical membrane of distal tubule cells) also causes hypokalemia (see Chapter 4, Table 4-3). Hyperkalemia also is a common electrolyte disorder and is seen in 1% to 10% of hospitalized patients. Hyperkalemia often is seen in patients with renal failure, in persons taking drugs such as angiotensin-converting enzyme inhibitors and K^+-sparing diuretics (see Chapter 10), in persons with hyperglycemia (i.e., high blood sugar), and in the elderly. **Pseudohyperkalemia**, a falsely high plasma $[K^+]$, is caused by traumatic lysis of red blood cells while blood is being drawn. Red blood cells, like all cells, contain K^+, and lysis of red blood cells releases K^+ into the plasma, artificially elevating the plasma $[K^+]$.

The large concentration difference of K^+ across cell membranes (approximately 146 mEq/L) is maintained by the operation of sodium–potassium–adenosine triphosphatase (Na^+-K^+-ATPase). This K^+ gradient is important in maintaining the potential difference across cell membranes. Thus K^+ is critical for the excitability of nerve and muscle cells and for the contractility of cardiac, skeletal, and smooth muscle cells (Figure 7-1).

IN THE CLINIC

Cardiac arrhythmias are produced by both hypokalemia and hyperkalemia. The electrocardiogram (ECG; Figure 7-2) monitors the electrical activity of the heart and is a quick and easy way to determine whether changes in plasma $[K^+]$ influence the heart and other excitable cells. In contrast, measurements of the plasma $[K^+]$ by the clinical laboratory require a blood sample, and values often are not immediately available. The first sign of hyperkalemia is the appearance of tall, thin T waves on the ECG. Further increases in the plasma $[K^+]$ prolong the PR interval, depress the ST segment, and lengthen the QRS interval on the ECG. Finally, as the plasma $[K^+]$ approaches 10 mEq/L, the P wave disappears, the QRS interval broadens, the ECG appears as a sine wave, and the ventricles fibrillate (i.e., manifest rapid, uncoordinated contractions of muscle fibers). Hypokalemia prolongs the QT interval, inverts the T wave, and lowers the ST segment on the ECG.

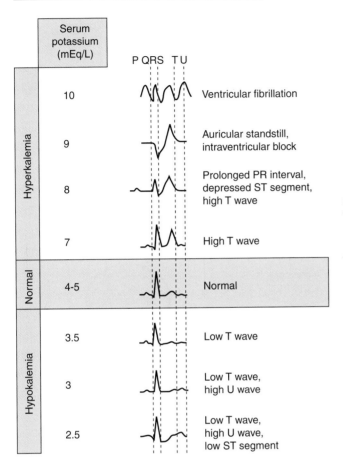

FIGURE 7-2 ■ Electrocardiograms from persons with varying plasma K⁺ concentrations. Hyperkalemia increases the height of the T wave, and hypokalemia inverts the T wave. *(Modified from Barker L, Burton J, Zieve P: Principles of ambulatory medicine, ed 5, Baltimore, 1999, Williams & Wilkins.)*

After a meal, the K^+ absorbed by the gastrointestinal tract enters the ECF within minutes (Figure 7-3). If the K^+ ingested during a normal meal ($\approx$33 mEq) were to remain in the ECF compartment (14 L), the plasma $[K^+]$ would increase by a potentially lethal 2.4 mEq/L (33 mEq added to 14 L of ECF):

$$33 \text{ mEq}/14 \text{ L} = 2.4 \text{ mEq/L} \qquad (7\text{-}1)$$

This rise in the plasma $[K^+]$ is prevented by the rapid uptake (within minutes) of K^+ into cells. Because the excretion of K^+ by the kidneys after a meal is relatively slow (within hours), the uptake of K^+ by cells is essential to prevent life-threatening hyperkalemia. Maintaining total body K^+ constant requires all the K^+ absorbed by the gastrointestinal tract to eventually be excreted by the kidneys. This process requires about 6 hours.

REGULATION OF PLASMA [K⁺]

As illustrated in Figure 7-3 and Box 7-1, several hormones, including epinephrine, insulin, and aldosterone, increase K^+ uptake into skeletal muscle, liver, bone, and red blood cells by stimulating Na^+-K^+-ATPase, the Na^+-K^+-$2Cl^-$ symporter, and the Na^+-Cl^- symporter in these cells. Acute stimulation of K^+ uptake (i.e., within minutes) is mediated by an increased turnover rate of existing Na^+-K^+-ATPase, Na^+-K^+-$2Cl^-$, and Na^+-Cl^- transporters, whereas the chronic increase in K^+ uptake (i.e., within hours to days) is mediated by an increase in the quantity of Na^+-K^+-ATPase. A rise in the plasma $[K^+]$ that follows K^+ absorption by the gastrointestinal tract stimulates insulin secretion from the pancreas, aldosterone release from the adrenal cortex, and epinephrine secretion from the adrenal medulla. In

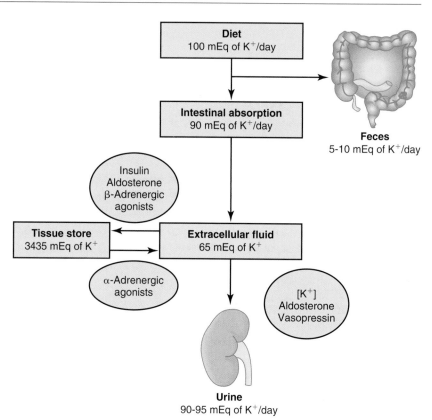

FIGURE 7-3 ■ Overview of potassium homeostasis. An increase in plasma insulin, β-adrenergic agonists, or aldosterone stimulates K$^+$ movement into cells and decreases plasma K$^+$ concentration ([K$^+$]), whereas a decrease in the plasma concentration of these hormones moves K$^+$ into cells and increases plasma [K$^+$]. α-Adrenergic agonists have the opposite effect. The amount of K$^+$ in the body is determined by the kidneys. A person is in K$^+$ balance when dietary intake and urinary output (plus output by the gastrointestinal tract) are equal. The excretion of K$^+$ by the kidneys is regulated by plasma [K$^+$], aldosterone, and arginine vasopressin.

contrast, a decrease in the plasma [K$^+$] inhibits the release of these hormones. Whereas insulin and epinephrine act within a few minutes, aldosterone requires about 1 hour to stimulate K$^+$ uptake into cells.

Epinephrine

Catecholamines affect the distribution of K$^+$ across cell membranes by activating α- and β$_2$-adrenergic receptors. The stimulation of α-adrenoceptors releases K$^+$ from cells, especially in the liver, whereas the stimulation of β$_2$-adrenceptors promotes K$^+$ uptake by cells. For example, the activation of β$_2$-adrenoceptors after exercise is important in preventing hyperkalemia. The rise in plasma [K$^+$] after a K$^+$-rich meal is greater if the patient has been pretreated with propranolol, a β$_2$-adrenoceptor antagonist. Furthermore, the release of epinephrine during stress (e.g., myocardial ischemia) can lower the plasma [K$^+$] rapidly.

Insulin

Insulin also stimulates K$^+$ uptake into cells. The importance of insulin is illustrated by two observations. First, the rise in plasma [K$^+$] after a K$^+$-rich meal is greater in patients with diabetes mellitus (i.e., insulin deficiency) than in healthy people. Second, insulin (and glucose to prevent insulin-induced hypoglycemia) can be infused to correct hyperkalemia. Insulin is the most important hormone that shifts K$^+$ into cells after the ingestion of K$^+$ in a meal.

Aldosterone

Aldosterone, like catecholamines and insulin, also promotes K$^+$ uptake into cells. A rise in aldosterone levels (e.g., primary aldosteronism) causes hypokalemia, whereas a fall in aldosterone levels (e.g., in persons with Addison disease) causes hyperkalemia. As discussed later, aldosterone also stimulates urinary K$^+$ excretion. Thus aldosterone alters the plasma [K$^+$] by

■ ■ ■ ■ ■ ■ ■ ■ ■ ■ ■ ■

BOX 7-1
MAJOR FACTORS, HORMONES, AND DRUGS INFLUENCING THE DISTRIBUTION OF K+ BETWEEN THE INTRACELLULAR AND EXTRACELLULAR FLUID COMPARTMENTS

PHYSIOLOGIC: KEEP PLASMA [K+] CONSTANT
Adrenergic receptor agonists
Insulin
Aldosterone

PATHOPHYSIOLOGIC: DISPLACE PLASMA [K+] FROM NORMAL
Acid-base disorders
Plasma osmolality
Cell lysis
Vigorous exercise

DRUGS THAT INDUCE HYPERKALEMIA
Dietary potassium supplements
Angiotensin-converting enzyme inhibitors
K+-sparing diuretics (see Chapter 10)
Heparin

acting on K+ uptake into cells and by altering urinary K+ excretion.

ALTERATIONS OF PLASMA [K+]

Several factors can alter the plasma [K+] (see Box 7-1). These factors are not involved in the regulation of the plasma [K+] but rather alter the movement of K+ between the intracellular fluid and ECF and thus cause the development of hypokalemia or hyperkalemia.

Acid-Base Balance

Metabolic acidosis increases the plasma [K+], whereas metabolic alkalosis decreases it. Respiratory alkalosis causes hypokalemia. Metabolic acidosis produced by the addition of inorganic acids (e.g., HCl and sulfuric acid) increases the plasma [K+] much more than an equivalent acidosis produced by the accumulation of organic acids (e.g., lactic acid, acetic acid, and keto acids). The reduced pH—that is, increased [H+]—promotes the movement of H+ into

cells and the reciprocal movement of K+ out of cells to maintain electroneutrality. This effect of acidosis occurs in part because acidosis inhibits the transporters that accumulate K+ inside cells, including the Na^+-K^+-ATPase and the Na^+-K^+-$2Cl^-$ symporter. In addition, the movement of H+ into cells occurs as the cells buffer changes in the [H+] of the ECF (see Chapter 8). As H+ moves across the cell membranes, K+ moves in the opposite direction; thus cations are neither gained nor lost across cell membranes. Metabolic alkalosis has the opposite effect; the plasma [K+] decreases as K+ moves into cells and H+ exits.

Although organic acids produce a metabolic acidosis, they do not cause significant hyperkalemia. Two explanations have been suggested for the reduced ability of organic acids to cause hyperkalemia. First, the organic anion may enter the cell with H+ and thereby eliminate the need for K+/H+ exchange across the membrane. Second, organic anions may stimulate insulin secretion, which moves K+ into cells. This movement may counteract the direct effect of the acidosis, which moves K+ out of cells.

Plasma Osmolality

The osmolality of the plasma also influences the distribution of K+ across cell membranes. An increase in the osmolality of the ECF enhances K+ release by cells and thus increases extracellular [K+]. The plasma [K+] may increase by 0.4 to 0.8 mEq/L for an elevation of 10 mOsm/kg H_2O in plasma osmolality. In patients with diabetes mellitus who do not take insulin, plasma K+ often is elevated in part because of the lack of insulin and in part because of the increase in the concentration of glucose in plasma (i.e., from a normal value of ~100 mg/dL to as high as ~1200 mg/dL), which increases plasma osmolality. Hypoosmolality has the opposite action. The alterations in plasma [K+] associated with changes in osmolality are related to changes in cell volume. For example, as plasma osmolality increases, water leaves cells because of the osmotic gradient across the plasma membrane (see Chapter 1). Water leaves cells until the intracellular osmolality equals that of the ECF. This loss of water shrinks cells and causes the cell [K+] to rise. The rise in intracellular [K+] provides a driving force for the exit of K+ from cells. This sequence increases plasma

[K+]. A fall in plasma osmolality has the opposite effect.

Cell Lysis

Cell lysis causes hyperkalemia, which results from the addition of intracellular K+ to the ECF. Severe trauma (e.g., burns) and some conditions such as **tumor lysis syndrome** (i.e., chemotherapy-induced destruction of tumor cells) and **rhabdomyolysis** (i.e., destruction of skeletal muscle) destroy cells and release K+ and other cell solutes into the ECF. In addition, gastric ulcers may cause the seepage of red blood cells into the gastrointestinal tract. The blood cells are digested, and the K+ released from the cells is absorbed and can cause hyperkalemia.

Exercise

During exercise, more K+ is released from skeletal muscle cells than during rest. The ensuing hyperkalemia depends on the degree of exercise. In people walking slowly, the plasma [K+] increases by 0.3 mEq/L. The plasma [K+] may increase by 2.0 mEq/L with vigorous exercise.

IN THE CLINIC

Exercise-induced changes in the plasma [K+] usually do not produce symptoms and are reversed after several minutes of rest. However, vigorous exercise can lead to life-threatening hyperkalemia in persons (1) who have endocrine disorders that affect the release of insulin, epinephrine (a β-adrenergic agonist), or aldosterone; (2) whose ability to excrete K+ is impaired (e.g., because of renal failure); or (3) who take certain medications, such as β₂-adrenergic blockers. For example, during vigorous exercise, the plasma [K+] may increase by at least 2 to 4 mEq/L in persons who take β₂-adrenergic receptor antagonists for hypertension.

Because acid-base balance, plasma osmolality, cell lysis, and exercise do not maintain the plasma [K+] at a normal value, they do not contribute to K+ homeostasis (see Box 7-1). The extent to which these pathophysiologic states alter the plasma [K+] depends on the integrity of the homeostatic mechanisms that regulate plasma [K+] (e.g., the secretion of epinephrine, insulin, and aldosterone).

K+ EXCRETION BY THE KIDNEYS

The kidneys play a major role in maintaining K+ balance. As illustrated in Figure 7-3, the kidneys excrete 90% to 95% of the K+ ingested in the diet. Excretion equals intake even when intake increases by as much as 10-fold. This balance of urinary excretion and dietary intake underscores the importance of the kidneys in maintaining K+ homeostasis. Although small amounts of K+ are lost each day in feces and sweat (approximately 5% to 10% of the K+ ingested in the diet), this amount is essentially constant (except during severe diarrhea), is not regulated, and therefore is relatively less important than the K+ excreted by the kidneys. K+ secretion from the blood into the tubular fluid by the cells of the distal tubule and collecting duct system is the key factor in determining urinary K+ excretion (Figure 7-4).

Because K+ is not bound to plasma proteins, it is freely filtered by the glomerulus. When individuals ingest 100 mEq of K+ per day, urinary K+ excretion is about 15% of the amount filtered. Accordingly, K+ must be reabsorbed along the nephron. When dietary K+ intake increases, however, K+ excretion can, in extreme circumstances, exceed the amount filtered. Thus K+ also can be secreted.

The proximal tubule reabsorbs about 67% of the filtered K+ under most conditions. Approximately 20% of the filtered K+ is reabsorbed by the loop of Henle, and, as with the proximal tubule, the amount reabsorbed is a constant fraction of the amount filtered. In contrast to these nephron segments, which can only reabsorb K+, the distal tubule and collecting duct are able to reabsorb or secrete K+. The rate of K+ reabsorption or secretion by the distal tubule and collecting duct depends on a variety of hormones and factors. When ingesting 100 mEq/day of K+, K+ is secreted by these nephron segments. A rise in dietary K+ intake increases K+ secretion. K+ secretion can increase the amount of K+ that appears in the urine so that it approaches 80% of the amount filtered (see Figure 7-4). In contrast, a low-K+ diet activates K+ reabsorption along the distal tubule and collecting duct so that urinary excretion falls to about 1% of the K+ filtered by the glomerulus (see Figure 7-4). Because the kidneys cannot reduce K+ excretion to the same low levels as they can for Na+ (i.e., 0.2%), hypokalemia can develop

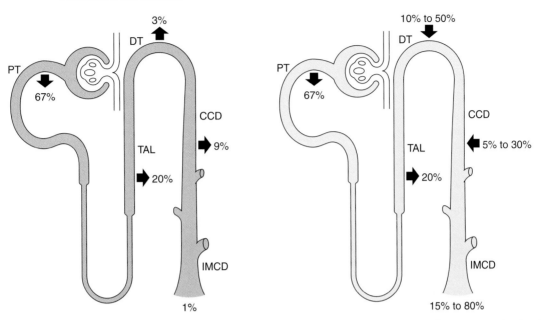

POTASSIUM DEPLETION

NORMAL AND INCREASED POTASSIUM INTAKE

FIGURE 7-4 ■ K$^+$ transport along the nephron. K$^+$ excretion depends on the rate and direction of K$^+$ transport by the distal tubule and collecting duct. Percentages refer to the amount of filtered K$^+$ reabsorbed or secreted by each nephron segment. *Left,* Dietary K$^+$ depletion. An amount of K$^+$ equal to 1% of the filtered load of K$^+$ is excreted. *Right,* Normal and increased dietary K$^+$ intake. An amount of K$^+$ equal to 15% to 80% of the filtered load is excreted. *CCD,* Cortical collecting duct; *DT,* distal tubule; *IMCD,* inner medullary collecting duct; *PT,* proximal tubule; *TAL,* thick ascending limb.

in persons who have a K$^+$-deficient diet. Because the magnitude and direction of K$^+$ transport by the distal tubule and collecting duct are variable, the overall rate of urinary K$^+$ excretion is determined by these tubular segments.

IN THE CLINIC

In persons with advanced **renal disease**, the kidneys are unable to eliminate K$^+$ from the body, and thus the plasma [K$^+$] rises. The resulting hyperkalemia reduces the resting membrane potential (i.e., the voltage becomes less negative), which decreases the excitability of neurons, cardiac cells, and muscle cells by inactivating fast Na$^+$ channels, which are critical for the depolarization phase of the action potential (see Figure 7-1). Severe, rapid increases in the plasma [K$^+$] can lead to cardiac arrest and death. In contrast, in patients taking diuretic drugs for hypertension, urinary K$^+$ excretion often exceeds dietary K$^+$ intake. Accordingly, the K$^+$ balance is negative, and hypokalemia develops. This decline in the extracellular [K$^+$] hyperpolarizes the resting cell membrane (i.e., the voltage becomes more negative) and reduces the excitability of neurons, cardiac cells, and muscle cells.

Severe hypokalemia can lead to paralysis, cardiac arrhythmias, and death. Hypokalemia also can impair the ability of the kidneys to concentrate the urine and can stimulate the renal production of ammonium, which affects acid-base balance (see Chapter 8). Therefore the maintenance of a high intracellular [K$^+$], a low extracellular [K$^+$], and a high K$^+$ concentration gradient across cell membranes is essential for a number of cellular functions.

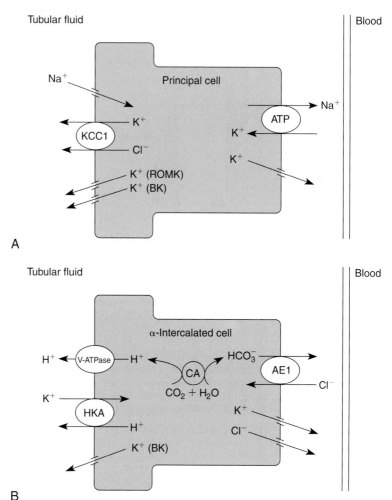

FIGURE 7-5 ■ Cellular mechanism of K⁺ secretion by principal cells (**A**) and α-intercalated cells (**B**) in the distal tubule and collecting duct. α-Intercalated cells contain very low levels of sodium-potassium adenosine triphosphatase in the basolateral membrane (not shown). K⁺ depletion increases K⁺ reabsorption by α-intercalated cells by stimulating H⁺-K⁺-adenosine triphosphatase (*HKA*). *AE1,* anion exchanger 1; *ATP,* adenosine triphosphate; *BK,* Ca⁺⁺-activated K⁺; *CA,* carbonic anhydrase; *HCO₃⁻,* bicarbonate; *KCC1,* K⁺-Cl⁻ symporter 1; *ROMK,* renal outer medullary K⁺; *V-ATPase,* vacuolar adenosine triphosphatase.

CELLULAR MECHANISMS OF K⁺ TRANSPORT BY PRINCIPAL CELLS AND INTERCALATED CELLS IN THE DISTAL TUBULE AND COLLECTING DUCT

Figure 7-5, *A*, illustrates the cellular mechanism of K⁺ secretion by principal cells in the distal tubule and collecting duct. Secretion from the blood into the tubule lumen is a two-step process: (1) K⁺ uptake from the blood across the basolateral membrane by Na⁺-K⁺-ATPase and (2) diffusion of K⁺ from the cell into the tubular fluid through K⁺ channels (the renal outer medullary K⁺ channel and the Ca⁺⁺-activated K⁺ [BK] channel). A K⁺-Cl⁻ symporter in the apical plasma membrane also secretes K⁺. Na⁺-K⁺-ATPase creates a high intracellular [K⁺], which provides the chemical driving force for K⁺ exit across the apical membrane through K⁺ channels. Although K⁺ channels also are present in the basolateral membrane, K⁺ preferentially leaves the cell across the apical membrane and enters the tubular fluid. K⁺ transport follows this route for two reasons. First, the electrochemical gradient of K⁺ across the apical membrane favors its downhill movement into the tubular fluid. Second, the permeability of the apical membrane to K⁺ is greater than that of the basolateral membrane. Therefore K⁺ preferentially diffuses across the apical membrane into the tubular fluid. K^+ secretion across the apical membrane via the K^+-Cl^- symporter is driven by the favorable concentration gradient of K^+ between the cell and tubular fluid. The three major factors that control the rate of K^+ secretion by the distal tubule and the collecting duct are:

1. The activity of Na^+-K^+-ATPase
2. The driving force (electrochemical gradient for K^+ channel and the chemical concentration gradient for the K^+-Cl^- symporter) for K^+ movement across the apical membrane
3. The permeability of the apical membrane to K^+

Every change in K^+ secretion by principal cells results from an alteration in one or more of these factors.

α-Intercalated cells reabsorb K^+ by an H^+-K^+-ATPase transport mechanism located in the apical membrane (see Figure 7-5, *B,* and Chapter 4). This transporter mediates K^+ uptake across the apical plasma membrane in exchange for H^+. K^+ exit from intercalated cells into the blood is mediated by a K^+ channel. The reabsorption of K^+ is activated by a low-K^+ diet. Intercalated cells also express the Ca^{++}-activated, BK channels in the apical plasma membrane. K^+ secretion by BK channels in intercalated cells (most likely α-intercalated cells) is activated by increased tubule flow rate, which enhances Ca^{++} uptake across the apical plasma membrane by activating a transient receptor potential channel also located in the apical plasma membrane (not shown in Figure 7-5, *B*). Increased intracellular Ca^{++} stimulates protein kinase C, which actives BK channels.

REGULATION OF K^+ SECRETION BY THE DISTAL TUBULE AND COLLECTING DUCT

The regulation of K^+ excretion is achieved mainly by alterations in K^+ secretion by principal cells of the distal tubule and collecting duct. Plasma $[K^+]$ and aldosterone are the major physiologic regulators of K^+ secretion. Ingestion of a K^+-rich meal also activates renal K^+ excretion by a mechanism involving an unknown gut-dependent mechanism. Arginine vasopressin (AVP) also stimulates K^+ secretion; however, it is less important than the plasma $[K^+]$ and aldosterone.

> **BOX 7-2**
> ### MAJOR FACTORS AND HORMONES INFLUENCING K^+ EXCRETION
>
> **PHYSIOLOGIC: KEEP K^+ BALANCE CONSTANT**
> Plasma $[K^+]$
> Aldosterone
> Arginine vasopressin
>
> **PATHOPHYSIOLOGIC: DISPLACE K^+ BALANCE**
> Flow rate of tubule fluid
> Acid-base disorders
> Glucocorticoids

Other factors, including the flow rate of tubular fluid and acid-base balance, influence K^+ secretion by the distal tubule and collecting duct. However, they are not homeostatic mechanisms because they disturb K^+ balance (Box 7-2).

Plasma $[K^+]$

Plasma $[K^+]$ is an important determinant of K^+ secretion by the distal tubule and collecting duct (Figure 7-6). Hyperkalemia (e.g., resulting from a high-K^+ diet or from rhabdomyolysis) stimulates K^+ secretion within minutes. Several mechanisms are involved. First, hyperkalemia stimulates Na^+-K^+-ATPase and thereby increases K^+ uptake across the basolateral membrane. This uptake raises the intracellular $[K^+]$ and increases the electrochemical driving force for K^+ exit across the apical membrane. Second, hyperkalemia also increases the permeability of the apical membrane to K^+. Third, hyperkalemia stimulates aldosterone secretion by the adrenal cortex, which acts synergistically with the plasma $[K^+]$ to stimulate K^+ secretion. Fourth, hyperkalemia also increases the flow rate of tubular fluid, which stimulates K^+ secretion by the distal tubule and collecting duct.

Hypokalemia (e.g., caused by a low-K^+ diet or K^+ loss in diarrhea) decreases K^+ secretion by actions opposite to those described for hyperkalemia. Hence hypokalemia inhibits Na^+-K^+-ATPase, decreases the electrochemical driving force for K^+ efflux across the apical membrane, reduces the permeability of the

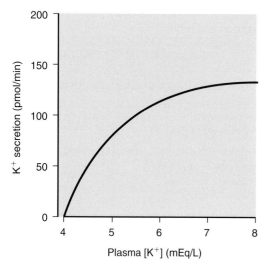

FIGURE 7-6 ■ The relationship between plasma K^+ concentration ($[K^+]$) and K^+ secretion by the distal tubule and the cortical collecting duct.

apical membrane to K^+, and reduces plasma aldosterone levels.

IN THE CLINIC

Chronic hypokalemia—that is, plasma K^+ concentration ($[K^+]$) <3.5 mEq/L—occurs most often in patients who receive diuretics for hypertension. Thus the excretion of K^+ by the kidneys exceeds the dietary intake of K^+. Hypokalemia also occurs in patients who vomit, have nasogastric suction, have diarrhea, abuse laxatives, or have hyperaldosteronism. Vomiting, nasogastric suction, diuretics, and diarrhea all can decrease the extracellular fluid volume, which in turn stimulates aldosterone secretion (see Chapter 6). Because aldosterone stimulates K^+ excretion by the kidneys, its action contributes to the development of hypokalemia.

Chronic hyperkalemia (plasma $[K^+]$ >5.0 mEq/L) occurs most frequently in persons with reduced urine flow, low plasma aldosterone levels, and renal disease in which the glomerular filtration rate falls below 20% of normal. In these persons, hyperkalemia occurs because the excretion of K^+ by the kidneys is less than the dietary intake of K^+. Less common causes for hyperkalemia occur in people with deficiencies of insulin, epinephrine, and aldosterone secretion or in people with metabolic acidosis caused by inorganic acids.

Aldosterone

A chronic (i.e., 24 hours or more) elevation in the plasma aldosterone concentration enhances K^+ secretion across principal cells in the distal tubule and collecting duct (Figure 7-7) by five mechanisms: (1) increasing the amount of Na^+-K^+-ATPase in the basolateral membrane; (2) increasing the expression of the sodium channel (ENaC) in the apical cell membrane; (3) elevating serum glucocorticoid stimulated kinase (Sgk1) levels, which also increases the expression of ENaC in the apical membrane and activates K^+ channels; (4) stimulating channel activating protease 1 (CAP1, also called **prostatin**), which directly activates ENaC; and (5) stimulating the permeability of the apical membrane to K^+.

The cellular mechanisms by which aldosterone affects the expression and activity of Na^+-K^+-ATPase and ENaC (preceding actions 1 to 4) have been described (see Chapter 4). Aldosterone increases the apical membrane K^+ permeability by increasing the number of K^+ channels in the membrane. However, the cellular mechanisms involved in this response are not completely known. Increased expression of Na^+-K^+-ATPase facilitates K^+ uptake across the basolateral membrane into cells and thereby elevates intracellular $[K^+]$. The increase in the number and activity of Na^+ channels enhances Na^+ entry into the cell from tubule fluid, an effect that depolarizes the apical membrane voltage. The depolarization of the apical membrane and increased intracellular $[K^+]$ enhance the electrochemical driving force for K^+ secretion from the cell into the tubule fluid. Taken together, these actions increase the cell $[K^+]$ and enhance the driving force for K^+ exit across the apical membrane. Aldosterone secretion is increased by hyperkalemia and by angiotensin II (after activation of the renin-angiotensin system). Aldosterone secretion is decreased by hypokalemia and natriuretic peptides released from the heart.

Although an acute increase in aldosterone levels (i.e., within hours) enhances the activity of Na^+-K^+-ATPase, K^+ excretion does not increase. The reason for this phenomenon is related to the effect of aldosterone on Na^+ reabsorption and tubular flow. Aldosterone stimulates Na^+ reabsorption and water reabsorption and thus decreases tubular flow. The decrease in flow in turn decreases K^+ secretion (discussed in more detail later in this chapter). However, chronic stimulation of

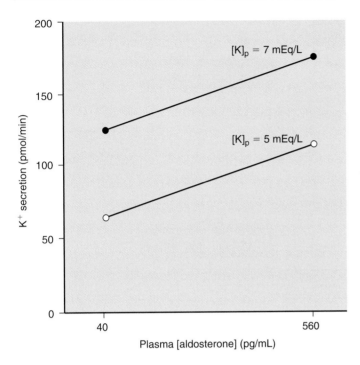

FIGURE 7-7 ■ The relationship between plasma aldosterone and K^+ secretion by the distal tubule and the cortical collecting duct. Note that K^+ secretion is increased further when the plasma K^+ concentration ($[K]_p$) is increased.

Na^+ reabsorption expands the ECF and thereby returns tubular flow to normal. These actions allow the direct stimulatory effect of aldosterone on the distal tubule and collecting duct to enhance K^+ excretion.

Arginine Vasopressin

Although AVP does not affect net urinary K^+ excretion, this hormone does stimulate K^+ secretion by the distal tubule and collecting duct (Figure 7-8). AVP increases the electrochemical driving force for K^+ exit across the apical membrane of principal cells by stimulating Na^+ uptake across the apical membrane of principal cells. The increased Na^+ uptake reduces the electrochemical driving force for K^+ exit across the apical membrane (i.e., the interior of the cell becomes less negatively charged). Despite this effect, AVP does not change K^+ secretion by these nephron segments. The reason for this phenomenon is related to the effect of AVP on tubular fluid flow. AVP decreases tubular fluid flow by stimulating water reabsorption. The decrease in tubular flow in turn reduces K^+ secretion (explained later in this chapter). The inhibitory effect of decreased flow of tubular fluid offsets the stimulatory effect of

AVP on the electrochemical driving force for K^+ exit across the apical membrane (see Figure 7-8). If AVP did not increase the electrochemical driving force favoring K^+ secretion, urinary K^+ excretion would decrease as AVP levels increase and urinary flow rates decrease. Hence K^+ balance would change in response to alterations in water balance. Thus the effects of AVP on the electrochemical driving force for K^+ exit across the apical membrane and tubule flow enable urinary K^+ excretion to be maintained constant despite wide fluctuations in water excretion.

FACTORS THAT PERTURB K^+ EXCRETION

Whereas plasma $[K^+]$, aldosterone, and AVP play important roles in regulating K^+ balance, the factors and hormones discussed next perturb K^+ balance (see Box 7-2).

Flow of Tubular Fluid

A rise in the flow of tubular fluid (e.g., with diuretic treatment and ECF volume expansion) stimulates K^+ secretion within minutes, whereas a fall (e.g., ECF

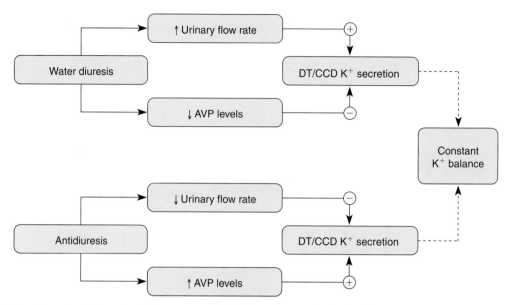

FIGURE 7-8 ■ Opposing effects of arginine vasopressin (*AVP*) on K⁺ secretion by the distal tubule (*DT*) and cortical collecting duct (*CCD*). Secretion is stimulated by an increase in the electrochemical gradient for K⁺ across the apical membrane and by an increase in the K⁺ permeability of the apical membrane. In contrast, secretion is reduced by a fall in the flow rate of tubular fluid. Because these effects oppose each other, net K⁺ secretion is not affected by AVP.

FIGURE 7-9 ■ Relationship between tubular flow rate and K⁺ secretion by the distal tubule and cortical collecting duct. A diet high in K⁺ increases the slope of the relationship between flow rate and secretion and increases the maximum rate of secretion. A diet low in K⁺ has the opposite effects. The shaded bar indicates the flow rate under most physiologic conditions.

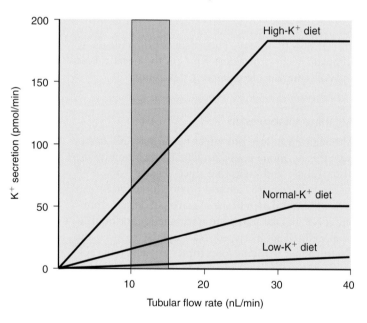

volume contraction caused by hemorrhage, severe vomiting, or diarrhea) reduces K⁺ secretion by the distal tubule and collecting duct (Figure 7-9). Increments in tubular fluid flow are more effective in stimulating K⁺ secretion as dietary K⁺ intake is increased. Studies of the primary cilium in principal cells have elucidated some of the mechanisms whereby increased flow stimulates K⁺ secretion. As described in Chapter 2, increased flow bends the primary cilium in principal cells, which activates the PKD1/PKD2 Ca⁺⁺ conducting channel complex. This mechanism allows more Ca^{++} to enter principal cells and increases intracellular $[Ca^{++}]$. The increase in $[Ca^{++}]$ activates BK channels in the apical plasma membrane, which enhances K^+ secretion from the cell into the tubule fluid. Increased flow also activates BK-mediated K^+ secretion by intercalated cells. Increased flow also may stimulate K^+ secretion by other mechanisms. As flow increases, for example, following the administration of diuretics or as the result of an increase in the ECF volume, so does the Na^+ concentration of tubule fluid. This increase in Na^+ concentration ($[Na^+]$) facilitates Na^+ entry across the apical membrane of distal tubule and collecting duct cells, thereby decreasing the interior negative membrane potential of the cell. This depolarization of the cell membrane potential increases the electrochemical driving force that promotes K^+ secretion across the apical cell membrane into tubule fluid. In addition, increased Na^+ uptake into cells activates the Na^+-K^+-ATPase in the basolateral membrane, thereby increasing K^+ uptake across the basolateral membrane and elevating cell $[K^+]$. However, it is important to note that an increase in flow rate during a water diuresis does not have a significant effect on K^+ excretion (see Figure 7-9), most likely because during a water diuresis the $[Na^+]$ of tubule fluid does not increase as flow rises.

Acid-Base Balance

Another factor that modulates K^+ secretion is the $[H^+]$ of the ECF (Figure 7-10). Acute alterations (within minutes to hours) in the pH of the plasma influence K^+ secretion by the distal tubule and collecting duct. Alkalosis (i.e., a plasma pH above normal) increases K^+ secretion, whereas acidosis (i.e., a plasma pH below normal) decreases it. An acute acidosis reduces K^+ secretion by two mechanisms: (1) it inhibits Na^+-K^+-ATPase and thereby reduces the cell $[K^+]$ and the electrochemical driving force for K^+ exit across the apical membrane, and (2) it reduces the permeability of the apical membrane to K^+. Alkalosis has the opposite effects.

The effect of a metabolic acidosis on K^+ excretion is time dependent. When metabolic acidosis lasts for several days, urinary K^+ excretion is stimulated (Figure 7-11). This stimulation occurs because chronic metabolic acidosis decreases the reabsorption of water and solutes (e.g., sodium chloride [NaCl]) by the

AT THE CELLULAR LEVEL

Renal outer medullary K^+ (**ROMK**) (*KCNJ1*) channels in the apical membrane of principal cells mediate K^+ secretion. Four ROMK subunits make up a single channel. Interestingly, knockout of the *KCNJ1* gene (ROMK) causes increased sodium chloride (NaCl) and K^+ excretion by the kidneys, leading to reduced extracellular fluid volume and hypokalemia. Although this effect is somewhat perplexing, it should be noted that ROMK also is expressed in the apical membrane of the thick ascending limb of Henle's loop, where it plays an important role in K^+ recycling across the apical membrane, an effect that is critical for the operation of the Na^+-K^+-$2Cl^-$ symporter (see Chapter 4). In the absence of ROMK, NaCl reabsorption by the thick ascending limb is reduced, which leads to NaCl loss in the urine. Reduction of NaCl reabsorption by the thick ascending limb also reduces the lumen-positive transepithelial voltage, which is the driving force for K^+ reabsorption by this nephron segment. Thus the reduction in paracellular K^+ reabsorption by the thick ascending limb increases urinary K^+ excretion, even when the cortical collecting duct is unable to secrete the normal amount of K^+ because of a lack of ROMK channels. The cortical collecting duct, however, does secrete K^+ even in ROMK knockout mice through the flow and Ca^{++}-dependent BK channels and by the operation of a K^+-Cl^- symporter expressed in the apical membrane of principal cells.

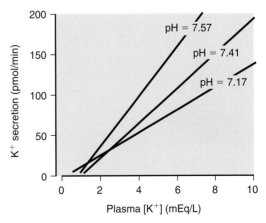

FIGURE 7-10 ■ Effect of plasma pH on the relationship between plasma K^+ concentration ($[K^+]$) and K^+ secretion by the distal tubule and collecting duct.

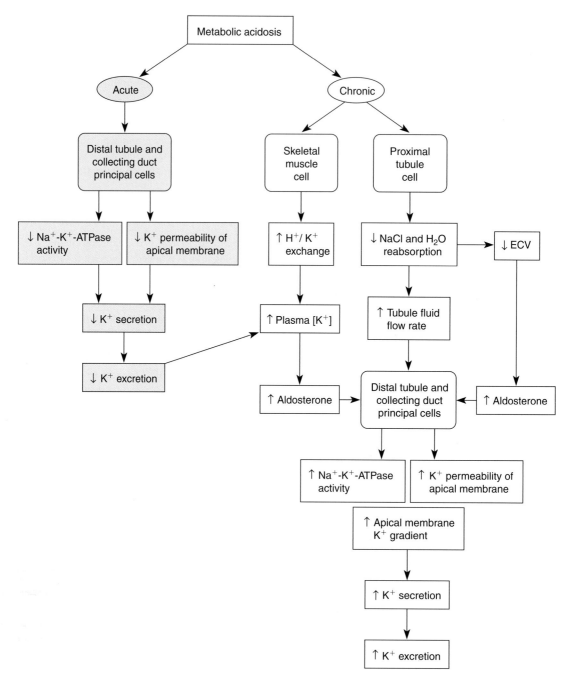

FIGURE 7-11 ■ Short-term versus long-term effect of metabolic acidosis on K⁺ excretion. *ECV*, Effective circulating volume; *NaCl*, sodium chloride; *Na⁺-K⁺-ATPase*, sodium–potassium–adenosine triphosphatase; *[K⁺]*, K⁺ concentration.

proximal tubule by inhibiting Na^+-K^+-ATPase. Hence the flow of tubular fluid is augmented along the distal tubule and collecting duct. The inhibition of proximal tubular water and NaCl reabsorption also decreases the ECF volume and thereby stimulates aldosterone secretion. In addition, chronic acidosis, caused by inorganic acids, increases the plasma $[K^+]$, which stimulates aldosterone secretion. The rise in tubular fluid flow, plasma $[K^+]$, and aldosterone levels offsets the effects of acidosis on the cell $[K^+]$ and apical membrane permeability, and K^+ secretion rises. Thus metabolic acidosis may either inhibit or stimulate K^+ excretion, depending on the duration of the disturbance.

AT THE CELLULAR LEVEL

The cellular mechanisms whereby changes in the K^+ content of the diet and acid-base balance regulate K^+ secretion by the distal tubule and collecting duct have been elucidated. Elevated K^+ intake increases K^+ secretion by several mechanisms, all related to increased serum K^+ concentration. Hyperkalemia increases the activity of the renal outer medullary K^+ (ROMK) channel in the apical plasma membrane of principal cells. Moreover, hyperkalemia inhibits proximal tubule sodium chloride (NaCl) and water reabsorption, thereby increasing distal tubule and collecting duct flow rate, a potent stimulus to K^+ secretion. Hyperkalemia also enhances aldosterone concentration, which increases K^+ secretion by three mechanisms. First, aldosterone increases the number of K^+ channels in the apical plasma membrane. Second, aldosterone stimulates K^+ uptake across the basolateral membrane by enhancing the number of Na^+-K^+-ATPase pumps, thereby enhancing the electrochemical gradient driving K^+ secretion across the apical membrane. Third, aldosterone increases Na^+ entry across the apical membrane, which depolarizes the apical plasma membrane voltage, thereby increasing the electrochemical gradient, promoting K^+ secretion. A low-K^+ diet dramatically reduces K^+ secretion by the distal tubule and collecting duct by increasing the activity of protein tyrosine kinase, which causes ROMK channels to be removed from the apical plasma membrane, thereby reducing K^+ secretion. Acidosis decreases K^+ secretion by inhibiting the activity of ROMK channels, whereas alkalosis stimulates K^+ secretion by enhancing ROMK channel activity.

As noted, acute metabolic alkalosis stimulates K^+ excretion. Chronic metabolic alkalosis, especially in association with ECF volume contraction, significantly increases renal K^+ excretion because of the associated increased levels of aldosterone.

Glucocorticoids

Glucocorticoids increase urinary K^+ excretion. This effect is in part mediated by an increase in the glomerular filtration rate, which enhances urinary flow rate, a potent stimulus of K^+ excretion, and by stimulating Sgk1 activity (discussed in a previous section).

As discussed earlier, the rate of urinary K^+ excretion is frequently determined by simultaneous changes in hormone levels, acid-base balance, or the flow rate of tubule fluid (Table 7-1). The powerful effect of flow often enhances or opposes the response of the distal tubule and collecting duct to hormones and changes in acid-base balance. This interaction can be beneficial in the case of hyperkalemia, in which the change in flow enhances K^+ excretion and thereby facilitates K^+ homeostasis. However, this interaction also can be detrimental, as in the case of alkalosis, in which changes in flow and acid-base status alter K^+ homeostasis.

TABLE 7-1
Effects of Hormones and Other Factors on K^+ Secretion by the Distal Tubule and Collecting Duct and on Urinary K^+ Excretion

CONDITION	DIRECT EFFECT ON DT/CD	TUBULAR FLOW RATE	URINARY EXCRETION
Hyperkalemia	Increase	Increase	Increase
Aldosterone			
Acute	Increase	Decrease	No change
Chronic	Increase	No change	Increase
Glucocorticoids	No change	Increase	Increase
AVP	Increase	Decrease	No change
Acidosis			
Acute	Decrease	No change	Decrease
Chronic	Decrease	Large increase	Increase
Alkalosis	Increase	Increase	Large increase

AVP, Arginine vasopressin; *CD*, collecting duct; *DT*, distal tubule.

SUMMARY

1. K$^+$ homeostasis is maintained by the kidneys, which adjust K$^+$ excretion to match dietary K$^+$ intake, and by the hormones insulin, epinephrine, and aldosterone, which regulate the distribution of K$^+$ between the intracellular fluid and ECF.
2. Other events, such as cell lysis, exercise, and changes in acid-base balance and plasma osmolality, disturb K$^+$ homeostasis and the plasma [K$^+$].
3. K$^+$ excretion by the kidneys is determined by the rate and direction of K$^+$ transport by the distal tubule and collecting duct. K$^+$ secretion by these tubular segments is regulated by the plasma [K$^+$], aldosterone, and AVP. In contrast, changes in tubular fluid flow and acid-base disturbances perturb K$^+$ excretion by the kidneys. In K$^+$-depleted states, K$^+$ secretion is inhibited and the distal tubule and collecting duct reabsorb K$^+$.

KEY WORDS AND CONCEPTS

- Hyperkalemia
- Hypokalemia
- Aldosterone
- Epinephrine
- Insulin

SELF-STUDY PROBLEMS

1. What would happen to the rise in plasma [K$^+$] following an intravenous K$^+$ load if the patient had a combination of sympathetic blockade and insulin deficiency?
2. What effect would aldosterone deficiency have on urinary K$^+$ excretion? What would happen to plasma [K$^+$], and what effect would aldosterone deficiency have on K$^+$ excretion?
3. Describe the homeostatic mechanisms involved in maintaining the plasma [K$^+$] following ingestion of a meal rich in K$^+$.
4. If the glomerular filtration rate declined by 50% (e.g., because of a loss of one kidney) and the amount of K$^+$ filtered across the glomerulus also declined by 50%, would the remaining kidney be able to maintain K$^+$ balance? If so, how would this maintenance of K$^+$ balance occur? If not, would the person become hyperkalemic?

8

REGULATION OF ACID-BASE BALANCE

. . . .

OBJECTIVES

Upon completion of this chapter, the student should be able to answer the following questions:

1. How does the bicarbonate (HCO_3^-) system operate as a buffer, and why is it an important buffer of the extracellular fluid?

2. How does metabolism of food produce acid and alkali, and what effect does the composition of the diet have on systemic acid-base balance?

3. What is the difference between volatile and nonvolatile acids?

4. How do the kidneys and lungs contribute to systemic acid-base balance?

5. Why are urinary buffers necessary for the excretion of acid by the kidneys?

6. What are the mechanisms for H^+ transport in the various segments of the nephron, and how are these mechanisms regulated?

7. How do the various segments of the nephron contribute to the process of reabsorbing the filtered HCO_3^-?

8. How do the kidneys produce new HCO_3^-?

9. How is ammonium produced by the kidneys, and how does its excretion contribute to renal acid excretion?

10. What are the major mechanisms by which the body defends itself against changes in acid-base balance?

11. What are the differences between simple metabolic and respiratory acid-base disorders, and how are they differentiated by blood gas measurements?

The concentration of H^+ in the body fluids is low compared with that of other ions. For example, Na^+ is present at a concentration some 3 million times greater than that of H^+ ([Na^+] = 140 mEq/L and [H^+] = 40 nEq/L). Because of the low [H^+] of the body fluids, it is commonly expressed as the negative logarithm, or pH.

Virtually all cellular, tissue, and organ processes are sensitive to pH. Indeed, life cannot exist outside a range of body fluid pH from 6.8 to 7.8 (160 to 16 nEq/L of H^+). Each day, acid and alkali are ingested in the diet. Also, cellular metabolism produces a number of substances that have an impact on the pH of body fluids. Without appropriate mechanisms to deal with this daily acid and alkali load and thereby maintain acid-base balance, many processes necessary for life could not occur. This chapter reviews the maintenance of whole-body acid-base balance. Although the emphasis is on the role of the kidneys in this process, the roles of the lungs and liver also are considered. In addition, the impact of diet and cellular metabolism on acid-base balance is presented. Finally, disorders of acid-base balance are considered, primarily to illustrate the physiologic processes involved. Throughout this chapter, **acid** is defined as any substance that adds H^+ to the body fluids, whereas **alkali** is defined as a substance that removes H^+ from the body fluids.

HCO_3^- BUFFER SYSTEM

Bicarbonate (HCO_3^-) is an important buffer of the extracellular fluid (ECF). With a normal plasma [HCO_3^-] of 23 to 25 mEq/L and a volume of 14 L (for a person weighing 70 kg), the ECF potentially can buffer 350 mEq of H^+. The HCO_3^- buffer system differs from the other buffer systems of the body (e.g., phosphate) because it is regulated by both the lungs and the kidneys. This situation is best appreciated by considering the following reaction.

$$CO_2 + H_2O + \xleftrightarrow{\text{slow}} H_2CO_3 \xleftrightarrow{\text{fast}} H^+ + HCO_3^- \quad (8\text{-}1)$$

As indicated, the first reaction (hydration/dehydration of CO_2) is the rate-limiting step. This normally slow reaction is greatly accelerated in the presence of carbonic anhydrase.* The second reaction, the ionization of carbonic acid (H_2CO_3) to H^+ and HCO_3^-, is virtually instantaneous.

The Henderson-Hasselbalch equation is used to quantitate how changes in CO_2 and HCO_3^- affect pH:

$$pH = pK' + \log \frac{HCO_3^-}{\alpha P_{CO_2}} \quad (8\text{-}2)$$

or

$$pH = 6.1 + \log \frac{HCO_3^-}{0.03\ P_{CO_2}} \quad (8\text{-}3)$$

In these equations, the amount of CO_2 is determined from the partial pressure of CO_2 (P_{CO_2}) and its solubility (α). For plasma at 37° C, α has a value of 0.03. Also, pK' is the negative logarithm of the overall dissociation constant for the reaction in equation 8-1 and has a value for plasma at 37° C of 6.1. Alternatively,

the relationships among HCO_3^-, CO_2, and [H^+] can be determined as follows:

$$[H^+] = \frac{24 \times P_{CO_2}}{[HCO_3^-]} \quad (8\text{-}4)$$

Inspection of equations 8-3 and 8-4 shows that the pH and the [H^+] vary when either the [HCO_3^-] or the P_{CO_2} is altered. Disturbances of acid-base balance that result from a change in the [HCO_3^-] are termed *metabolic acid-base disorders*, whereas those that result from a change in the P_{CO_2} are termed *respiratory acid-base disorders*. These disorders are considered in more detail in a subsequent section. The kidneys are primarily responsible for regulating the [HCO_3^-] of the ECF, whereas the lungs control the P_{CO_2}.

OVERVIEW OF ACID-BASE BALANCE

The diet of humans contains many constituents that are either acid or alkali. In addition, cellular metabolism produces acid and alkali. Finally, alkali is normally lost each day in the feces. As described later in this chapter, the net effect of these processes is the addition of acid to the body fluids. For acid-base balance to be maintained, acid must be excreted from the body at a rate equivalent to its addition. If acid addition exceeds excretion, **acidosis** results. Conversely, if acid excretion exceeds addition, **alkalosis** results.

As summarized in Figure 8-1, the major constituents of the diet are carbohydrates and fats. When tissue perfusion is adequate, O_2 is available to tissues, and insulin is present at normal levels, carbohydrates and fats are metabolized to CO_2 and H_2O. On a daily basis, 15 to 20 moles of CO_2 are generated through this process. Normally, this large quantity of CO_2 is effectively eliminated from the body by the lungs. Therefore this metabolically derived CO_2 has no impact on acid-base balance. CO_2 usually is termed **volatile acid**, reflecting the fact that it has the potential to generate H^+ after hydration with H_2O (see equation 8-1). Acid not derived directly from the hydration of CO_2 is termed **nonvolatile acid** (e.g., lactic acid).

The cellular metabolism of other dietary constituents also has an impact on acid-base balance (see Figure 8-1). For example, cysteine and methionine, which are

---

*Carbonic anhydrase actually catalyzes the following reaction: $H_2O \rightarrow H^+ + OH^- + CO_2 \rightarrow HCO_3^- + H^+ \rightarrow H_2CO_3$.

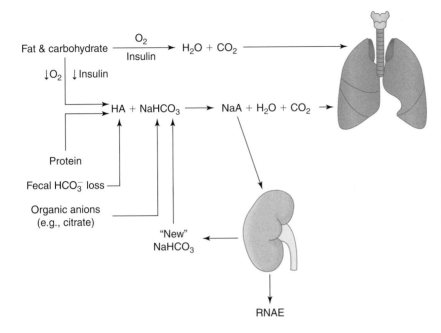

FIGURE 8-1 ■ Overview of the role of the kidneys in acid-base balance. HA represents nonvolatile acids and is referred to as net endogenous acid production. HCO_3^-, bicarbonate; *NaA*, sodium salt of nonvolatile acid; *NaHCO₃*, sodium bicarbonate; *RNAE*, renal net acid excretion.

sulfur-containing amino acids, yield sulfuric acid when metabolized, whereas hydrochloric acid results from the metabolism of lysine, arginine, and histidine. A portion of this nonvolatile acid load is offset by the production of HCO_3^- through the metabolism of the amino acids aspartate and glutamate. On average, the metabolism of dietary amino acids yields net nonvolatile acid production. The metabolism of certain organic anions (e.g., citrate) results in the production of HCO_3^-, which offsets nonvolatile acid production to some degree. Overall, in persons who ingest a diet containing meat, acid production exceeds HCO_3^- production. In addition to the metabolically derived acids and alkalis, the foods ingested contain acid and alkali. For example, the presence of phosphate ($H_2PO_4^-$) in ingested food increases the dietary acid load. Finally, during digestion, some HCO_3^- is normally lost in the feces. This loss is equivalent to the addition of nonvolatile acid to the body. Together, dietary intake, cellular metabolism, and fecal HCO_3^- loss result in the addition of approximately 1 mEq/kg body weight of nonvolatile acid to the body each day (50 to 100 mEq/day for most adults). This acid, referred to as **net endogenous acid production** (NEAP), results in an equivalent loss of HCO_3^- from the body that must be replaced. Importantly, the kidneys excrete acid and in that process generate HCO_3^-.

IN THE CLINIC

When insulin levels are normal, carbohydrates and fats are completely metabolized to $CO_2 + H_2O$. However, if insulin levels are abnormally low (e.g., in persons with **diabetes mellitus**), the metabolism of carbohydrates leads to the production of several organic keto acids (e.g., β-hydroxybutyric acid).

In the absence of adequate levels of O_2 (**hypoxia**), anaerobic metabolism by cells also can lead to the production of organic acids (e.g., lactic acid) rather than $CO_2 + H_2O$. This phenomenon frequently occurs in healthy persons during vigorous exercise. Poor tissue perfusion, such as occurs with reduced cardiac output, also can lead to anaerobic metabolism by cells and thus to acidosis. In these conditions, the organic acids accumulate and the pH of the body fluids decreases (acidosis). Treatment (e.g., administration of insulin in the case of diabetes) or improved delivery of adequate levels of O_2 to the tissues (e.g., in the case of poor tissue perfusion) results in the metabolism of these organic acids to $CO_2 + H_2O$, which consumes H^+ and thereby helps correct the acid-base disorder.

Nonvolatile acids do not circulate throughout the body but are immediately neutralized by the HCO_3^- in the ECF:

$$H_2SO_4 + 2NaHCO_3 \leftrightarrow$$
$$Na_2SO_4 + 2CO_2 + 2H_2O \qquad (8\text{-}5)$$

$$HCl + NaHCO_3 \leftrightarrow NaCl + CO_2 + H_2O \qquad (8\text{-}6)$$

This neutralization process yields the Na^+ salts of the strong acids and removes HCO_3^- from the ECF. Thus HCO_3^- minimizes the effect of these strong acids on the pH of the ECF. As noted previously, the ECF contains approximately 350 mEq of HCO_3^-. If this HCO_3^- was not replenished, the daily production of nonvolatile acids ($\approx$70 mEq/day) would deplete the ECF of HCO_3^- within 5 days. Systemic acid-base balance is maintained when **renal net acid excretion** (RNAE) equals NEAP.

RENAL NET ACID EXCRETION

Under normal conditions, the kidneys excrete an amount of acid equal to NEAP and in so doing replenish the HCO_3^- that is lost by neutralization of the nonvolatile acids. In addition, the kidneys must prevent the loss of HCO_3^- in the urine. The latter task is quantitatively more important because the filtered load of HCO_3^- is approximately 4320 mEq/day (24 mEq/L × 180 L/day = 4320 mEq/day), compared with only 50 to 100 mEq/day needed to balance NEAP.

Both the reabsorption of filtered HCO_3^- and the excretion of acid are accomplished by H^+ secretion by the nephrons. Thus in a single day the nephrons must secrete approximately 4390 mEq of H^+ into the tubular fluid. Most of the secreted H^+ serves to reabsorb the filtered load of HCO_3^-. Only 50 to 100 mEq of H^+, an amount equivalent to nonvolatile acid production, is excreted in the urine. As a result of this acid excretion, the urine is normally acidic.

The kidneys cannot excrete urine more acidic than pH 4.0 to 4.5. Even at a pH of 4.0, only 0.1 mEq/L of H^+ can be excreted. Thus to excrete sufficient acid, the kidneys excrete H^+ with urinary buffers such as inorganic phosphate (P_i).* Other constituents of the urine also can serve as buffers (e.g., creatinine), although their role is less important than that of P_i. Collectively, the various urinary buffers are termed *titratable acid*. This term is derived from the method by which these buffers are quantitated in the laboratory. Typically, alkali (OH^-) is added to a urine sample to titrate its pH to that of plasma (i.e., 7.4). The amount of alkali added is equal to the H^+ titrated by these urine buffers and is termed titratable acid.

The excretion of H^+ as a titratable acid is insufficient to balance NEAP. An additional and important mechanism by which the kidneys contribute to the maintenance of acid-base balance is through the synthesis and excretion of **ammonium** (NH_4^+). The mechanisms involved in this process are discussed in more detail later in this chapter. With regard to the renal regulation of acid-base balance, each NH_4^+ excreted in the urine results in the return of one HCO_3^- to the systemic circulation, which replenishes the HCO_3^- lost during neutralization of the nonvolatile acids. Thus the production and excretion of NH_4^+, like the excretion of titratable acid, are equivalent to the excretion of acid by the kidneys.

In brief, the kidneys contribute to acid-base homeostasis by reabsorbing the filtered load of HCO_3^- and excreting an amount of acid equivalent to NEAP. This overall process is termed RNAE, and it can be quantitated as follows:

$$RNAE = [(U_{NH_4^+} \times \dot{V}) + (U_{TA} \times \dot{V})]$$
$$- (U_{HCO_3^-} \times \dot{V}) \qquad (8\text{-}7)$$

where $(U_{NH_4^+} \times \dot{V})$ and $(U_{TA} \times \dot{V})$ are the rates of excretion (mEq/day) of NH_4^+ and titratable acid and $(U_{HCO_3^-} \times \dot{V})$ is the amount of HCO_3^- lost in the urine (equivalent to adding H^+ to the body).† Again, maintenance of acid-base balance means that RNAE must equal NEAP. Under most conditions, very little HCO_3^- is excreted in the urine. Thus RNAE essentially reflects titratable acid and NH_4^+ excretion. Quantitatively, TA accounts for approximately one third and NH_4^+ for two thirds of RNAE.

---

*The titration reaction is $HPO_4^{-2} + H^+ \leftrightarrow H_2PO_4^-$. This reaction has a pK of approximately 6.8.

†This equation ignores the small amount of free H^+ excreted in the urine. As already noted, urine with pH = 4.0 contains only 0.1 mEq/L of H^+.

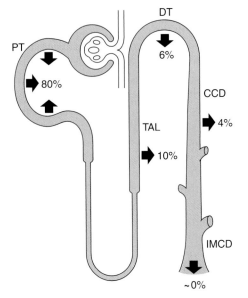

FIGURE 8-2 ■ Segmental reabsorption of bicarbonate (HCO₃⁻). The fraction of the filtered HCO_3^- reabsorbed by the various segments of the nephron is shown. Normally, the entire filtered HCO_3^- is reabsorbed and little or no HCO_3^- appears in the urine. *CCD,* Cortical collecting duct; *DT,* distal tubule; *IMCD,* inner medullary collecting duct; *PT,* proximal tubule; *TAL,* thick ascending limb.

HCO₃⁻ REABSORPTION ALONG THE NEPHRON

As indicated by equation 8-7, RNAE is maximized when little or no HCO_3^- is excreted in the urine. Indeed, under most circumstances, very little HCO_3^- appears in the urine. Because HCO_3^- is freely filtered at the glomerulus, approximately 4320 mEq/day are delivered to the nephrons and are then reabsorbed. Figure 8-2 summarizes the contribution of each nephron segment to the reabsorption of the filtered HCO_3^-.

The proximal tubule reabsorbs the largest portion of the filtered load of HCO_3^-. Figure 8-3 summarizes the primary transport processes involved. H⁺ secretion across the apical membrane of the cell occurs by both a Na⁺-H⁺ antiporter and H⁺–adenosine triphosphatase (H⁺-ATPase). The Na⁺-H⁺ antiporter (NHE3) is the predominant pathway for H⁺ secretion (accounts for approximately two thirds of HCO_3^- reabsorption) and uses the lumen-to-cell [Na⁺] gradient to drive this process (i.e., secondary active secretion of H⁺). Within the cell, H⁺ and HCO_3^- are produced in a reaction catalyzed by carbonic anhydrase (CA-II). The H⁺ is secreted into the tubular fluid, whereas the HCO_3^- exits the cell across the basolateral membrane and returns to the peritubular blood. HCO_3^- movement out of the cell across the basolateral membrane is coupled to other ions. The majority of HCO_3^- exits

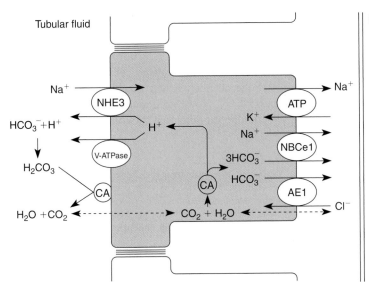

FIGURE 8-3 ■ Cellular mechanism for the reabsorption of filtered bicarbonate (HCO₃⁻) by cells of the proximal tubule. Carbonic anhydrase (*CA*) also is expressed on the basolateral surface (not shown). *AE1,* anion exchanger 1; *ATP,* Adenosine triphosphate; *H₂CO₃,* carbonic acid; *NBCe1,* sodium bicarbonate symporter; *NHE3,* Na⁺-H⁺ antiporter; *V-ATPase,* vacuolar adenosine triphosphatase.

through a symporter that couples the efflux of Na^+ with $3HCO_3^-$ (sodium bicarbonate cotransporter, NBCe1). In addition, some of the HCO_3^- may exit in exchange for Cl^- (via a Cl^--HCO_3^- antiporter; AE1). As noted in Figure 8-3, CA-IV also is present in the brush border of the proximal tubule cells. This enzyme catalyzes the dehydration of H_2CO_3 in the luminal fluid and thereby facilitates the reabsorption of HCO_3^-. CA-IV also is present in the basolateral membrane (not shown in Figure 8-3), where it may facilitate the exit of HCO_3^- from the cell.

AT THE CELLULAR LEVEL

Carbonic anhydrases (CAs) are zinc-containing enzymes that catalyze the hydration of CO_2 (see equation 8-1). The isoform CA-I is found in red blood cells and is critical for the cells' ability to carry CO_2. Two isoforms, CA-II and CA-IV, play important roles in urine acidification. The CA-II isoform is localized to the cytoplasm of many cells along the nephron, including the proximal tubule, thick ascending limb of Henle's loop, and intercalated cells of the distal tubule and collecting duct. The CA-IV isoform is membrane bound and exposed to the contents of the tubular fluid. It is found in the apical membrane of both the proximal tubule and thick ascending limb of Henle's loop, where it facilitates the reabsorption of the large amount of HCO_3^- reabsorbed by these segments. CA-IV has also been demonstrated in the basolateral membrane of the proximal tubule and thick ascending limb of Henle's loop. Its function at this site is thought to facilitate the exit of HCO_3^- from the cell.

The cellular mechanism for HCO_3^- reabsorption by the thick ascending limb of the loop of Henle is very similar to that in the proximal tubule. H^+ is secreted by an Na^+-H^+ antiporter and a vacuolar H^+-ATPase. As in the proximal tubule, the Na^+-H^+ antiporter is the predominant pathway for H^+ secretion. HCO_3^- exit from the cell involves both a Na^+-HCO_3^- symporter and a Cl^--HCO_3^- antiporter. However, the isoforms for these transporters differ from those in the proximal tubule. The Na^+-HCO_3^- symporter is electrically neutral, exchanging equal numbers of Na^+ for HCO_3^-. The Cl^--HCO_3^- antiporter is the anion exchanger 2. Recently, evidence has been obtained for the presence of a K^+-HCO_3^- symporter in the

basolateral membrane, which also may contribute to HCO_3^- exit from the cell.

The distal tubule* and collecting duct reabsorb the small amount of HCO_3^- that escapes reabsorption by the proximal tubule and loop of Henle. Figure 8-4 shows the cellular mechanism of HCO_3^- reabsorption by the collecting duct, where H^+ secretion occurs through the intercalated cell (see Chapter 2). Within the cell, H^+ and HCO_3^- are produced by the hydration of CO_2; this reaction is catalyzed by carbonic anhydrase (CA-II). H^+ is secreted into the tubular fluid by two mechanisms. The first mechanism involves an apical membrane vacuolar H^+-ATPase. The second mechanism couples the secretion of H^+ with the reabsorption of K^+ through an H^+-K^+-ATPase similar to that found in the stomach. The HCO_3^- exits the cell across the basolateral membrane in exchange for Cl^- (through a Cl^--HCO_3^- antiporter, anion exchanger-1) and enters the peritubular capillary blood. Cl^- exit from the cell across the basolateral membrane occurs via a Cl^- channel, and perhaps also via a K^+-Cl^- symporter (KCC4).

A second population of intercalated cells within the collecting duct secretes HCO_3^- rather than H^+ into the tubular fluid.† In these intercalated cells, in contrast to the intercalated cells previously described, the H^+-ATPase is located in the basolateral membrane (and to some degree also in the apical membrane), and a Cl^--HCO_3^- antiporter is located in the apical membrane (see Figure 8-4). The apical membrane Cl^--HCO_3^- antiporter is different from the one found in the basolateral membrane of the H^+-secreting intercalated cell and has been identified as pendrin. The activity of the HCO_3^--secreting intercalated cell is increased during metabolic alkalosis, when the kidneys must excrete excess HCO_3^-. However, under normal conditions, H^+ secretion predominates in the collecting duct.

---

*Here and in the remainder of the chapter the focus is on the function of intercalated cells. The early portion of the distal tubule, which does not contain intercalated cells, also reabsorbs HCO_3^-. The cellular mechanism is similar to that already described for the thick ascending limb of Henle's loop, although transporter isoforms may be different.

†The HCO_3^--secreting intercalated cells are termed either *type B* (or β-intercalated cells), or simply *non–type-A intercalated cells*. The H^+ secreting intercalated cells are termed *type A* (or α-intercalated cells).

H$^+$-secreting cell

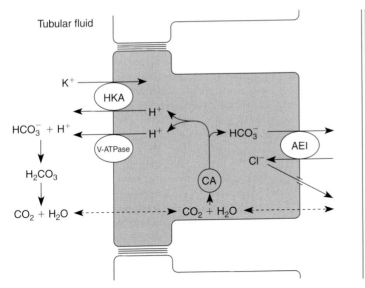

HCO$_3^-$-secreting cell

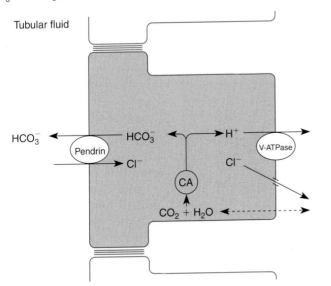

FIGURE 8-4 ■ Cellular mechanisms for the reabsorption and secretion of HCO$_3^-$ by intercalated cells of the collecting duct. Cl$^-$ also may exit the cell across the basolateral membrane via a K$^+$-Cl$^-$ symporter (not shown). *AE1,* anion exchanger 1; *CA,* carbonic anhydrase; *HCO$_3^-$,* bicarbonate; *H$_2$CO$_3$,* carbonic acid; *HKA,* H$^+$-K$^+$–adenosine triphosphatase; *V-ATPase,* vacuolar adenosine triphosphatase.

The apical membrane of collecting duct cells is not very permeable to H$^+$, and thus the pH of the tubular fluid can become quite acidic. Indeed, the most acidic tubular fluid along the nephron (pH = 4.0 to 4.5) is produced there. In comparison, the permeability of the proximal tubule to H$^+$ and HCO$_3^-$ is much higher, and the tubular fluid pH falls to only 6.5 in this segment. As explained later, the ability of the collecting duct to lower the pH of the tubular fluid is critically important for the excretion of urinary titratable acids and NH$_4^+$.

REGULATION OF H⁺ SECRETION

A number of factors regulate the secretion of H⁺, and thus the reabsorption of HCO_3^-, by the cells of the nephron. From a physiologic perspective, the primary factor that regulates H⁺ secretion by the nephron is a change in systemic acid-base balance. Thus acidosis stimulates RNAE, whereas RNAE is reduced during alkalosis.

The response of the kidneys to metabolic acidosis has been extensively studied and includes both immediate changes in the activity or number of transporters in the membrane, or both, and longer term changes in the synthesis of transporters. For example, with metabolic acidosis, the pH of the cells of the nephron decreases. This decrease stimulates H⁺ secretion by multiple mechanisms, depending on the particular nephron segment. First, the decrease in intracellular pH creates a more favorable cell-to-tubular fluid H⁺ gradient and thereby makes the secretion of H⁺ across the apical membrane more energetically favorable. Second, the decrease in pH can lead to allosteric changes in transport proteins, thereby altering their kinetics. Lastly, transporters may be shuttled to the plasma membrane from intracellular vesicles. With long-term acidosis, the abundance of transporters is increased, either by increased transcription of appropriate transporter genes or by increased translation of transporter messenger ribonucleic acid.

Although some of the effects just described may be attributable directly to the decrease in intracellular pH that occurs with metabolic acidosis, most of these changes in cellular H⁺ transport are mediated by hormones or other factors. Three known mediators of the renal response to acidosis are endothelin (ET-1), cortisol, and angiotensin-II. ET-1 is produced by endothelial and proximal tubule cells. With acidosis, ET-1 secretion is enhanced. In the proximal tubule ET-1 stimulates the phosphorylation and subsequent insertion into the apical membrane of the Na⁺-H⁺ antiporter and insertion of the Na^+-$3HCO_3^-$ symporter into the basolateral membrane. ET-1 may mediate the response to acidosis in other nephron segments as well. With acidosis, the secretion of the glucocorticoid hormone cortisol by the adrenal cortex is stimulated. It, in turn, acts on the kidneys to increase the transcription of the Na⁺-H⁺ antiporter and Na^+-$3HCO_3^-$ symporter genes in the proximal tubule. Angiotensin

AT THE CELLULAR LEVEL

In response to metabolic acidosis, H⁺ secretion along the nephron is increased. Several mechanisms responsible for the increase in H⁺ secretion have been elucidated. For example, the intracellular acidification that occurs during metabolic acidosis has been reported to lead to allosteric changes in the Na⁺-H⁺ antiporter (NHE3) in the proximal tubule, thereby increasing its transport kinetics. Transporters also are shuttled to the plasma membrane from intracellular vesicles. This mechanism occurs in both the intercalated cells of the collecting duct, where acidosis stimulates the exocytic insertion of H⁺ adenosine triphosphatase (H⁺-ATPase) into the apical membrane, and in the proximal tubule, where apical membrane insertion of the Na⁺-H⁺ antiporter and H⁺-ATPase has been reported, as has insertion of the Na^+-$3HCO_3^-$ symporter (NBCe1) into the basolateral membrane. With long-term acidosis, the abundance of transporters is increased, either by increased transcription of appropriate transporter genes or by increased translation of transporter messenger ribonucleic acid. Examples of this phenomenon include NHE3 and NBCe1 in the proximal tubule and the H⁺-ATPase and Cl⁻-HCO_3^- antiporter (anion exchanger 1) in the acid-secreting intercalated cells. Additionally, acidosis reduces the expression of pendrin in the HCO_3^--secreting intercalated cells.

II increases with acidosis and stimulates H⁺ secretion by increasing the activity of the Na⁺-H⁺ antiporter throughout the nephron. In the proximal tubule, angiotensin II also stimulates ammonium production and its secretion into the tubular fluid, which, as described later in this chapter, is an important component of the kidneys' response to acidosis.

Acidosis also stimulates the secretion of parathyroid hormone. The increased levels of parathyroid hormone act on the proximal tubule to inhibit phosphate reabsorption (see Chapter 9). In so doing, more phosphate is delivered to the distal nephron, where it can serve as a urinary buffer and thus increase the capacity of the kidneys to excrete titratable acid.

As noted, the response of the kidneys to alkalosis is less well characterized. Clearly RNAE is decreased, which occurs in part by increased HCO_3^- excretion but also by a decrease in the excretion of ammonium and titratable acid. The signals that regulate this response are not well characterized.

AT THE CELLULAR LEVEL

Cells in the kidney and many other organs express H^+ and HCO_3^- receptors that play key roles in the adaptive response to changes in acid base balance. For example, G protein–coupled receptors that are regulated by extracellular $[H^+]$ (i.e., they are inactive when the pH is >7.5 and maximally activated when the pH is 6.8) recently have been identified (OGR1, GPR4, and TDAG8). When activated by extracellular acidification, these receptors increase the production of cyclic adenosine monophosphate (via stimulation of adenylyl cyclase) and/or IP3 and diacylglycerol (via stimulation of phospholipase C), which regulate a variety of acid-base transporters. By contrast, Pyk2 is activated by intracellular acidification, and its activation in the proximal tubule increases H^+ secretion via the Na^+-H^+ antiporter (NHE3) located in the apical membrane and HCO_3^- absorption via NBCe1 across the basolateral membrane. Two signaling enzymes, soluble adenylyl cyclase and guanylyl cyclase-D, are regulated by changes in intracellular HCO_3^-. When activated, soluble adenylyl cyclase increases cyclic adenosine monophosphate production, which activates protein kinase A, an effect that increases the amount of H^+-ATPase in the apical membrane of α-intercalated cells in the kidney collecting duct.

Other factors not necessarily related to the maintenance of acid-base balance can influence the secretion of H^+ by the cells of the nephron. Because a significant H^+ transporter in the nephron is the Na^+-H^+ antiporter, factors that alter Na^+ reabsorption can secondarily affect H^+ secretion. For example, with volume contraction (negative Na^+ balance), Na^+ reabsorption by the nephron is increased (see Chapter 6), including reabsorption of Na^+ via the Na^+-H^+ antiporter. As a result, H^+ secretion is enhanced. This phenomenon occurs by several mechanisms. One mechanism involves the renin-angiotensin-aldosterone system, which is activated by volume contraction. Angiotensin

II acts on the proximal tubule to stimulate the apical membrane Na^+-H^+ antiporter and the basolateral Na^+-$3HCO_3^-$ symporter. This stimulatory effect includes increased activity of the transporters and insertion of transporters into the membrane. To a lesser degree, angiotensin II stimulates H^+ secretion in the thick ascending limb of Henle's loop and the early portion of the distal tubule, a process also mediated by the Na^+-H^+ antiporter. The primary action of aldosterone on the distal tubule and collecting duct is to stimulate Na^+ reabsorption by principal cells (see Chapter 6). However, it also stimulates intercalated cells in these segments to secrete H^+. This effect is both indirect and direct. By stimulating Na^+ reabsorption by principal cells, aldosterone hyperpolarizes the transepithelial voltage (i.e., the lumen becomes more electrically negative). This change in transepithelial voltage then facilitates the secretion of H^+ by the intercalated cells. In addition to this indirect effect, aldosterone (and angiotensin II) acts directly on intercalated cells to stimulate H^+ secretion via the H^+-ATPase. The precise mechanisms for this stimulatory effect are not fully understood.

Another mechanism by which ECF volume contraction enhances H^+ secretion (HCO_3^- reabsorption) is through changes in peritubular capillary Starling forces. As described in Chapters 4 and 6, ECF volume contraction alters the peritubular capillary Starling forces such that overall proximal tubule reabsorption is enhanced. With this enhanced reabsorption, more of the filtered load of HCO_3^- is reabsorbed.

Potassium balance influences the secretion of H^+ by the proximal tubule. H^+ secretion is stimulated by hypokalemia and inhibited by hyperkalemia. It is thought that K^+-induced changes in intracellular pH are responsible, at least in part, for this effect, with the cells being acidified by hypokalemia and alkalinized by hyperkalemia. Hypokalemia also stimulates H^+ secretion by the collecting duct, which occurs as a result of increased expression of the H^+-K^+-ATPase in intercalated cells.

FORMATION OF NEW HCO_3^-

As discussed previously, reabsorption of the filtered HCO_3^- is important for maximizing RNAE. However, HCO_3^- reabsorption alone does not replenish

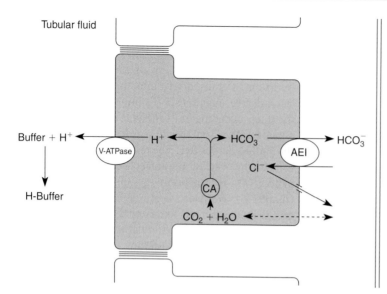

Tubular fluid

Blood

FIGURE 8-5 ■ General scheme for the excretion of H^+ with non-bicarbonate (non-HCO_3^-) urinary buffers (titratable acid). The primary urinary buffer is phosphate (HPO_4^{-2}). An H^+-secreting intercalated cell is shown. For simplicity, only the H^+ adenosine triphosphatase (V-ATPase) is depicted. H^+ secretion by H^+-K^+-ATPase also titrates luminal buffers. *AE1*, anion exchanger 1; *CA*, carbonic anhydrase; *V-ATPase*, vacuolar adenosine triphosphatase.

the HCO_3^- lost during the buffering of the nonvolatile acids produced during metabolism. To maintain acid-base balance, the kidneys must replace this lost HCO_3^- with new HCO_3^-. A portion of the new HCO_3^- is produced when urinary buffers (primarily P_i) are excreted as titratable acid. This process is illustrated in Figure 8-5. In the distal tubule and collecting duct, where the tubular fluid contains little or no HCO_3^- because of "upstream" reabsorption, H^+ secreted into the tubular fluid combines with a urinary buffer. Thus H^+ secretion results in the excretion of H^+ with a buffer, and the HCO_3^- produced in the cell from the hydration of CO_2 is added to the blood. The amount of P_i excreted each day and thus available to serve as a urinary buffer is not sufficient to allow adequate generation of new HCO_3^-. However, as noted, increased excretion of P_i does occur with acidosis and therefore contributes to the kidneys' response to the acidosis. Nevertheless, this amount of P_i is inadequate to allow the kidneys to excrete sufficient net acid. In comparison, NH_4^+ is produced by the kidneys and its synthesis, and subsequent excretion adds HCO_3^- to the ECF. In addition, the synthesis of NH_4^+ and the subsequent production of HCO_3^- are regulated in response to the acid-base requirements of the body. Because of this process, NH_4^+ excretion is critically involved in the formation of new HCO_3^-.

NH_4^+ is produced in the kidneys through the metabolism of **glutamine**. Essentially, the kidneys metabolize glutamine, excrete NH_4^+, and add HCO_3^- to the body. However, the formation of new HCO_3^- by this process depends on the kidneys' ability to excrete NH_4^+ in the urine. If NH_4^+ is not excreted in the urine but enters the systemic circulation instead, it is converted into urea by the liver. This conversion process generates H^+, which is then buffered by HCO_3^-. Thus the production of urea from renally generated NH_4^+ consumes HCO_3^- and negates the formation of HCO_3^- through the synthesis and excretion of NH_4^+ by the kidneys. However, normally, the kidneys excrete NH_4^+ in the urine and thereby produce new HCO_3^-.

The process by which the kidneys excrete NH_4^+ is complex. Figure 8-6 illustrates the essential features of this process. NH_4^+ is produced from glutamine in the cells of the proximal tubule, a process termed **ammoniagenesis**. Each glutamine molecule produces two molecules of NH_4^+ and the divalent anion 2-oxoglutarate^{-2}. The metabolism of this anion ultimately provides two molecules of HCO_3^-. The HCO_3^- exits the cell across the basolateral membrane and enters the peritubular blood as new HCO_3^-. NH_4^+ exits the cell across the apical membrane and enters the tubular fluid. The primary mechanism for the secretion of NH_4^+ into the tubular fluid involves the Na^+-H^+ antiporter, with NH_4^+ substituting for H^+. In addition, NH_3 can diffuse out of the

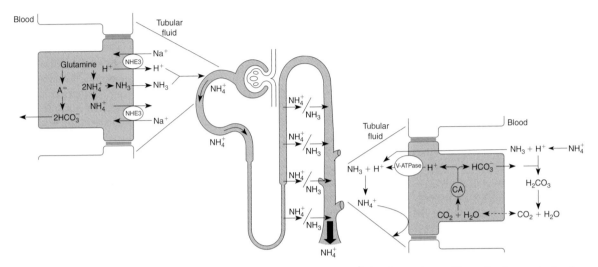

FIGURE 8-6 ■ Production, transport, and excretion of ammonium (NH_4^+) by the nephron. Glutamine is metabolized to NH_4^+ and bicarbonate (HCO_3^-) in the proximal tubule. The NH_4^+ is secreted into the lumen, and the HCO_3^- enters the blood. The secreted NH_4^+ is reabsorbed in Henle's loop primarily by the thick ascending limb and accumulates in the medullary interstitium, where it exists as both NH_4^+ and ammonia (NH_3) (pKa $\approx$9.0). NH_4^+ diffuses into the tubular fluid of the collecting duct via RhCG and RhBG (not shown), and H^+ secretion by the collecting duct leads to accumulation of NH_4^+ in the lumen by the processes of nonionic diffusion and diffusion trapping. For each molecule of NH_4^+ excreted in the urine, a molecule of "new" HCO_3^- is added back to the extracellular fluid. *CA,* Carbonic anhydrase; *V-ATPase,* vacuolar adenosine triphosphatase.

cell across the plasma membrane into the tubular fluid, where it is protonated to NH_4^+.

A significant portion of the NH_4^+ secreted by the proximal tubule is reabsorbed by the loop of Henle. The thick ascending limb is the primary site of this NH_4^+ reabsorption, with NH_4^+ substituting for K^+ on the Na^+-K^+-$2Cl^-$ symporter. In addition, the lumen-positive transepithelial voltage in this segment drives the paracellular reabsorption of NH_4^+ (see Chapter 4).

The NH_4^+ reabsorbed by the thick ascending limb of the loop of Henle accumulates in the medullary interstitium, where it exists in chemical equilibrium with NH_3 (pK = 9.0). NH_4^+ is then secreted into the tubular fluid of the collecting duct. The mechanisms by which NH_4^+ is secreted by the collecting duct include (1) transport into intercalated cells by the Na^+-K^+-ATPase (NH_4^+ substituting for K^+) and exit from the cell across the apical membrane of intercalated cells by the H^+-K^+-ATPase (NH_4^+ substituting for H^+) and (2) the process of **nonionic diffusion** and **diffusion trapping**. Of these mechanisms for NH_4^+ secretion, quantitatively the

most important is nonionic diffusion and diffusion trapping. By this mechanism, NH_3 diffuses from the medullary interstitium into the lumen of the collecting duct. As previously described, H^+ secretion by the intercalated cells of the collecting duct acidifies the luminal fluid (a luminal fluid pH as low as 4.0 to 4.5 can be achieved). Consequently, NH_3 diffusing from the medullary interstitium into the collecting duct lumen (nonionic diffusion) is protonated to NH_4^+ by the acidic tubular fluid. Because the collecting duct is less permeable to NH_4^+ than to NH_3, NH_4^+ is trapped in the tubule lumen (diffusion trapping) and eliminated from the body in the urine. Ammonia diffusion across the collecting duct occurs via Rh glycoproteins.* Two Rh glycoproteins have been identified thus far in the kidney (RhBG and RhCG) and are localized to the dis-

---

*Rh glycoproteins, or rhesus glycoproteins, are so named because of their homology to the rhesus proteins found on red blood cells, which are responsible for hemolytic disease of the newborn. They are a class of membrane proteins that transport NH_3 and perhaps NH_4^+.

tal tubule and collecting duct. RhBG is localized to the basolateral membrane, whereas RhCG is found in both the apical and basolateral membranes. Both RhBG and RhCG are expressed to a greater degree in intercalated cells versus principal cells.

IN THE CLINIC

Assessing NH_4^+ excretion by the kidneys is done indirectly because assays of urine NH_4^+ are not routinely available. In metabolic acidosis, the appropriate renal response is to increase net acid excretion. Accordingly, little or no HCO_3^- appears in the urine, the urine is acidic, and NH_4^+ excretion is increased. To assess NH_4^+ production, and especially the amount of NH_4^+ excreted, the urinary net charge, or urine anion gap, can be calculated by measuring the urinary concentrations of Na^+, K^+, and Cl^-:

$$\text{Urine anion gap} = ([Na^+] + [K^+]) - [Cl^-] \quad (8\text{-}8)$$

The concept of urine anion gap during a metabolic acidosis assumes that the major cations in the urine are Na^+, K^+, and NH_4^+ and that the major anion is Cl^- (with urine pH less than 6.5, virtually no HCO_3^- is present). As a result, the urine anion gap yields a negative value when adequate amounts of NH_4^+ are being excreted and thereby reflects the amount of NH_4^+ excreted in the urine. Indeed, the absence of a urine anion gap or the existence of a positive value indicates a renal defect in NH_4^+ production and excretion.

H^+ secretion by the collecting duct is critical for the excretion of NH_4^+. If collecting duct H^+ secretion is inhibited, the NH_4^+ reabsorbed by the thick ascending limb of Henle's loop is not excreted in the urine. Instead, it is returned to the systemic circulation, where, as described previously, it is converted to urea by the liver, consuming HCO_3^- in the process. Thus new HCO_3^- is produced during the metabolism of glutamine by cells of the proximal tubule. However, the overall process is not complete until the NH_4^+ is excreted (i.e., the production of urea from NH_4^+ by the liver is prevented). Thus NH_4^+ excretion in the urine can be used as a "marker" of glutamine metabolism in the proximal tubule. In the net, one new HCO_3^- is returned to the systemic circulation for each NH_4^+ excreted in the urine.

IN THE CLINIC

Renal tubule acidosis (RTA) refers to conditions in which net acid excretion by the kidneys is impaired. Under these conditions, the kidneys are unable to excrete a sufficient amount of net acid (renal net acid excretion [RNAE]) to balance net endogenous acid production, and acidosis results. RTA can be caused by a defect in H^+ secretion in the proximal tubule (**proximal RTA**) or distal tubule (**distal RTA**) or by inadequate production and excretion of NH_4^+.

Proximal RTA can be caused by a variety of hereditary and acquired conditions (e.g., **cystinosis**, **Fanconi syndrome**, or administration of carbonic anhydrase inhibitors). The majority of cases of proximal RTA result from generalized tubule dysfunction rather than a selective defect in one of the proximal tubule acid-base transporters. However, autosomal recessive and autosomal dominant forms of proximal RTA have been identified. An autosomal recessive form of proximal RTA results from a mutation in the Na^+-HCO_3^- symporter (NBCe1). Because this transporter also is expressed in the eye, these patients also have ocular abnormalities. Another autosomal recessive form of proximal RTA occurs in persons who lack carbonic anhydrase (CA-II). Because CA-II is required for normal distal acidification, this defect includes a distal RTA component as well. Finally, an autosomal dominant form of proximal RTA has been identified. However, the transporter involved has not been identified. Regardless of the cause, if H^+ secretion by the cells of the proximal tubule is impaired, there is decreased reabsorption of the filtered HCO_3^-. Consequently, HCO_3^- is lost in the urine, the plasma $[HCO_3^-]$ decreases, and acidosis ensues.

Distal RTA also occurs in a number of hereditary and acquired conditions (e.g., **medullary sponge kidney**, certain drugs such as **amphotericin B**, and conditions secondary to urinary obstruction). Both autosomal dominant and autosomal recessive forms of distal RTA have been identified. An autosomal dominant form results from mutations in the gene coding for the Cl^--HCO_3^- antiporter (anion exchanger-1) in the basolateral membrane of the acid-secreting intercalated cell. Autosomal recessive forms are caused by mutations in various subunits of vacuolar $[H^+]$-adenosine triphosphatase (H^+-ATPase). In some patients with Sjögren syndrome, an autoimmune disease, distal RTA develops as a result of antibodies directed against H^+-ATPase. Lastly, H^+ secretion by the distal tubule and the collecting duct may be normal, but the permeability of the cells to H^+ is increased. This effect occurs with the antifungal drug amphotericin B, the administration of which leads to the development of distal RTA. Regardless of the cause of distal RTA, the ability to acidify the tubular fluid in the distal tubule and collecting duct is impaired. Consequently, titratable acid excretion is reduced, and nonionic diffusion and diffusion trapping of NH_4^+ are impaired. This situation, in turn, decreases RNAE, with the subsequent development of acidosis.

Failure to produce and excrete sufficient quantities of NH_4^+ also can reduce net acid excretion by the kidneys. This situation occurs as a result of generalized dysfunction of the distal tubule and collecting duct with impaired H^+, NH_4^+, and K^+ secretion. Generalized distal nephron dysfunction is seen in persons with loss of function mutations in the Na^+ channel (ENaC), which are inherited in an autosomal recessive pattern. An autosomal dominant form also is seen with loss of function mutations in the mineralocorticoid receptor. More commonly, NH_4^+ production and excretion are impaired in patients with hyporeninemic hypoaldosteronism. These patients typically have moderate degrees of renal failure with reduced levels of renin and, thus, aldosterone. As a result, distal tubule and collecting duct function is impaired. Finally, a number of drugs also can result in distal tubule and collecting duct dysfunction. These drugs block the Na^+ channel (e.g., amiloride), block the production or action of angiotensin II (angiotensin-converting enzyme inhibitor, angiotensin I receptor blockers), or block the action of aldosterone (e.g., spironolactone). Regardless of the cause, the impaired function of the distal tubule and collecting duct results in the development of hyperkalemia, which in turn impairs ammoniagenesis by the proximal tubule. H^+ secretion by the distal tubule and collecting duct and thus NH_4^+ secretion also are impaired by these drugs. Thus RNAE is less than net endogenous acid production, and metabolic acidosis develops.

If the acidosis that results from any of these forms of RTA is severe, individuals must ingest alkali (e.g., baking soda or a solution containing citrate*) to maintain acid-base balance. In this way, the HCO_3^- lost each day in the buffering of nonvolatile acid is replenished by the extra HCO_3^- ingested in the diet.

*One of the byproducts of citrate metabolism is HCO_3^-. Ingestion of drinks containing citrate often is more palatable to patients than ingesting baking soda.

An important feature of the renal NH_4^+ system is that it can be regulated by systemic acid-base balance. As already noted, cortisol levels increase during acidosis and cortisol stimulates ammoniagenesis (i.e., NH_4^+ production from glutamine). Angiotensin II also stimulates ammoniagenesis and secretion of NH_4^+ into the tubular fluid. The expression of RhCG in the distal tubule and collecting duct is increased with acidosis (in some species, expression of RhBG is also increased). Thus in response to acidosis, both NH_4^+ production and excretion are stimulated. Because this response involves the synthesis of new enzymes, it requires several days for complete adaptation.

Other factors can alter renal NH_4^+ excretion. For example, the $[K^+]$ of the ECF alters NH_4^+ production. Hyperkalemia inhibits NH_4^+ production, whereas hypokalemia stimulates NH_4^+ production. The mechanism by which plasma $[K^+]$ alters NH_4^+ production is not fully understood. Alterations in the plasma $[K^+]$ may change the intracellular pH of proximal tubule cells and in that way influence glutamine metabolism. By this mechanism, hyperkalemia would raise intracellular pH and thereby inhibit glutamine metabolism. The opposite would occur during hypokalemia.

RESPONSE TO ACID-BASE DISORDERS

The pH of the ECF is maintained within a very narrow range (7.35 to 7.45).* Inspection of equation 8-3 shows

---

*For simplicity of presentation in this chapter, the value of 7.40 for body fluid pH is used as normal, even though the normal range is from 7.35 to 7.45. Similarly, the normal range for Pco_2 is 35 to 45 mm Hg. However, a Pco_2 of 40 mm Hg is used as the normal value. Finally, a value of 24 mEq/L is considered a normal ECF $[HCO_3^-]$, even though the normal range is 22 to 28 mEq/L.

that the pH of the ECF varies when either the $[HCO_3^-]$ or P_{CO_2} is altered. As already noted, disturbances of acid-base balance that result from a change in the $[HCO_3^-]$ of the ECF are termed **metabolic acid-base disorders**, whereas those resulting from a change in the P_{CO_2} are termed **respiratory acid-base disorders**. The kidneys are primarily responsible for regulating the $[HCO_3^-]$, whereas the lungs regulate the P_{CO_2}.

When an acid-base disturbance develops, the body uses a series of mechanisms to defend against the change in the pH of the ECF. These defense mechanisms do not correct the acid-base disturbance but merely minimize the change in pH imposed by the disturbance. Restoration of the blood pH to its normal value requires correction of the underlying process or processes that produced the acid-base disorder. The body has three general mechanisms to compensate for, or defend against, changes in body fluid pH produced by acid-base disturbances: (1) extracellular and intracellular buffering, (2) adjustments in blood P_{CO_2} by alterations in the ventilatory rate of the lungs, and (3) adjustments in the RNAE.

Extracellular and Intracellular Buffers

The first line of defense against acid-base disorders is extracellular and intracellular buffering. The response of the extracellular buffers is virtually instantaneous, whereas the response to intracellular buffering is slower and can take several minutes.

Metabolic disorders that result from the addition of nonvolatile acid or alkali to the body fluids are buffered in both the extracellular and intracellular compartments. The HCO_3^- buffer system is the principal ECF buffer. When nonvolatile acid is added to the body fluids (or alkali is lost from the body), HCO_3^- is consumed during the process of neutralizing the acid load, and the $[HCO_3^-]$ of the ECF is reduced. Conversely, when nonvolatile alkali is added to the body fluids (or acid is lost from the body), H^+ is consumed, causing more HCO_3^- to be produced from the dissociation of H_2CO_3. Consequently, the $[HCO_3^-]$ increases.

Although the HCO_3^- buffer system is the principal ECF buffer, P_i and plasma proteins provide additional extracellular buffering. The combined action of the ECF buffering processes for HCO_3^-, P_i, and

plasma protein accounts for approximately 50% of the buffering of a nonvolatile acid load and 70% of that of a nonvolatile alkali load. The remainder of the buffering under these two conditions occurs intracellularly. Intracellular buffering involves the movement of H^+ into cells (during buffering of nonvolatile acid) or the movement of H^+ out of cells (during buffering of nonvolatile alkali). H^+ is titrated inside the cell by HCO_3^-, P_i, and the histidine groups on proteins.

Bone represents an additional source of extracellular buffering. With acidosis, buffering by bone results in its demineralization because Ca^{++} is released from bone as salts containing Ca^{++} bind H^+ in exchange for Ca^{++}.

When respiratory acid-base disorders occur, the pH of body fluids changes as a result of alterations in the P_{CO_2}. Virtually all buffering in respiratory acid-base disorders occurs intracellularly. When the P_{CO_2} rises (respiratory acidosis), CO_2 moves into the cell, where it combines with H_2O to form H_2CO_3. H_2CO_3 then dissociates to H^+ and HCO_3^-. Some of the H^+ is buffered by cellular protein, and HCO_3^- exits the cell and raises the plasma $[HCO_3^-]$. This process is reversed when the P_{CO_2} is reduced (respiratory alkalosis). Under this condition, the hydration reaction ($H_2O + CO_2 \leftrightarrow H_2CO_3$) is shifted to the left by the decrease in P_{CO_2}. As a result, the dissociation reaction ($H_2CO_3 \leftrightarrow H^+ + HCO_3^-$) also shifts to the left, thereby reducing the plasma $[HCO_3^-]$.

Respiratory Compensation

The lungs are the second line of defense against acid-base disorders. As indicated by the Henderson-Hasselbalch equation (see equation 8-3), changes in the P_{CO_2} alter the blood pH; a rise decreases the pH, and a reduction increases the pH.

The ventilatory rate determines the P_{CO_2}. Increased ventilation decreases P_{CO_2}, whereas decreased ventilation increases it. The blood P_{CO_2} and pH are important regulators of the ventilatory rate. Chemoreceptors located in the brainstem (ventral surface of the medulla) and periphery (carotid and aortic bodies) sense changes in P_{CO_2} and $[H^+]$ and alter the ventilatory rate appropriately. Thus when metabolic acidosis occurs, a rise in the $[H^+]$ (decrease in pH) increases the ventilatory rate. Conversely, during metabolic alkalosis, a decreased [H⁺] (increase in pH) leads to a reduced ventilatory rate. With maximal hyperventilation, the P_{CO_2} can be reduced to approximately 10 mm Hg. Because hypoxia, a potent stimulator of ventilation,

also develops with hypoventilation, the degree to which the P_{CO_2} can be increased is limited. In an otherwise healthy person, hypoventilation cannot raise the P_{CO_2} above 60 mm Hg. The respiratory response to metabolic acid-base disturbances may be initiated within minutes but may require several hours to complete.

IN THE CLINIC

Metabolic acidosis can develop in patients with insulin-dependent diabetes (secondary to the production of keto acids) if insulin dosages are not adequate. As a compensatory response to this acidosis, deep and rapid breathing develops. This breathing pattern is termed **Kussmaul respiration**. With prolonged Kussmaul respiration, the muscles involved can become fatigued. When this muscle fatigue happens, respiratory compensation is impaired, and the acidosis can become more severe.

IN THE CLINIC

Loss of gastric contents from the body (i.e., through vomiting or nasogastric suction) produces metabolic alkalosis as a result of the loss of HCl. If the loss of gastric fluid is significant, extracellular fluid volume contraction occurs. Under this condition, the kidneys cannot excrete sufficient quantities of HCO_3^- to compensate for the metabolic alkalosis. Bicarbonate (HCO_3^-) is not excreted because the volume contraction enhances Na^+ reabsorption by the proximal tubule and increases angiotensin II and aldosterone levels (see Chapter 6). These responses in turn limit HCO_3^- excretion because a significant amount of Na^+ reabsorption in the proximal tubule is coupled to H^+ secretion through the Na^+-H^+ antiporter. As a result, HCO_3^- reabsorption is increased because of the need to reduce Na^+ excretion. In addition, the elevated aldosterone levels stimulate H^+ secretion by the distal tubule and collecting duct. Thus in persons who lose gastric contents, metabolic alkalosis and, paradoxically, acidic urine characteristically occur. Correction of the alkalosis occurs only when euvolemia is reestablished. With restoration of euvolemia, by the addition of sodium chloride (NaCl) with fluid (e.g., isotonic saline), HCO_3^- reabsorption by the proximal tubule decreases, as does H^+ secretion by the distal tubule and collecting duct. As a result, HCO_3^- excretion increases, and the plasma concentration of HCO_3^- ([HCO_3^-]) returns to normal.

IN THE CLINIC

When nonvolatile acid is added to the body fluids, as in **diabetic ketoacidosis**, the concentration of H^+ ([H^+]) increases (pH decreases) and the concentration of HCO_3^- ([HCO_3^-]) decreases. In addition, the concentration of the anion associated with the nonvolatile acid increases. This change in the anion concentration provides a convenient way to analyze the cause of a metabolic acidosis by calculating what is termed the **anion gap**. The anion gap represents the difference between the concentration of the major extracellular fluid cation (Na^+) and the major extracellular fluid anions (Cl^- and HCO_3^-):

$$\text{Anion gap} = [Na^+] - ([Cl^-] + [HCO_3^-]) \quad (8\text{-}9)$$

Under normal conditions, the anion gap ranges from 8 to 16 mEq/L. It is important to recognize that an anion gap does not actually exist. All cations are balanced by anions. The gap simply reflects the parameters that are measured. In reality:

$$[Na^+] + [\text{unmeasured cations}] =$$
$$[Cl^-] + [HCO_3^-] + [\text{unmeasured anions}] \quad (8\text{-}10)$$

If the anion of the nonvolatile acid is Cl^-, the anion gap is normal; that is, the decrease in the [HCO_3^-] is matched by an increase in [Cl^-]. The metabolic acidosis associated with diarrhea or renal tubular acidosis has a normal anion gap. In contrast, if the anion of the nonvolatile acid is not Cl^- (e.g., lactate and β-hydroxybutyrate), the anion gap increase (i.e., the decrease in the [HCO_3^-] is not matched by an increase in the [Cl^-] but rather by an increase in the concentration of the unmeasured anion). The anion gap is increased in metabolic acidosis associated with renal failure, diabetes mellitus (ketoacidosis), lactic acidosis, and the ingestion of large quantities of aspirin. Thus calculation of the anion gap is a useful way to identify the etiology of metabolic acidosis in the clinical setting.

Renal Compensation

The third and final line of defense against acid-base disorders is the kidneys. In response to an alteration in the plasma pH and Pco_2, the kidneys make appropriate adjustments in the excretion of HCO_3^- and net acid. The renal response may require several days to reach completion because it takes hours to days to increase the synthesis and activity of key H^+ and HCO_3^- transporters and the proximal tubule enzymes involved in NH_4^+ production. In the case of acidosis (increased $[H^+]$ or Pco_2), the secretion of H^+ by the nephron is stimulated, and the entire filtered load of HCO_3^- is reabsorbed. Titratable acid excretion is increased, the production and excretion of NH_4^+ are also stimulated, and thus RNAE is increased (see equation 8-7 and Figure 8-7). The new HCO_3^- generated during the process of net acid excretion is added to the body, and the plasma $[HCO_3^-]$ increases.

When alkalosis exists (decreased $[H^+]$ or Pco_2), the secretion of H^+ by the nephron is inhibited. As a result, HCO_3^- reabsorption is reduced, as is the excretion of both titratable acid and NH_4^+. Thus RNAE is decreased and HCO_3^- appears in the urine. Also, some HCO_3^- is secreted into the urine by the HCO_3^--secreting intercalated cells of the distal tubule and collecting duct. With enhanced excretion of HCO_3^-, the plasma $[HCO_3^-]$ decreases.

SIMPLE ACID-BASE DISORDERS

Table 8-1 summarizes the primary alterations and the subsequent compensatory or defense mechanisms of the various simple acid-base disorders. In all acid-base disorders the compensatory response does not correct the underlying disorder but simply reduces the magnitude of the change in pH. Correction of the acid-base disorder requires treatment of its cause.

Metabolic Acidosis

Metabolic acidosis is characterized by a decreased ECF $[HCO_3^-]$ and pH. It can develop through addition of nonvolatile acid to the body (e.g., diabetic ketoacidosis), loss of nonvolatile alkali (e.g., HCO_3^- loss caused by diarrhea), or failure of the kidneys to excrete sufficient net acid to replenish the HCO_3^- used to neutralize nonvolatile acids (e.g., renal tubular acidosis and renal failure). As previously described, the buffering of H^+ occurs in both the ECF and intracellular fluid (ICF) compartments. When the pH falls, the respiratory centers are stimulated, and the ventilatory rate is increased (respiratory compensation). This process reduces the Pco_2, which further minimizes the decrease in plasma pH. In general, a decrease of 1.2 mm Hg occurs in the Pco_2 for every 1 mEq/L decrease in ECF $[HCO_3^-]$. Thus

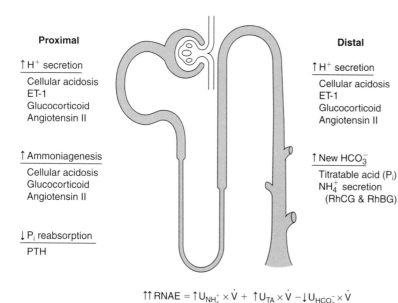

Proximal

↑H^+ secretion
  Cellular acidosis
  ET-1
  Glucocorticoid
  Angiotensin II

↑Ammoniagenesis
  Cellular acidosis
  Glucocorticoid
  Angiotensin II

↓P_i reabsorption
  PTH

Distal

↑H^+ secretion
  Cellular acidosis
  ET-1
  Glucocorticoid
  Angiotensin II

↑New HCO_3^-
  Titratable acid (P_i)
  NH_4^+ secretion
  (RhCG & RhBG)

FIGURE 8-7 ■ Response of the nephron to acidosis. *ET-1,* Endothelin; *HCO_3^-,* bicarbonate; *NH_4^+,* ammonium; *P_i,* phosphate; *PTH,* parathyroid hormone; *RhCG & RhBG,* rhesus glycoproteins; *RNAE,* renal net acid excretion; *TA,* titratable acid; *$\dot{V}$,* urine flow rate.

$$\uparrow\uparrow RNAE = \uparrow U_{NH_4^+} \times \dot{V} + \uparrow U_{TA} \times \dot{V} - \downarrow U_{HCO_3^-} \times \dot{V}$$

if the $[HCO_3^-]$ was reduced to 14 mEq/L from a normal value of 24 mEq/L, the expected decrease in Pco_2 would be 12 mm Hg and the measured Pco_2 would decrease to 28 mm Hg (normal $Pco_2 = 40$ mm Hg).

Finally, in metabolic acidosis, RNAE is increased. This increase occurs through the elimination of all HCO_3^- from the urine (enhanced reabsorption of filtered HCO_3^-) and through increased titratable acid and NH_4^+ excretion (enhanced production of new HCO_3^-). If the process that initiated the acid-base disturbance is corrected, the enhanced net acid excretion by the kidneys ultimately returns the pH and $[HCO_3^-]$ to normal. After correction of the pH, the ventilatory rate also returns to normal.

Metabolic Alkalosis

Metabolic alkalosis is characterized by an increased ECF $[HCO_3^-]$ and pH. It can occur through the addition of nonvolatile alkali to the body (e.g., ingestion of antacids), as a result of volume contraction (e.g., hemorrhage), or, more commonly, from the loss of nonvolatile acid (e.g., loss of gastric HCl because of prolonged vomiting). Buffering occurs predominantly in the ECF compartment and to a lesser degree in the ICF compartment. The increase in the pH inhibits the respiratory centers, the ventilatory rate is reduced, and thus the Pco_2 is elevated (respiratory compensation). With appropriate respiratory compensation, a 0.7 mm Hg increase in Pco_2 is expected for every 1 mEq/L rise in ECF $[HCO_3^-]$.

The renal compensatory response to metabolic alkalosis is to increase the excretion of HCO_3^- by reducing its reabsorption along the nephron. Normally, this process occurs quite rapidly (within minutes to hours) and effectively. However, as already noted, when alkalosis occurs with ECF volume contraction (e.g., vomiting in which fluid loss occurs with H^+ loss), HCO_3^- is not excreted. In volume-depleted individuals, renal excretion of HCO_3^- is impaired and alkalosis is corrected, only with restoration of euvolemia. Enhanced renal excretion of HCO_3^- eventually returns the pH and $[HCO_3^-]$ to normal, provided that the underlying cause of the initial acid-base disturbance is corrected. When the pH is corrected, the ventilatory rate also returns to normal.

Respiratory Acidosis

Respiratory acidosis is characterized by an elevated Pco_2 and reduced ECF pH. It results from decreased gas exchange across the alveoli as a result of either inadequate ventilation (e.g., drug-induced depression of the respiratory centers) or impaired gas diffusion (e.g., pulmonary edema, such as that which occurs in cardiovascular or lung disease). In contrast to metabolic acid-base disorders, buffering during respiratory acidosis occurs almost entirely in the ICF compartment. The increase in the Pco_2 and the decrease in pH stimulate both HCO_3^- reabsorption by the nephron and titratable acid and NH_4^+ excretion (renal compensation). Together, these responses increase RNAE and generate new HCO_3^-. The renal compensatory response takes several days to develop fully. Consequently, respiratory acid-base disorders are commonly divided into acute and chronic phases. In the acute phase, the time for the renal compensatory response is not sufficient, and the body relies on ICF buffering to minimize the change in pH. During this phase, and because of the buffering, a 1 mEq/L increase in ECF $[HCO_3^-]$ occurs for every 10 mm Hg rise in Pco_2. In the chronic phase, renal compensation occurs, and a 3.5 mEq/L increase in ECF $[HCO_3^-]$ occurs for each 10 mm Hg rise in Pco_2. Correction of the underlying disorder returns the Pco_2 to normal, and renal net acid excretion decreases to its initial level.

TABLE 8-1			
Characteristics of Simple Acid-Base Disorders			
DISORDER	**PLASMA pH**	**PRIMARY ALTERATION**	**DEFENSE MECHANISMS**
Metabolic acidosis	↓	↓ ECF $[HCO_3^-]$	ICF and ECF buffers Hyperventilation (↓ Pco_2) ↑RNAE
Metabolic alkalosis	↑	↑ ECF $[HCO_3^-]$	ICF and ECF buffers Hypoventilation (↑ Pco_2) ↓RNAE
Respiratory acidosis	↓	↑ Pco_2	ICF buffers ↑ RNAE
Respiratory alkalosis	↑	↓Pco_2	ICF buffers ↓ RNAE

ECF, Extracellular fluid; *ICF,* intracellular fluid; *Pco_2,* partial pressure of CO_2; *RNAE,* renal net acid excretion.

Respiratory Alkalosis

Respiratory alkalosis is characterized by a reduced Pco_2 and an increased ECF pH. It results from increased gas exchange in the lungs, usually caused by increased ventilation from stimulation of the respiratory centers (e.g., by drugs or disorders of the central nervous system). Hyperventilation also occurs at high altitude and as a result of anxiety, pain, or fear. As noted, buffering is primarily in the ICF compartment. As with respiratory acidosis, respiratory alkalosis has both acute and chronic phases reflecting the time required for renal compensation to occur. In the acute phase of respiratory alkalosis, which reflects intracellular buffering, the ECF $[HCO_3^-]$ decreases 2 mEq/L for every 10 mm Hg decrease in Pco_2. With renal compensation, the elevated pH and reduced Pco_2 inhibit HCO_3^- reabsorption by the nephron and reduce TA and NH_4^+ excretion. As a result of these two effects, net acid excretion is reduced. With complete renal compensation, an expected 5 mEq/L decrease in ECF $[HCO_3^-]$ occurs for every 10 mm Hg reduction in Pco_2. Correction of the underlying disorder returns the Pco_2 to normal, and renal excretion of acid then increases to its initial level.

ANALYSIS OF ACID-BASE DISORDERS

The analysis of an acid-base disorder is directed at identifying the underlying cause so that appropriate therapy can be initiated. The patient's medical history and associated physical findings often provide valuable clues about the nature and origin of an acid-base disorder. In addition, the analysis of an arterial blood sample is frequently required. Such an analysis is straightforward if approached systematically. For example, consider the following data:

pH	7.35
$[HCO_3^-]$	16 mEq/L
Pco_2	30 mm Hg

The acid-base disorder represented by these values, or any other set of values, can be determined using the following three-step approach (Figure 8-8):

1. *Examination of the pH:* When the pH is considered first, the underlying disorder can be classified as either an acidosis or an alkalosis. The defense mechanisms of the body cannot correct an acid-base disorder by themselves. Thus even if the defense mechanisms are completely operative, the change in pH indicates the acid-base disorder. In the example provided, the pH of 7.35 indicates acidosis.

2. *Determination of metabolic versus respiratory disorder:* Simple acid-base disorders are either metabolic or respiratory. To determine which disorder is present, the clinician must next examine the ECF $[HCO_3^-]$ and Pco_2. As previously discussed, acidosis could be the result of a decrease in the $[HCO_3^-]$ (metabolic) or an increase in the Pco_2 (respiratory). Alternatively, alkalosis could be the result of an increase in the ECF $[HCO_3^-]$ (metabolic) or a decrease in the Pco_2 (respiratory). For the example provided, the ECF $[HCO_3^-]$ is reduced from normal (normal = 24 mEq/L), as is the Pco_2 (normal = 40 mm Hg). The disorder therefore must be metabolic acidosis; it cannot be a respiratory acidosis because the Pco_2 is reduced.

3. *Analysis of a compensatory response:* Metabolic disorders result in compensatory changes in ventilation and thus in the Pco_2, whereas respiratory disorders result in compensatory changes in RNAE and thus in the ECF $[HCO_3^-]$. In an appropriately compensated metabolic acidosis, the Pco_2 is decreased, whereas it is elevated in compensated metabolic alkalosis. With respiratory acidosis, compensation results in an elevation of the $[HCO_3^-]$. Conversely, the ECF $[HCO_3^-]$ is reduced in response to respiratory alkalosis. In this example, the Pco_2 is reduced from normal, and the magnitude of this reduction (10 mm Hg decrease in Pco_2 for an 8 mEq/L increase in ECF $[HCO_3^-]$) is as expected (see Figure 8-8). Therefore the acid-base disorder is a simple metabolic acidosis with appropriate respiratory compensation.

If the appropriate compensatory response is not present, a **mixed acid-base disorder** should be suspected. Such a disorder reflects the presence of two or more underlying causes for the acid-base disturbance. A mixed disorder should be suspected when analysis of the arterial blood gas indicates that appropriate

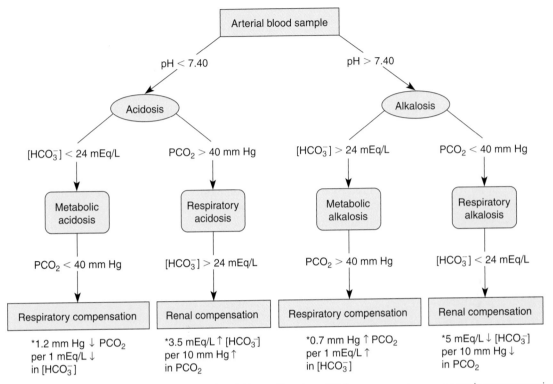

FIGURE 8-8 ■ Approach for the analysis of simple acid-base disorders. *If the compensatory response is not appropriate, a mixed acid-base disorder should be suspected. HCO_3^-, bicarbonate; Pco_2, partial pressure of carbon dioxide.

compensation has not occurred. For example, consider the following data:

pH	6.96
$[HCO_3^-]$	12 mEq/L
Pco_2	55 mm Hg

When the three-step approach is followed, it is evident that the disturbance is an acidosis that has both a metabolic component (ECF $[HCO_3^-]$ <24 mEq/L) and a respiratory component (Pco_2 >40 mm Hg). Thus this disorder is mixed. Mixed acid-base disorders can occur, for example, in a person who has a history of a chronic pulmonary disease such as emphysema (i.e., chronic respiratory acidosis) and who experiences an acute gastrointestinal illness with

diarrhea. Because diarrhea fluid contains HCO_3^-, its loss from the body results in the development of metabolic acidosis.

A mixed acid-base disorder also is indicated when a patient has abnormal Pco_2 and ECF $[HCO_3^-]$ values but the pH is normal. Such a condition can develop in a patient who has ingested a large quantity of aspirin. The salicylic acid (which is the active ingredient in aspirin) produces metabolic acidosis, and at the same time it stimulates the respiratory centers, causing hyperventilation and respiratory alkalosis. Thus the patient has a reduced ECF $[HCO_3^-]$ and a reduced Pco_2. (Note: The Pco_2 is lower than would occur with normal respiratory compensation of a metabolic acidosis.)

SUMMARY

1. The pH of the body fluids is maintained within a narrow range by the coordinated function of the lungs and kidneys. These organs maintain acid-base balance by balancing the excretion of acid and alkali with the amounts ingested in the diet and produced by metabolism.

2. The kidneys maintain acid-base balance through the excretion of an amount of acid equal to the amount of nonvolatile acid produced by metabolism and the quantity ingested in the diet. The kidneys also prevent the loss of HCO_3^- in the urine by reabsorbing virtually all the HCO_3^- filtered at the glomeruli. Both the reabsorption of filtered HCO_3^- and the excretion of acid are accomplished by the secretion of H^+ by the nephrons.

3. RNAE is quantitated as:

$$RNAE = [(U_{NH_4^+} \times \dot{V}) + (U_{TA} \times \dot{V})]$$
$$- (U_{HCO_3^-} \times \dot{V})$$

where $(U_{NH_4^+} \times \dot{V})$ and $(U_{TA} \times \dot{V})$ are the rates of excretion (mEq/day) of NH_4^+ and titratable acid and $(U_{HCO_3^-} \times \dot{V})$ is the amount of HCO_3^- lost in the urine (equivalent to adding H^+ to the body).

4. The primary titratable urinary buffer is P_i (titratable acid). The excretion of titratable acid together with the production (from glutamine metabolism) and excretion of NH_4^+ are critical to the generation of new HCO_3^- by the kidneys.

5. The body uses three lines of defense to minimize the impact of acid-base disorders on body fluid pH: (1) ECF and ICF buffering, (2) respiratory compensation, and (3) renal compensation.

6. Metabolic acid-base disorders result from primary alterations in the ECF $[HCO_3^-]$, which in turn results from the addition of acid to or loss of alkali from the body. In response to metabolic acidosis, pulmonary ventilation is increased, which decreases the P_{CO_2}, and renal net acid excretion is increased. An increase in the ECF $[HCO_3^-]$ causes alkalosis. This condition decreases pulmonary ventilation, which elevates the P_{CO_2}. Renal net acid excretion is decreased, and net alkali excretion results. The pulmonary response to metabolic acid-base disorders occurs in a matter of minutes. The renal response may take several days to develop fully.

7. Respiratory acid-base disorders result from primary alterations in the P_{CO_2}. Elevation of the P_{CO_2} produces acidosis, and the kidneys respond with an increase in net acid excretion. Conversely, reduction of the P_{CO_2} produces alkalosis, and renal net acid excretion is reduced. The kidneys respond to respiratory acid-base disorders over several hours to days.

KEY WORDS AND CONCEPTS

- Over3
- Acid
- Alkali
- HCO_3^- buffer system
- Carbonic anhydrase (CA)
- Henderson-Hasselbalch equation
- Acidosis
- Alkalosis
- Volatile acid
- Nonvolatile acid
- Net endogenous acid production (NEAP)
- Diabetes mellitus
- Hypoxia
- Intercalated cell
- Titratable acids
- Ammonium (NH_4^+)
- Renal net acid excretion (RNAE)
- Formation of new HCO_3^-
- Nonionic diffusion
- Diffusion trapping (of ammonia)
- Metabolic acid-base disorder
- Respiratory acid-base disorder
- Chemoreceptors
- Extracellular fluid (ECF) and intracellular fluid (ICF) buffering
- Respiratory compensation
- Plasma anion gap
- Urinary net charge (urine anion gap)
- Renal compensation
- Simple acid-base disorders

SELF-STUDY PROBLEMS

1. If there were no urinary buffers, how much urine (L/day) would the kidneys have to produce to excrete net acid equal to the amount of nonvolatile acid produced from metabolism? Assume that nonvolatile acid production is 70 mEq/day and the minimum urine pH is 4.0.

2. In the accompanying table, indicate the simple acid-base disorder that exists for the laboratory data given. Use the following as normal values: pH = 7.40; $[HCO_3^-]$ = 24 mEq/L; P_{CO_2} = 40 mm Hg.

pH	$[HCO_3^-]$ (mEq/L)	P_{CO_2} (mm Hg)	Disorder
7.23	10	25	_____
7.46	30	44	_____
7.37	28	50	_____
7.66	22	20	_____
7.34	26	50	_____
7.54	18	22	_____

3. A previously healthy person experiences a gastrointestinal illness with nausea and vomiting. The following laboratory data are obtained after 12 hours of this illness:

Body weight:	70 kg
Blood pressure:	120/80 mm Hg
Plasma pH:	7.48
P_{CO_2}:	44 mm Hg
Plasma $[HCO_3^-]$:	32 mEq/L
Urine pH:	7.5

a. What is the acid-base disorder of this person? What was its origin? The illness continues, and 48 hours later the following laboratory data are obtained:

Body weight:	68 kg
Blood pressure:	80/40 mm Hg
Plasma pH:	7.50
P_{CO_2}:	48 mm Hg
Plasma $[HCO_3^-]$:	36 mEq/L
Urine pH:	6.0

b. Has the acid-base disturbance changed? How do you explain the paradoxical decrease in urine pH?

4. What would happen to urinary HCO_3^- excretion if a drug that inhibits carbonic anhydrase is administered, and by what mechanism would this effect occur? What type of acid-base disorder could result from the use of this drug?

5. A previously healthy 28-year-old man with severe right flank pain is seen in the emergency department. Shortly after arrival, he passes a kidney stone. He reports that several people in his family also have had kidney stones. The following laboratory data are obtained (see Appendix B for normal values):

Serum $[Na^+]$:	137 mEq/L
Serum $[K^+]$:	3.1 mEq/L
Serum $[Cl^-]$:	111 mEq/L
Serum $[HCO_3^-]$:	13 mEq/L
Arterial pH:	7.28
Arterial P_{CO_2}:	28 mm Hg
Urine pH:	7.10

a. What is the acid-base disorder, and what is the plasma anion gap?

b. How do you explain his urine pH value, and how did this contribute to the formation of his kidney stone?

9

REGULATION OF CALCIUM AND PHOSPHATE HOMEOSTASIS

O B J E C T I V E S

Upon completion of this chapter, the student should be able to answer the following questions:

1. What is the physiologic importance of Ca^{++} and inorganic phosphate (P_i)?

2. How does the body maintain Ca^{++} and P_i homeostasis?

3. What roles do the kidneys, intestinal tract, and bone play in maintaining plasma Ca^{++} and P_i levels?

4. What hormones and factors regulate plasma Ca^{++} and P_i levels?

5. What are the cellular mechanisms responsible for Ca^{++} and P_i reabsorption along the nephron?

6. What hormones regulate renal Ca^{++} and P_i excretion by the kidneys?

7. What is the role of the calcium-sensing receptor?

8. What are some of the more common clinical disorders of Ca^{++} and P_i homeostasis?

9. What is the role of the kidneys in the production of calcitriol (active form of vitamin D)?

10. What effects do loop and thiazide diuretics have on Ca^{++} excretion?

Ca^{++} and inorganic phosphate (P_i)* are multivalent ions that subserve many complex and vital functions. Ca^{++} is an important cofactor in many enzymatic reactions, it is a key second messenger in numerous signaling pathways, it plays an important role in the excitability of nerve and muscle, signal transduction, blood clotting, and muscle contraction, and it is a critical component of the extracellular matrix, cartilage, teeth, and bone. P_i, like Ca^{++}, is a key component of bone. P_i is important for metabolic processes, including formation of adenosine triphosphate, and it is an important component of nucleotides, nucleosides, and phospholipids. Phosphorylation of proteins is an important mechanism of cellular signaling, and P_i is an important buffer in cells, plasma, and urine.

In adults, the kidneys play important roles in regulating total body Ca^{++} and P_i by excreting the amount of Ca^{++} and P_i that is absorbed by the intestinal tract (normal bone remodeling results in no net addition of Ca^{++} and P_i to the bone or Ca^{++} and P_i release from the bone). If the plasma concentrations of Ca^{++} and P_i decline substantially, intestinal absorption, bone

---

*At physiologic pH, inorganic phosphate exists as HPO_4^{-2} and $H_2PO_4^-$ (pK = 6.8). For simplicity, these ion species are collectively refered to as P_i.

resorption (i.e., the loss of Ca^{++} and P_i from bone), and renal tubular reabsorption increase and return plasma concentrations of Ca^{++} and P_i to normal levels. During growth and pregnancy, intestinal absorption exceeds urinary excretion, and these ions accumulate in newly formed fetal tissue and bone. In contrast, bone disease (e.g., osteoporosis) or a decline in lean body mass increases urinary Ca^{++} and P_i loss without a change in intestinal absorption. These conditions produce a net loss of Ca^{++} and P_i from the body. Finally, during chronic renal failure, P_i accumulates in the body because absorption by the intestinal tract exceeds excretion in the urine. This situation can lead to the accumulation of P_i in the body and changes in bone (see In The Clinic on page 157).

The kidneys, in conjunction with the intestinal tract and bone, play a major role in maintaining plasma Ca^{++} and P_i levels as well as Ca^{++} and P_i balance. Accordingly, this chapter discusses Ca^{++} and P_i handling by the kidneys, with an emphasis on the hormones and factors that regulate urinary excretion.

CALCIUM

Cellular processes in which Ca^{++} plays an important role include bone formation, cell division and growth, blood coagulation, hormone-response coupling, and electrical stimulus-response coupling (e.g., muscle contraction and neurotransmitter release). A total of 99% of Ca^{++} is stored in bone and teeth, approximately 1% is found in the intracellular fluid (ICF), and 0.1% is located in the extracellular fluid (ECF). The total Ca^{++} concentration ([Ca^{++}]) in plasma is 10 mg/dL (2.5 mmol/L, or 5 mEq/L), and its concentration is normally maintained within very narrow limits. Approximately 50% of the Ca^{++} in plasma is ionized, 40% is bound to plasma proteins (mainly albumin), and 10% is complexed to several anions, including P_i, bicarbonate (HCO_3^-), citrate, and $SO_4^=$ (Figure 9-1). The pH of plasma influences this distribution (Figure 9-2). Acidemia increases the percentage of ionized Ca^{++} at the expense of Ca^{++} bound to proteins, whereas alkalemia decreases the percentage of ionized Ca^{++}, again by altering the Ca^{++} bound to proteins. Persons with alkalemia are susceptible to **tetany** (tonic muscular spasms), whereas persons with acidemia are less susceptible to tetany, even when total plasma Ca^{++} levels

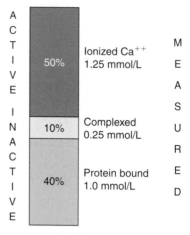

Distribution of Ca^{++} in plasma

ACTIVE — INACTIVE

MEASURED

Ionized Ca^{++} 1.25 mmol/L — 50%

Complexed 0.25 mmol/L — 10%

Protein bound 1.0 mmol/L — 40%

FIGURE 9-1 ■ Distribution of Ca^{++} in plasma.

are reduced. The increase in [H^+] in patients with metabolic acidosis causes more H^+ to bind to plasma proteins, P_i, HCO_3^-, citrate, and $SO_4^=$, thereby displacing Ca^{++}. This displacement increases the plasma concentration of ionized Ca^{++}. In alkalemia, the [H^+] of plasma decreases. Some H^+ ions dissociate from plasma proteins, P_i, HCO_3^-, citrate, and $SO_4^=$ in exchange for Ca^{++}, thereby decreasing the plasma concentration of ionized Ca^{++}. In addition, the plasma albumin concentration also affects ionized plasma [Ca^{++}]. **Hypoalbuminemia** increases the ionized [Ca^{++}], whereas **hyperalbuminemia** decreases ionized plasma [Ca^{++}]. The total measured plasma [Ca^{++}] does not reflect the total ionized [Ca^{++}], which is the physiologic relevant measure of plasma [Ca^{++}]. A low ionized plasma [Ca^{++}] **(hypocalcemia)** increases the excitability of nerve and muscle cells and can lead to hypocalcemic tetany. Tetany associated with hypocalcemia occurs because hypocalcemia causes the threshold potential to shift to more negative values (i.e., closer to the resting membrane voltage; see Figure 9-3). An elevated ionized plasma [Ca^{++}] **(hypercalcemia)** may decrease neuromuscular excitability or produce cardiac arrhythmias, lethargy, disorientation, and even death.* This effect of

---

*In clinical practice, the terms "hypercalcemia" and "hypocalcemia" often are used to describe a high or low total plasma [Ca^{++}], respectively, even though this usage is not the physiologically correct usage of hypercalcemia and hypocalcemia.

Effect of pH on Plasma [Ca^{++}]

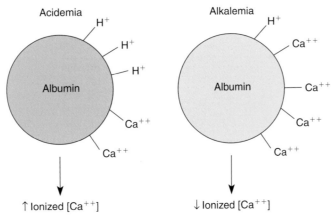

FIGURE 9-2 ■ Effect of pH on plasma concentration of Ca^{++} ([Ca^{++}]).

Effect of Ca^{++} on nerve and muscle excitability

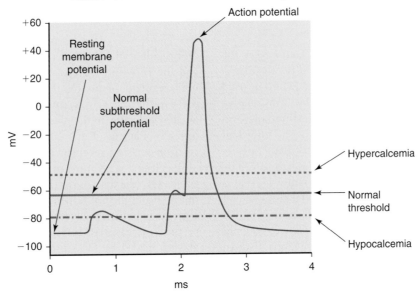

FIGURE 9-3 ■ Effect of Ca^{++} on nerve and muscle excitability.

hypercalcemia occurs because an elevated plasma [Ca^{++}] causes the threshold potential to shift to less negative values (i.e., further from the resting membrane voltage). Plasma [Ca^{++}] is regulated within a very narrow range primarily by **parathyroid hormone** (PTH), **calcitriol** (1,25-dihydroxyvitamin D), the active metabolite of vitamin D$_3$, and plasma Ca^{++}.

Within cells, Ca^{++} is sequestered in the endoplasmic reticulum and mitochondria, or it is bound to proteins. Thus the free intracellular [Ca^{++}] is very low (~100 nmol). The large concentration gradient for [Ca^{++}] across cell membranes is maintained by a Ca^{++}–adenosine triphosphatase (ATPase) pump (PMCa1b) in all cells and by a 3Na$^+$-Ca^{++} exchanger (NCX1) in some cells.

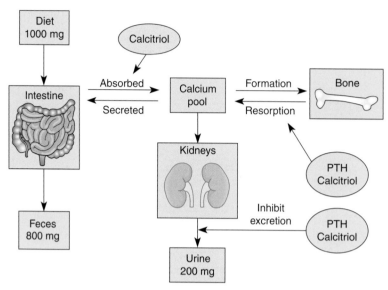

FIGURE 9-4 ■ Overview of Ca^{++} homeostasis. *PTH,* Parathyroid hormone.

Overview of Ca^{++} Homeostasis

Ca^{++} homeostasis depends on two factors: (1) the total amount of Ca^{++} in the body and (2) the distribution of Ca^{++} between bone and the ECF. The total body Ca^{++} level is determined by the relative amounts of Ca^{++} absorbed by the intestinal tract and excreted by the kidneys (Figure 9-4). The intestinal tract absorbs Ca^{++} through an active, carrier-mediated transport mechanism that is stimulated by calcitriol, the active metabolite of vitamin D$_3$ that is produced in the proximal tubule of the kidneys. Net Ca^{++} absorption by the intestine is normally 200 mg/day (5 mmol/day), but it can increase to 600 mg/day (15 mmol/day) when calcitriol levels rise. In adults, Ca^{++} excretion by the kidneys equals the amount absorbed by the gastrointestinal tract (200 mg/day), and it changes in parallel with intestinal absorption. Thus in adults, Ca^{++} balance is maintained because the amount of Ca^{++} ingested in an average diet (1000 mg/day or 25 mmol/day) equals the amount lost in the feces (800 mg/day or 20 mmol/day), the amount that escapes absorption by the intestinal tract, plus the amount excreted in the urine (200 mg/day).

The second factor that controls Ca^{++} homeostasis is the distribution of Ca^{++} between bone and the ECF

(see Figure 9-4). Two hormones (PTH and calcitriol*) regulate the distribution of Ca^{++} between bone and the ECF and thereby, in concert with the kidneys, regulate the plasma [Ca^{++}]. PTH is secreted by the parathyroid glands, and its secretion is stimulated by a decline in the plasma [Ca^{++}] (i.e., hypocalcemia). Plasma Ca^{++} is an agonist of the **calcium-sensing receptor** (CaSR), which is located in the plasma membrane of chief cells in parathyroid glands (see the discussion that follows). Hypercalcemia activates the CaSR, which decreases PTH release, whereas hypocalcemia reduces CaSR activity, which in turn increases PTH release. PTH increases the plasma [Ca^{++}] by (1) stimulating bone resorption, (2) increasing Ca^{++} reabsorption by the distal tubule of the kidney, and (3) stimulating the production of calcitriol, which in turn increases Ca^{++} absorption by the intestinal tract and facilitates PTH-mediated

---

*Calcitonin is secreted by thyroid C-cells (also known as parafollicular cells), and its secretion is stimulated by hypercalcemia. Calcitonin decreases the plasma [Ca^{++}] mainly by stimulating bone formation (i.e., deposition of Ca^{++} in bone). Although calcitonin plays an important role in Ca^{++} homeostasis in lower vertebrates, it plays only a minor role in Ca^{++} homeostasis in humans and thus is not discussed further in this book.

bone resorption. The production of calcitriol in the kidney is stimulated by hypocalcemia and hypophosphatemia. Calcitriol increases the plasma [Ca^{++}] primarily by stimulating Ca^{++} absorption from the intestinal tract. It also facilitates the action of PTH on bone and enhances Ca^{++} reabsorption in the kidneys by increasing the expression of key Ca^{++} transport and binding proteins in the kidneys. In addition, hypercalcemia activates the CaSR in the thick ascending limb of Henle's loop, inhibiting Ca^{++} reabsorption in this segment, which results in an increase in urinary Ca^{++} excretion and thereby reduces plasma [Ca^{++}]. Hypocalcemia has the opposite effect. Importantly, regulation of Ca^{++} excretion by the kidneys is one of the major ways that the body regulates plasma [Ca^{++}].

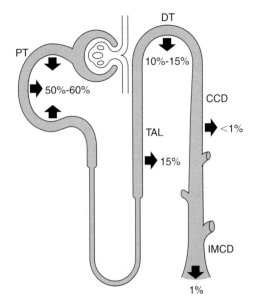

FIGURE 9-5 ■ Overview of Ca^{++} transport along the nephron. Percentages refer to the amount of the filtered Ca^{++} reabsorbed by each segment. *CCD,* Cortical collecting duct; *DT,* distal tubule; *IMCD,* inner medullary collecting duct; *PT,* proximal tubule; *TAL,* thick ascending limb.

IN THE CLINIC

Conditions that lower parathyroid hormone (PTH) levels (e.g., hypoparathyroidism after parathyroidectomy for an adenoma) reduce plasma [Ca^{++}], which can cause **hypocalcemic tetany** (intermittent muscular contractions). In severe cases, hypocalcemic tetany can cause death by asphyxiation. Hypercalcemia also can cause lethal cardiac arrhythmias and decreased neuromuscular excitability. Clinically, the most common causes of hypercalcemia are primary hyperparathyroidism and malignancy-associated hypercalcemia. Primary hyperparathyroidism results most often from the overproduction of PTH caused by a benign tumor of the parathyroid glands. In contrast, malignancy-associated hypercalcemia, which occurs in 10% to 20% of all patients with cancer, is caused by the secretion of **parathyroid hormone–related peptide,** a PTH-like hormone secreted by carcinomas in various organs. Increased levels of PTH and parathyroid hormone–related peptide cause hypercalcemia and hypercalciuria.

Ca^{++} Transport Along the Nephron

The Ca^{++} available for glomerular filtration consists of the ionized fraction and the amount complexed with anions. Thus about 60% of the Ca^{++} in the plasma is available for glomerular filtration. Normally, 99% of the filtered Ca^{++} is reabsorbed by the nephron (Figure 9-5). The proximal tubule reabsorbs about 50% to 60% of the filtered Ca^{++}. Another 15% is reabsorbed in the loop of Henle (mainly the cortical portion of the thick ascending limb), about 10% to 15% is reabsorbed by the distal tubule, and <1% is reabsorbed by the collecting duct. About 1% (200 mg/day) is excreted in the urine. This fraction is equal to the net amount absorbed daily by the intestinal tract.

Ca^{++} reabsorption by the proximal tubule occurs primarily via the paracellular pathway (see Figure 4-1). This passive, paracellular reabsorption of Ca^{++} is driven by the lumen-positive transepithelial voltage across the second half of the proximal tubule and by a favorable concentration gradient of Ca^{++}, both of which are established by transcellular sodium and water reabsorption in the first half of the proximal tubule.

Ca^{++} reabsorption by the loop of Henle also occurs primarily via the paracellular pathway. Like the proximal tubule, Ca^{++} and Na$^+$ reabsorption in the thick ascending limb parallel each other. These processes are parallel because of the significant component of Ca^{++} reabsorption that occurs via passive, paracellular reabsorption secondary to Na^+ reabsorption that generates a lumen-positive transepithelial voltage. Loop diuretics inhibit Na^+ reabsorption by the thick ascending limb of the loop of Henle, and in so doing reduce the magnitude of the lumen-positive transepithelial voltage (see Chapter 10). This action in turn inhibits the reabsorption of Ca^{++} via the paracellular pathway. Thus loop diuretics are used to increase renal Ca^{++} excretion in patients with hypercalcemia.

In the distal tubule, where the voltage in the tubule lumen is electrically negative with respect to the blood, Ca^{++} reabsorption is entirely active because Ca^{++} is reabsorbed against its electrochemical gradient (Figure 9-6). Thus Ca^{++} reabsorption by the distal tubule is exclusively transcellular. Calcium enters the cell across the apical membrane by a Ca^{++}-permeable ion channel (TRPV5). Inside the cell, Ca^{++} binds to calbindin-D_{28k}. The calbindin-Ca^{++} complex carries Ca^{++} across the cell and delivers it to the basolateral membrane, where it is extruded from the cell primarily by the $3Na^+/Ca^{++}$ antiporter (NCX1); however, the

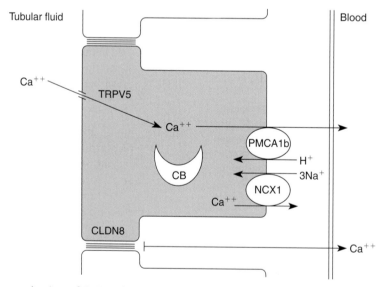

FIGURE 9-6 ■ Cellular mechanism of Ca^{++} reabsorption by the distal tubule. Ca^{++} is reabsorbed exclusively by a cellular pathway. Ca^{++} enters the cell across the apical membrane via a Ca^{++}-permeable ion channel (*TRPV5*). Inside cells, Ca^{++} binds to calbindin (calbindin-D_{28K} [*CB*]), and the Ca^{++}-calbindin complex diffuses across the cell to deliver Ca^{++} to the basolateral membrane. Ca^{++} is transported across the basolateral membrane primarily by a 3 (or 4) Na^+-Ca^{++} antiporter (*NCX1*), and also by a Ca^{++}-H^+ adenosine triphosphatase (*PMCA1b*). Claudin-8 (*CLDN8*) is a tight junction protein that is impermeable to Ca^{++} and thereby prevents the backdiffusion of Ca^{++} across the tight junction into the tubule lumen, which is electrically negative compared with the blood side of the cell.

Ca^{++} ATPase (PMCA1b) also may contribute. Urinary Na^+ and Ca^{++} excretion usually change in parallel. However, excretion of these ions does not always change in parallel because the reabsorption of Ca^{++} and Na^+ by the distal tubule is independent and is differentially regulated. For example, **thiazide diuretics** inhibit Na^+ reabsorption by the distal tubule and stimulate Ca^{++} reabsorption by this segment. Accordingly, the net effects of thiazide diuretics are to increase urinary Na^+ excretion and reduce urinary Ca^{++} excretion (see Chapter 10). Accordingly, because thiazide diuretics reduce urinary Ca^{++} excretion, they often are given to reduce the urinary $[Ca^{++}]$ in persons who produce kidney stones that contain Ca^{++}.

Regulation of Urinary Ca⁺⁺ Excretion

Several hormones and factors influence urinary Ca^{++} excretion (Table 9-1). Of these hormones and factors, PTH exerts the most powerful control on renal Ca^{++} excretion, and it is the primary hormone/factor responsible for maintaining Ca^{++} homeostasis. Overall, this hormone stimulates Ca^{++} reabsorption by the

kidneys (i.e., reduces Ca^{++} excretion). Although PTH inhibits the reabsorption of NaCl and fluid, and therefore Ca^{++} reabsorption by the proximal tubule, PTH stimulates Ca^{++} reabsorption by the thick ascending limb of the loop of Henle and the distal tubule. Thus the net effect of PTH is to enhance renal Ca^{++} reabsorption. Changes in the plasma $[Ca^{++}]$ also regulate urinary Ca^{++} excretion, with hypercalcemia increasing excretion and hypocalcemia decreasing excretion. Hypercalcemia increases urinary Ca^{++} excretion by (1) reducing proximal tubule Ca^{++} reabsorption (reduced paracellular reabsorption due to increased interstitial fluid $[Ca^{++}]$); (2) inhibiting Ca^{++} reabsorption by the thick ascending limb of the loop of Henle via activation of the CaSR located in the basolateral membrane of these cells (NaCl reabsorption is decreased, thereby reducing the magnitude of the lumen-positive transepithelial voltage); and (3) suppressing Ca^{++} reabsorption by the distal tubule by reducing PTH levels. As a result, urinary Ca^{++} excretion increases. Hypocalcemia has the opposite effect on urinary Ca^{++} excretion, primarily by increasing Ca^{++} reabsorption by the proximal tubule and thick ascending limb. Calcitriol

TABLE 9-1			
Summary of Hormones, Factors, and Diuretics Affecting Ca⁺⁺ Reabsorption			
	NEPHRON LOCATION		
FACTOR/HORMONE	**PROXIMAL TUBULE**	**TAL**	**DISTAL TUBULE**
PTH (PTHrP)*	Decrease	Increase	Increase
Calcitriol			Increase
Volume expansion	Decrease	No change	Decrease
Hypercalcemia	Decrease	Decrease (CaSR)	Decrease (via PTH)
Hypocalcemia	Increase	Increase	
Phosphate loading (hyperphosphatemia)			Increase (via PTH)
Phosphate depletion (hypophosphatemia)	Decrease		Decrease (via PTH)
Acidemia			Decrease
Alkalemia			Increase
Loop diuretics		Decrease	
Thiazide diuretics			Increase

*PTH inhibits Ca^{++} reabsorption by the proximal tubule but stimulates reabsorption by the TAL and distal tubule. Overall, the net effect is to increase Ca^{++} reabsorption and thereby reduce urinary Ca^{++} excretion.
CaSR, Calcium-sensing receptor; *PTH*, parathyroid hormone; *PTHrP*, parathyroid hormone–related peptide; *TAL*, thick ascending limb.
Modified from Mount DB, Yu ASL: Transport of inorganic solutes: sodium, chloride, potassium, magnesium, calcium and phosphate. In Brenner BM, editor: *Brenner and Rector's the kidney*, ed 8, Philadelphia, 2008, Saunders Elsevier.

enhances Ca^{++} reabsorption by the distal tubule, but it is less effective than PTH.

Several factors disturb Ca^{++} excretion. An increase in the plasma $[P_i]$ (e.g., caused by a dramatic increase in the dietary intake of P_i or by reduced kidney function) elevates PTH levels both directly and by decreasing the ionized plasma $[Ca^{++}]$, and thereby decreases Ca^{++} excretion. A decline in the plasma $[P_i]$ (e.g., caused by dietary P_i depletion) has the opposite effect. (Note: With normal kidney function, changes in dietary P_i intake over a sevenfold range have no effect on plasma $[P_i]$.) Changes in the ECF volume alter Ca^{++} excretion mainly by affecting sodium chloride (NaCl) and fluid reabsorption in the proximal tubule. Volume contraction increases NaCl and water reabsorption by the proximal tubule and thereby enhances Ca^{++} reabsorption. Accordingly, urinary Ca^{++} excretion declines. Volume expansion has the opposite effect. Acidemia increases Ca^{++} excretion, whereas alkalemia decreases excretion. The regulation of Ca^{++} reabsorption by pH occurs primarily in the distal tubule. Alkalosis stimulates the apical membrane Ca^{++} channel (TRPV5), thereby increasing Ca^{++} reabsorption. By contrast, acidosis inhibits the same channel, thereby reducing Ca^{++} reabsorption. Finally, as previously noted, loop diuretics inhibit Ca^{++} reabsorption by the thick ascending limb (TAL), and thiazide diuretics stimulate Ca^{++} reabsorption by the distal tubule.

Calcium-Sensing Receptor

The CaSR is a receptor expressed in the plasma membrane of cells involved in regulating Ca^{++} homeostasis. The CaSR senses small changes in extracellular $[Ca^{++}]$. Ca^{++} binds to CaSR receptors in PTH-secreting cells of the parathyroid gland and calcitriol-producing cells of the proximal tubule. Activation of the receptor by an increase in plasma $[Ca^{++}]$ results in inhibition of PTH secretion and the production of calcitriol by the proximal tubule. Moreover, the reduction in PTH secretion also contributes to decreased production of calcitriol because PTH is a potent stimulus of calcitriol synthesis. By contrast, a decrease in plasma $[Ca^{++}]$ has the opposite effect on PTH and calcitriol secretion.

The CaSR also maintains Ca^{++} homeostasis by directly regulating Ca^{++} excretion by the kidneys.

CaSRs in the thick ascending limb respond directly to changes in plasma $[Ca^{++}]$ and regulate Ca^+ absorption. An increase in plasma $[Ca^{++}]$ activates CaSR in the TAL and inhibits Ca^{++} absorption, thereby stimulating urinary Ca^{++} excretion. By contrast, a decrease in plasma $[Ca^{++}]$ leads to an increase in Ca^{++} absorption by the TAL and a corresponding decrease in urinary Ca^{++} excretion. Thus the direct effect of plasma $[Ca^{++}]$ on CaSRs in the TAL acts in concert with changes in PTH, which regulates Ca^{++} reabsorption by the distal tubule to regulate urinary Ca^{++} excretion and thereby maintain Ca^{++} homeostasis.

IN THE CLINIC

Mutations in the gene coding for the calcium-sensing receptor (**CaSR**) cause disorders in Ca^{++} homeostasis. **Familial hypocalciuric hypercalcemia** is an autosomal dominant disease caused by an inactivating mutation of CaSR. The hypercalcemia is caused by deranged Ca^{++}-regulated parathyroid hormone (PTH) secretion; that is, the set point for Ca^{++}-regulated PTH secretion is shifted such that PTH levels are elevated at any level of plasma $[Ca^{++}]$ and are not suppressed in the setting of hypercalcemia. The hypocalciuria is caused by enhanced Ca^{++} reabsorption in the thick ascending limb and distal tubule as a result of elevated PTH levels and defective CaSR regulation of Ca^{++} transport in the kidneys. **Autosomal dominant hypoparathyroidism** is caused by an activating mutation in CaSR. Activation of CaSRs causes deranged Ca^{++}-regulated PTH secretion (i.e., the set point for Ca^{++}-regulated PTH secretion is shifted such that PTH levels are decreased at any level of plasma $[Ca^{++}]$). Hypercalciuria results and is caused by decreased PTH levels and defective CaSR-regulated Ca^{++} transport in the kidneys.

PHOSPHATE

P_i is an important component of many organic molecules, including deoxyribonucleic acid, ribonucleic acid, adenosine triphosphate, nucleotides, nucleosides, and phospholipids and intermediates of metabolic pathways . Like Ca^{++}, P_i is a major constituent of bone. Its concentration in plasma is an important determinant of bone formation and resorption. In addition, urinary P_i is an important buffer (titratable acid) involved in the maintenance of acid-base balance (see Chapter 8). Eighty-five percent of P_i is located in bone and teeth, approximately 14% is located in the ICF, and 1% is located in the ECF. The normal plasma $[P_i]$ is 3 to 4 mg/dL (1-1.5 mmol/L). P_i in the plasma is ionized (45%), complexed (30%), and bound to protein (25%). Phosphate deficiency causes muscle weakness, rhabdomyolysis, and reduced bone mineralization, resulting in **rickets** (in children) and **osteomalacia** (in adults).

Overview of P_i Homeostasis

A general scheme of P_i homeostasis is shown in Figure 9-7. The maintenance of P_i homeostasis depends on two factors: (1) the amount of P_i in the body and (2) the distribution of P_i between the ICF and ECF compartments. Total body P_i levels are determined by the relative amount of P_i absorbed by the intestinal tract versus the amount excreted by the kidneys. P_i absorption by the intestinal tract occurs via active and passive mechanisms; P_i absorption increases as dietary P_i rises, and it is stimulated by calcitriol. Despite variations in P_i intake between 800 and 1500 mg/day, in adults (i.e., the steady state), the kidneys maintain total body P_i balance constant by excreting an amount of P_i in the urine equal to the amount absorbed by the intestinal

tract (normal bone remodeling results in no net addition of P_i to, or P_i release from, the bone). By contrast, during growth, P_i is accumulated in the body. Renal P_i excretion is the primary mechanism by which the body regulates P_i balance and thereby P_i homeostasis.

The second factor that maintains P_i homeostasis is the distribution of P_i among bone and the ICF and ECF compartments. Two hormones, PTH and calcitriol, in concert with the kidneys, regulate plasma $[P_i]$ (see Figures 9-7 and 9-8). The release of P_i from bone is stimulated by the same hormones (i.e., PTH and calcitriol) that release Ca^{++} from this pool. Thus the release of P_i is always accompanied by a release of Ca^{++}.

The kidneys also make an important contribution to maintaining plasma $[P_i]$ within a narrow range (1-1.5 mmol/L). P_i excretion by the kidneys is regulated by PTH and calcitriol (see Figure 9-7).

PTH increases P_i excretion, whereas calcitriol inhibits P_i excretion. Plasma $[P_i]$ is determined by (1) intestinal absorption, (2) storage in bone, and (3) P_i excretion by the kidneys. Maintenance of plasma $[P_i]$ is essential for optimal Ca^{++}-P_i complex formation required for bone mineralization without deposition of Ca^{++}-P_i in vascular and other soft tissues.

A rise in the plasma $[P_i]$ directly stimulates PTH synthesis and release and also decreases the ionized

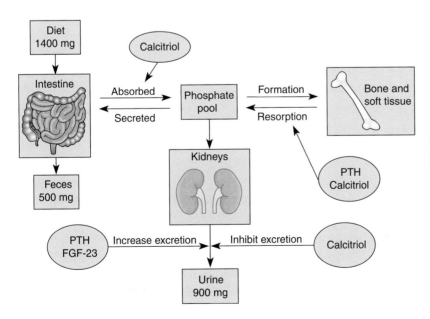

FIGURE 9-7 ■ Overview of inorganic phosphate homeostasis. *FGF-23,* Fibroblast growth factor 23; *PTH,* parathyroid hormone.

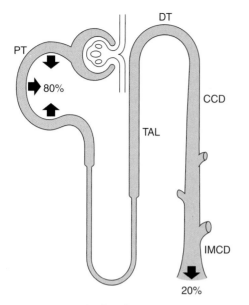

FIGURE 9-8 ■ Inorganic phosphate (P$_i$) transport along the nephron. P$_i$ is reabsorbed primarily by the proximal tubule. Percentages refer to the amount of the filtered P$_i$ reabsorbed by each nephron segment. Approximately 20% of the filtered P$_i$ is excreted. *CCD,* Cortical collecting duct; *DT,* distal tubule; *IMCD,* inner medullary collecting duct; *PT,* proximal tubule; *TAL,* thick ascending limb.

[Ca^{++}], which stimulates PTH release by its interaction with CaSR. PTH enhances urinary P$_i$ excretion by inhibiting proximal tubule P$_i$ reabsorption. Hyperphosphatemia also decreases calcitriol production by the proximal tubule, which leads to a reduction in P$_i$ absorption by the intestine. Both the increase in PTH and the decrease in calcitriol reduce plasma [P$_i$].

P$_i$ Transport Along the Nephron

Figure 9-8 summarizes P$_i$ transport by the various portions of the nephron. The proximal tubule reabsorbs 80% of the P$_i$ filtered by the glomerulus, and the loop of Henle, distal tubule, and the collecting duct reabsorb negligible amounts of P$_i$. Therefore approximately 20% of the Pi filtered across the glomerular capillaries is excreted in the urine.

P$_i$ reabsorption by the proximal tubule occurs by a transcellular route (Figure 9-9). P$_i$ uptake across the apical membrane of the proximal tubule occurs via two Na$^+$-P$_i$ symporters (IIa and IIc). Type IIa transports 3Na$^+$ with one divalent P$_i$ (HPO$_4^{-2}$), and carries positive charge into the cell. Type IIc transports 2Na$^+$ with one monovalent P$_i$ (H$_2$PO$_4^-$) and is electrically neutral. P$_i$ exits across the basolateral membrane by a P$_i$-inorganic anion antiporter that has not been characterized.

FIGURE 9-9 ■ Cellular mechanisms of inorganic phosphate (P$_i$) reabsorption by the proximal tubule. The apical transport pathway contains two Na$^+$-P$_i$ symporters, one that transports three Na$^+$ for each P$_i$ (IIa) and one that transports two Na$^+$ for each P$_i$ (IIc). P$_i$ leaves the cell across the basolateral membrane by an unknown mechanism. *ATP,* Adenosine triphosphate.

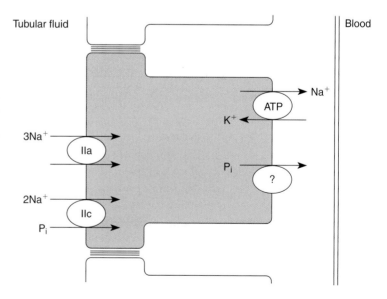

Regulation of Urinary P_i Excretion

Several hormones and factors regulate urinary P_i excretion (Table 9-2 and Figure 9-10). PTH, the most important hormone that controls P_i excretion, inhibits P_i reabsorption by the proximal tubule and thereby increases P_i excretion. PTH reduces P_i reabsorption by stimulating the endocytic removal of Na^+-P_i transporters from the brush border membrane of the proximal tubule. Dietary P_i intake also regulates P_i excretion by mechanisms unrelated to changes in PTH levels. P_i loading increases excretion, whereas P_i depletion decreases it. Changes in dietary P_i intake modulate P_i transport by altering the transport rate of each Na^+-P_i symporter and the number of symporters in the apical membrane of the proximal tubule.

IN THE CLINIC

In patients with **chronic renal failure**, the kidneys cannot excrete inorganic phosphate (P_i). Because of continued P_i absorption by the intestinal tract, P_i accumulates in the body, and the plasma $[P_i]$ rises. The excess P_i complexes with Ca^{++} and reduces the ionized plasma concentration of Ca^{++} ($[Ca^{++}]$). P_i accumulation also decreases the production of calcitriol. This response reduces Ca^{++} absorption by the intestine, an effect that further reduces the plasma $[Ca^{++}]$. This reduction in plasma $[Ca^{++}]$ increases parathyroid hormone secretion and Ca^{++} release from bone. These actions result in **renal osteodystrophy** (i.e., increased bone resorption with replacement by fibrous tissue, which renders bone more susceptible to fracture). Chronic hyperparathyroidism (i.e., elevated parathyroid hormone levels due to the decrease in plasma $[Ca^{++}]$) during chronic renal failure can lead to metastatic calcifications in which Ca^{++} and P_i precipitate in arteries, soft tissues, and viscera. The deposition of Ca^{++} and P_i in the heart may cause myocardial failure. The prevention and treatment of hyperparathyroidism and P_i retention include a low-P_i diet or the administration of a "phosphate binder" (i.e., an agent that forms insoluble P_i salts and thereby renders P_i unavailable for absorption by the intestinal tract) in the diet. Supplemental Ca^{++} and calcitriol also are prescribed to increase plasma $[Ca^{++}]$.

ECF volume also affects P_i excretion. Expansion of the ECF enhances P_i excretion by (1) increasing glomerular filtration rate and thus the filtered load of P_i; (2) decreasing Na-P_i coupled reabsorption, which reduces the ECF volume; and (3) reducing the plasma $[Ca^{++}]$, thereby increasing PTH, which inhibits P_i reabsorption in the proximal tubule. Acid-base balance also influences P_i excretion; chronic acidosis

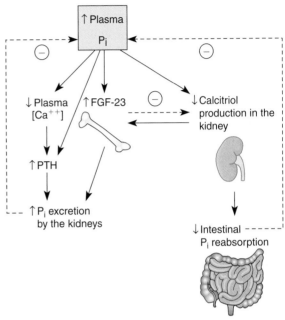

FIGURE 9-10 ■ Overview of the major hormones regulating plasma concentration of P_i. *Dashed lines* indicate negative feedback. *FGF-23*, Fibroblast growth factor 23; *PTH*, parathyroid hormone.

TABLE 9-2

Summary of Hormones and Factors Affecting P_i Reabsorption by the Proximal Tubule

FACTOR/HORMONE	PROXIMAL TUBULE REABSORPTION
PTH	Decrease
FGF-23	Decrease
Phosphate loading	Decrease
Phosphate depletion	Increase
Metabolic acidosis: chronic	Decrease
Metabolic alkalosis: chronic	Increase
ECFV expansion	Decrease
Growth hormone	Increase
Glucocorticoids	Decrease

ECFV, extracellular fluid volume; *FGF-23*, fibroblast growth factor 23; *P_i*, inorganic phosphate; *PTH*, parathyroid hormone.

increases Pi excretion, and chronic alkalosis decreases it. These effects of acid-base balance, like the effect of PTH, are mediated by changes of expression of the $Na-P_i$ symporters in the apical membrane. As described in Chapter 8, systemic acidosis causes glucocorticoid secretion, and these glucocorticoids increase the excretion of P_i by inhibiting P_i reabsorption by the proximal tubule. This inhibition, together with the direct effect of acidosis on P_i reabsorption by the proximal tubule, enables the distal tubule and collecting duct to secrete

---

IN THE CLINIC

In the absence of glucocorticoids (e.g., in **Addison disease**), inorganic phosphate (P_i) excretion is depressed, as is the ability of the kidneys to excrete titratable acid and to generate new bicarbonate (HCO_3^-). Growth hormone also has an important effect on P_i homeostasis. Growth hormone increases the reabsorption of P_i by the proximal tubule. As a result, growing children are in positive P_i balance and have a higher plasma $[P_i]$ than do adults, and this elevated $[P_i]$ is important for the formation of bone.

IN THE CLINIC

Phosphate homeostasis is altered by mutations in the fibroblast growth factor 23 (FGF-23) gene by mutations in **PHEX**, an endopeptidase, and by tumors that produce excess amounts of FGF-23. For example, in **tumor-induced osteomalacia**, excessive production of FGF-23 leads to hypophosphatemia, renal phosphate wasting, and a defect in bone mineralization. This phenotype also is observed in patients with autosomal dominant hypophosphatemic rickets (caused by mutations in the FGF-23 gene that make FGF-23 resistant to proteolysis), autosomal recessive hypophosphatemic rickets (caused by elevated levels of FGF-23), and X-linked hypophosphatemic rickets (caused by inactivating mutations in PHEX). In contrast, an inactivating mutation in the FGF-23 gene causes hyperphosphatemia, hypophosphaturia, and calcification of soft tissues.

---

more H^+ as titratable acid and to generate more HCO_3^- because P_i is an important urinary buffer. Growth hormone decreases P_i excretion.

Fibroblast growth factor 23 (FGF-23) regulates renal P_i excretion and thereby contributes to the regulation of plasma $[P_i]$. FGF-23 is secreted by osteocytes and osteoblasts and inhibits P_i reabsorption and calcitriol production by the proximal tubule (see Figure 9-8). Secretion of FGF-23 is stimulated by sustained hyperphosphatemia, PTH, and calcitriol. Activating mutations in the FGF-23 gene cause hypophosphatemia, low plasma calcitriol, and rickets/osteomalacia, whereas inactivating mutations cause hyperphosphatemia, high serum calcitriol, and calcification of soft tissue.

INTEGRATIVE REVIEW OF PARATHYROID HORMONE AND CALCITRIOL ON CA^{++} AND P$_i$ HOMEOSTASIS

Hypocalcemia is the major stimulus of PTH secretion. As summarized in Figure 9-11, PTH has numerous effects on Ca^{++} and P_i homeostasis. PTH stimulates bone resorption, increases urinary P_i excretion, decreases urinary Ca^{++} excretion, and stimulates the production of calcitriol, which stimulates Ca^{++} and P_i absorption by the intestine. Because changes in P_i handling in bone, the intestines, and the kidneys tend to balance out, PTH increases the plasma $[Ca^{++}]$ while having little effect on the plasma $[P_i]$. Overall, a rise in the plasma PTH levels in response to hypocalcemia returns the plasma $[Ca^{++}]$ to the normal range. A decline in plasma $[Ca^{++}]$ has the opposite effect.

Calcitriol (the active form of vitamin D) also plays an important role in Ca^{++} and P_i homeostasis (see Figure 9-12). The primary action of calcitriol is to stimulate Ca^{++} and P_i absorption by the intestine. To a lesser degree it acts with PTH to release Ca^{++} and P_i from the bone and decreases Ca^{++} excretion by the kidneys. The net effect of calcitriol is to increase the plasma $[Ca^{++}]$ and $[P_i]$. Thus the major stimuli of calcitriol production are hypocalcemia via PTH and hypophosphatemia (i.e., a low plasma $[P_i]$).

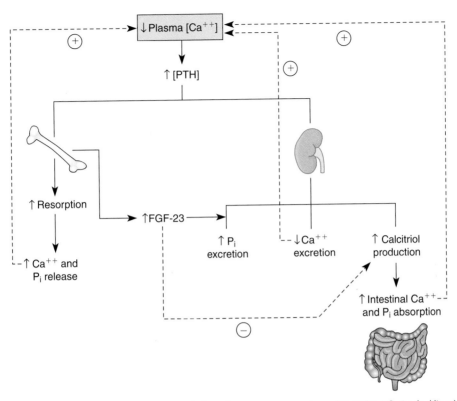

FIGURE 9-11 ■ Overview of the major hormones regulating plasma concentration of Ca^{++} [Ca^{++}]. *Dashed lines* indicate negative feedback. *FGF-23*, Fibroblast growth factor 23; P_i, inorganic phosphate; *PTH*, parathyroid hormone.

SUMMARY

1. The kidneys, in conjunction with the intestinal tract and bone, play a vital role in regulating the plasma [Ca^{++}] and [P_i].

2. Plasma Ca^{++} is regulated by PTH and calcitriol. Calcitonin is not a major regulatory hormone in humans. Ca^{++} excretion by the kidneys is regulated by PTH, plasma [Ca^{++}], and calcitriol, and is altered by changes in acid-base status, extracellular fluid volume, and plasma P_i.

3. Ca^{++} reabsorption by the thick ascending limb and distal tubule are regulated by PTH and calcitriol,

both of which stimulate Ca^{++} reabsorption, and by plasma [Ca^{++}].

4. The plasma [P_i] is regulated by PTH, FGF-23, and calcitriol. P_i excretion is regulated by PTH, FGF-23, dietary phosphate, and growth hormone, and it is altered by acid-base balance, ECFV expansion, and glucocorticoids. Bone tumors secrete FGF-23, which enhances renal P_i excretion and thereby causes hypophosphatemia, hyperphosphatemia, and a defect in bone mineralization (i.e., osteomalacia).

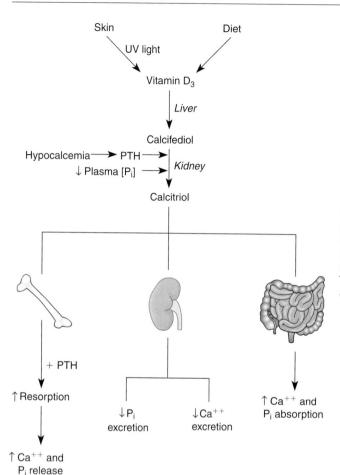

FIGURE 9-12 ■ Activation of vitamin D_3 and its effect on Ca^{++} and inorganic phosphate (P_i) homeostasis. Hypocalcemia, via parathyroid hormone (*PTH*), and hypophosphatemia are the major stimuli of the metabolism of calcifediol to calcitriol in the kidneys. The net effect of calcitriol is to increase plasma concentrations of Ca^{++} and P_i. *UV,* Ultraviolet.

KEY WORDS AND CONCEPTS

- Hypocalcemia
- Hypercalcemia
- Calcitriol
- Vitamin D_3
- Calcium-sensing receptor (CaSR)
- Na^+-P_i symporter
- Parathyroid hormone (PTH)
- Phosphatonins
- Fibroblast growth factor 23 (FGF-23)
- Parathyroid hormone–related peptide
- Claudin-16

SELF-STUDY PROBLEMS

1. How is Ca^{++} reabsorption in the proximal tubule dependent on Na^+ reabsorption? What would happen to Ca^{++} excretion if a subject was given a diuretic, such as mannitol, that inhibits sodium and water reabsorption by the proximal tubule?
2. Why would furosemide, an inhibitor of Na^+ reabsorption by the thick ascending limb of Henle's loop, increase urinary Ca^{++} excretion?
3. How is P_i excretion by the kidneys regulated?

10

PHYSIOLOGY OF DIURETIC ACTION

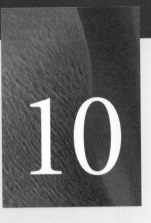

Diuretics, as the name implies, are drugs that cause an increase in urine output. It is important, however, to distinguish this diuresis from that which occurs after the ingestion of large volumes of water. In the latter case, the urine is primarily made up of water, and solute excretion is not increased. In contrast, diuretics result in the enhanced excretion of both solute and water.

All diuretics (with the exception of aquaretics, which will be discussed) have as their common mode of action the primary inhibition of Na$^+$ reabsorption by the nephron. Consequently, they cause an increase in the excretion of Na$^+$, termed **natriuresis**. However, the effects of diuretics are not limited to Na$^+$ handling.

The renal handling of many other solutes also is influenced, usually as a consequence of alterations in Na$^+$ transport. Recently, drugs have been developed that block the action of arginine vasopressin (AVP) on the distal tubule and collecting duct. These drugs, called **aquaretics**, cause a **water diuresis**. This chapter reviews the cellular mechanisms of action of various diuretics and the nephron sites at which these diuretics act. In addition to their effects on Na$^+$ handling by the nephron, their effects on the renal handling of other solutes (e.g., K$^+$, Ca^{++}, inorganic phosphate [P$_i$], and bicarbonate [HCO$_3^-$]) and of water are considered. The effects of aquaretics on water excretion also are discussed.

GENERAL PRINCIPLES OF DIURETIC ACTION

The primary action of diuretics is to increase the excretion of Na^+. As described in Chapter 6, alterations in Na^+ excretion by the kidneys result in alterations in the volume of the extracellular fluid (ECF) compartment. Consequently, diuretics decrease the volume of the ECF. Indeed, diuretics commonly are given in clinical situations when the ECF compartment is expanded, with the intent of reducing its volume. Because the ECF volume also determines blood volume and pressure, diuretics commonly are used in the therapy of hypertension.

Although generally predictable for a particular class of diuretics, the effects of diuretic administration can be quite variable. Several factors are important in determining the overall effect of a particular diuretic:

1. The nephron segment where the diuretic acts
2. The response of nephron segments not directly affected by the diuretic
3. The delivery of sufficient quantities of the diuretic to its site of action
4. The volume of the ECF

Sites of Action of Diuretics

Figure 10-1 depicts the nephron sites at which the different classes of diuretics act. The osmotic diuretics act along the proximal tubule and portions of the thin descending limb of Henle's loop (i.e., those portions of the nephron that have a high water permeability). The carbonic anhydrase inhibitors act primarily in the proximal tubule. The thick ascending limb of Henle's loop is the site of action of the loop diuretics. The early portion of the distal tubule is the site of action of the thiazide diuretics, and the K^+-sparing diuretics act primarily on the late portion of the distal tubule and the cortical portion of the collecting duct where they not only inhibit Na^+ reabsorption but also K^+ secretion. This same class of diuretics also can inhibit Na^+ reabsorption in portions of the collecting duct that do not secrete K^+.

The site of action of a diuretic in turn determines the magnitude of the associated natriuresis (Table 10-1). For example, diuretics acting on the thick

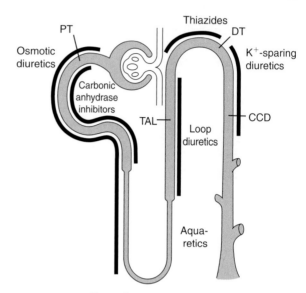

FIGURE 10-1 ■ Sites of action of diuretics and aquaretics along the nephron. *CCD*, Cortical collecting duct; *DT*, distal tubule; *PT*, proximal tubule; *TAL*, thick ascending limb.

ascending limb of Henle's loop cause a larger diuresis than diuretics acting on the early portion of the distal tubule, because a larger portion of the filtered Na^+ is absorbed by the thick ascending limb (see Chapters 4 and 6). The effect diuretics have on the handling of solutes other than Na^+ also depends on the site of action. Examples illustrating this point are given in subsequent sections.

Response of Other Nephron Segments

When a diuretic inhibits Na^+ reabsorption at one nephron site, it causes increased delivery of Na^+ and water to more distal segments. The function of these more distal segments and their ability or inability to handle this increased load ultimately determine the overall effect of the diuretic on urinary solute and water excretion. Examples of this phenomenon are considered in detail with discussion of each of the various diuretics. In addition, diuretic-induced changes in ECF volume (discussed later in this chapter) may modulate Na^+ transport in segments of the nephron not directly affected by the diuretic and thereby influence the degree of natriuresis.

TABLE 10-1
Diuretic Effects on Renal Excretion

DIURETIC	Na$^+$ EXCRETION*	K$^+$EXCRETION	HCO$_3^-$ EXCRETION	Ca^{++} EXCRETION	FREE WATER EXCRETION	FREE WATER REABSORPTION
Osmotic diuretic	10%	↑	↑	↑	↑	↑
Cai	5%-10%	↑	↑	↑	↑	↑
Loop diuretic	25%	↑	↓	↑	↓	↓
Thiazide diuretic	5%-10%	↑	↓	↓	↓	NC
K$^+$-sparing diuretic	3%-5%	↓	↑	NC	NC	NC
Aquaretics	0%	NC	NC	NC	↑	↓

All the effects (except HCO$_3^-$ excretion) reflect the initial effect of the diuretic. The effects of loop and thiazide diuretics on HCO$_3^-$ excretion occur with prolonged use of these drugs and are secondary to the diuretic-induced decrease in extracellular fluid volume.
*Percentage of filtered Na$^+$ excreted into the urine.
Cai, Carbonic anhydrase inhibitor; *NC,* no change.

Adequate Delivery of Diuretics to Their Site of Action

The effect of a diuretic on Na$^+$ excretion also depends on the delivery of adequate quantities of the drug to its site of action. With the exception of the aldosterone antagonists, which act intracellularly, diuretics act from the lumen of the nephron (carbonic anhydrase inhibitors have both luminal and intracellular sites of action). Diuretics gain access to the lumen by glomerular filtration and through secretion by the organic anion and organic cation secretory systems located in the proximal tubule (see Chapter 4). Because some diuretics are bound to plasma proteins (e.g., loop diuretics), their secretion by the proximal tubule is the primary mechanism for delivery of the diuretic to its site of action in the lumen of the nephron. Thus the effect of a diuretic can be blunted if, for example, it is administered with another drug that competes for the same organic anion and organic cation secretory mechanism.

Volume of the Extracellular Fluid

The effect of a diuretic also depends on the volume of the ECF. As described in Chapter 6, when the volume of the ECF is decreased, the glomerular filtration rate (GFR) is reduced, thereby reducing the amount of filtered Na$^+$. In addition, Na$^+$ reabsorption by the nephron is enhanced. Thus the effect of a diuretic that acts on the distal tubule would be blunted if administered in the setting of a reduced ECF volume. Under this condition, the decreased GFR (i.e., decreased filtered Na$^+$), together with enhanced Na$^+$ reabsorption by the proximal tubule, would result in the delivery of a smaller quantity of Na$^+$ to the distal tubule. Thus even if the diuretic completely inhibited Na$^+$ reabsorption in the distal tubule, the associated natriuresis would be less than would occur if the ECF volume were normal.

DIURETIC BRAKING PHENOMENON

As illustrated in Figure 10-2, administration of a diuretic to a person with fixed Na$^+$ intake results in a short-lived natriuresis. The transient response, called the **diuretic braking phenomenon,** reflects several changes in renal function that are both a direct effect of the diuretic and secondary to changes in the volume of the ECF. One component of this response is that diuretic-induced inhibition of Na$^+$ reabsorption in the targeted nephron segment increases Na$^+$ delivery to more distal nephron segments and simulates Na$^+$ reabsorption at these sites. A second important component of this response is that loss of sodium chloride (NaCl) and water from the body as a result of diuretic action decreases the volume of the ECF. This decrease in turn is sensed by the body's vascular baroreceptors

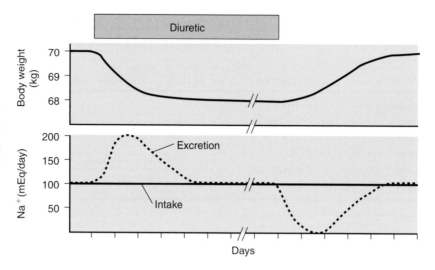

FIGURE 10-2 ■ Effect of long-term diuretic therapy on renal Na⁺ excretion. Because diuretics induce a natriuresis, extracellular fluid volume is reduced, which is detected as a decrease in body weight.

and effector mechanisms, prompting them to increase NaCl and water conservation by the kidneys (see Chapter 6 for details).

AT THE CELLULAR LEVEL

Studies in experimental animals have shown that loop and thiazide diuretics increase the expression of the transporters they inhibit. For example, loop diuretics, which inhibit the Na^+-K^+-$2Cl^-$ cotransporter (NKCC2) in the apical membrane of the cells of the thick ascending limb of Henle's loop, also increase the expression of the transporter in this segment. Similarly, thiazide diuretics, which inhibit the Na^+-Cl^- symporter (NCC) in the apical membrane of the early portion of the distal tubule, also increase the expression of these transporters in this segment. In addition, both loop and thiazide diuretics increase the expression of the Na^+ channel (epithelial sodium channel [ENaC]) in the late portion of the distal tubule and collecting duct. Thiazide diuretics also increase the expression of aquaporin-2 in the principal cells of the late portion of the distal tubule and the collecting duct. Whether this effect is direct or indirect (i.e., related to changes in ECF volume) is uncertain. Regardless of the mechanism, the increased expression of aquaporin-2 is expected to increase water reabsorption by the arginine vasopressin (AVP)-sensitive nephron segments.

With the diuretic-induced decrease in the ECF volume, the renin-angiotensin-aldosterone system is activated, renal sympathetic nerve activity is increased, and AVP secretion is stimulated, which in combination act to reduce urinary sodium chloride (NaCl) and water excretion (see Chapter 6 for details). At the cellular level, angiotensin II increases the expression of the Na^+-Cl^- symporter in the early portion of the distal tubule, and aldosterone increases the expression of ENaC in the late distal tubule and collecting duct. AVP also increases the expression of key transporters. Specifically, AVP increases the expression of NKCC2 in the thick ascending limb of Henle's loop, NCC in the early portion of the distal tubule, and ENaC in the late distal tubule and collecting duct. Finally, angiotensin II increases the abundance of the Na^+-H^+ antiporter (NHE3) in the proximal tubule. Upregulation of these transporters by diuretics reduces their efficacy, and when the diuretic administration is terminated, results in a rapid increase in NaCl reabsorption.

As a result of the braking phenomenon, a new steady state is reached where even with continued administration of the diuretic, urinary Na^+ excretion once again equals intake. However, this steady state occurs at a reduced ECF volume, which is detected as a decrease in body weight. When diuretic therapy is discontinued, renal Na^+ excretion is reduced. After a period of positive Na^+ balance, during which the ECF returns to normal (i.e., return of body weight to its original value), a new steady state is again achieved.

The concept of steady state deserves special emphasis. Normally, persons are in steady-state balance with regard to solute (e.g., Na^+) and water, with intake equaling excretion. Administration of a diuretic temporarily disrupts this balance by increasing solute and water excretion, and a negative balance exists. However, solute and water excretion cannot exceed intake indefinitely, and a new steady state eventually is achieved. In this new steady state, intake and excretion are again balanced, but the ECF volume is reduced as a result of diuretic-induced excretion of NaCl and water. In general, when a person has been taking a diuretic for several days or longer, a new steady state is achieved. If Na^+ intake is not increased, the ECF volume is decreased in proportion to the degree of negative Na^+ balance.

MECHANISMS OF ACTION OF DIURETICS

Osmotic Diuretics

Osmotic diuretics, as the name implies, are agents that inhibit the reabsorption of solute and water by altering osmotic driving forces along the nephron. Unlike the other classes of diuretics, osmotic diuretics do not inhibit a specific membrane transport protein; they simply affect water transport across the cells of the nephron through the generation of an osmotic pressure gradient. The best example of an exogenous osmotic diuretic is the sugar mannitol. When present in abnormally high concentrations, freely filtered endogenous substances such as glucose (i.e., in patients with diabetes mellitus) and urea (i.e., in patients with renal disease whose plasma urea levels are elevated) also can act as osmotic diuretics.

Osmotic diuretics (e.g., mannitol) gain access to the proximal tubular fluid by glomerular filtration. Because they are not reabsorbed or are only poorly reabsorbed, they remain within the tubular lumen, where they can exert an osmotic pressure that inhibits tubular fluid reabsorption. Osmotic diuretics affect fluid reabsorption in the segments that have high permeability to water (i.e., the proximal tubule and portions of the thin descending limb of Henle's loop). Because of the large volumes of filtrate reabsorbed in the proximal tubule (60% to 70% of the filtrate), this nephron site is most important when considering the action of osmotic diuretics.

As described in Chapter 4, reabsorption of tubular fluid by the proximal tubule is essentially an isosmotic process (i.e., the osmolality of the reabsorbed fluid is only slightly hyperosmotic compared with that of tubular fluid). Solute (primarily NaCl) is actively reabsorbed by the proximal tubule cells. This reabsorption sets up a small osmotic pressure difference across the tubule, with the tubular fluid being 3 to 5 mOsm/kg H_2O hypoosmotic with respect to the interstitial fluid. Given the fact that water is readily able to cross the proximal tubule, this small osmotic pressure gradient is sufficient to cause water reabsorption. Also, as water flows from the lumen to the interstitium, it brings additional solute with it by solvent drag.

When an osmotic diuretic is present in the tubular fluid, its concentration increases progressively as a result of NaCl and water reabsorption by the nephron. With this increase in concentration, an osmotic gradient develops opposite to the normal gradient generated by NaCl reabsorption. As a result, both NaCl (solvent drag component) and water reabsorption are reduced. With an osmotic diuresis, an increase in blood flow to the medulla of the kidney also occurs. This increase in blood flow dissipates the standing interstitial osmotic gradient (see Chapter 5) and thus also impairs water reabsorption by the descending limb of Henle's loop and the medullary collecting duct.

Some of the Na^+ that is not reabsorbed by the proximal tubule is reabsorbed downstream by the thick ascending limb, distal tubule, and collecting duct. Thus the degree of natriuresis seen with osmotic diuretics is less than expected on the basis of the magnitude of proximal tubule reabsorption. Although Na^+ excretion rates as high as 60% of the filtered Na^+ have been seen in experimental situations, the usual natriuresis seen in persons treated with osmotic diuretics is only about 10% of the filtered Na^+.

Carbonic Anhydrase Inhibitors

Carbonic anhydrase inhibitors (e.g., acetazolamide) reduce Na^+ reabsorption by their effect on carbonic anhydrase. This enzyme is abundant in the proximal tubule and therefore represents the major site of action of these diuretics. Carbonic anhydrase also is present in other cells along the nephron (e.g., thick ascending limb of Henle's loop and intercalated cells of the collecting duct), and administration of carbonic anhydrase inhibitors affects the activity of the enzyme at these sites as well. However, the effects of these diuretics are almost entirely attributed to their inhibition of the enzyme in the proximal tubule. This phenomenon reflects the fact that approximately one third of proximal tubule Na^+ reabsorption occurs in exchange for H^+ (through the Na^+-H^+ antiporter) and thus depends on the activity of carbonic anhydrase (see Chapter 8).

Even though one third of proximal tubule Na^+ reabsorption is coupled to the secretion of H^+, inhibition of this process by the carbonic anhydrase inhibitors does not result in a large natriuresis for several reasons. First, even with complete inhibition of carbonic anhydrase, some Na^+ reabsorption (linked to bicarbonate reabsorption) still occurs. Second, downstream nephron segments increase their reabsorption of Na^+ (e.g., the thick ascending limb, distal tubule, and collecting duct), and third, increased delivery of Na^+ to the macula densa leads to a reduction in the GFR by the tubuloglomerular feedback mechanism. Finally, with long-term administration, a metabolic acidosis develops, which further decreases the effect of carbonic anhydrase inhibitors by reducing the filtration of HCO_3^- (i.e., the percentage of Na^+ reabsorbed with HCO_3^- in the proximal tubule is reduced). Typically, administration of carbonic anhydrase inhibitors results in Na^+ excretion rates that are 5% to 10% of the filtered Na^+.

Loop Diuretics

Loop diuretics (e.g., furosemide, bumetanide, torsemide, and ethacrynic acid) are organic anions that enter the tubular lumen primarily through secretion by the organic anion secretory system of the proximal tubule (see Chapter 4). They directly inhibit Na^+ reabsorption by the thick ascending limb of Henle's loop by blocking the Na^+-K^+-$2Cl^-$ symporter located in the apical membrane of these cells (see Chapter 4). By this action, they not only inhibit Na^+ reabsorption but also disrupt the ability of the kidneys to dilute and concentrate the urine. Dilution is impaired because solute

(NaCl) reabsorption by the water-impermeable thick ascending limb of Henle's loop is inhibited. NaCl reabsorption by the medullary portion of the thick ascending limb also is critical for the generation and maintenance of an elevated medullary interstitial fluid osmolality. Therefore inhibition of NaCl transport by loop diuretics results in a decrease in the osmolality of the medullary interstitial fluid. With a decrease in medullary interstitial fluid osmolality, water reabsorption from the collecting duct is impaired, and the concentrating ability of the kidneys is reduced. Water reabsorption from some portions of the thin descending limb of Henle's loop also is impaired by loop diuretics, again because of the decrease in medullary interstitial fluid osmolality. This decrease in thin descending limb water reabsorption accounts in part for the increase in water excretion seen with loop diuretics.

Loop diuretics are the most potent diuretics available, increasing the excretion of Na^+ to as much as 25% of the amount filtered. This large natriuresis reflects the fact that the thick ascending limb normally reabsorbs approximately 20% to 25% of the filtered Na^+ and that downstream segments of the nephron have a limited ability to reabsorb the excess Na^+ delivered as a consequence of loop diuretic action.

Thiazide Diuretics

Like the loop diuretics, thiazide diuretics (e.g., hydrochlorothiazide, chlorthalidone, and metolazone)* are organic anions. Because they largely are bound to plasma proteins, they gain access to the tubular lumen primarily by secretion in the proximal tubule. They act to inhibit Na^+ reabsorption in the early portion of the distal tubule by blocking the Na^+-Cl^- symporter in the apical membrane of these cells (see Chapter 4). Because water cannot cross this portion of the nephron, it is a site where the urine is diluted. Therefore thiazides reduce the ability to dilute the urine maximally by inhibiting NaCl reabsorption. Because thiazide diuretics act in the cortex and not the medulla, they do not

---

*Metolazone and chlorthalidone are not in the same chemical class of drugs as the thiazides. However, because their site of action is the same, they are grouped with this class of drugs and often are referred to as "thiazidelike" diuretics.

affect the ability of the kidneys to concentrate the urine maximally. Natriuresis with thiazide diuretics is 5% to 10% of the filtered Na^+.

K^+-Sparing Diuretics

K^+-sparing diuretics act on the region of the nephron where K^+ secretion occurs (i.e., the late portion of the distal tubule and cortical collecting duct). They produce a small natriuresis (3% to 5% of the filtered Na^+), reflecting the amount of Na^+ reabsorbed by this region of the nephron. As the name implies, their utility lies in their ability to inhibit K^+ secretion by this region of the nephron.

There are two classes of K^+-sparing diuretics: one acts by antagonizing the action of aldosterone on the principal cell (e.g., spironolactone and eplerenone), whereas the other class blocks the entry of Na^+ into the same cells through the Na^+-selective channels (epithelial sodium channels [ENaC]) in the apical membrane (e.g., amiloride and triamterene). Amiloride and triamterene are organic cations that enter the tubular lumen primarily by secretion by the organic cation secretory system of the proximal tubule (see Chapter 4).

As described in detail in Chapters 6 and 7, aldosterone stimulates both Na^+ reabsorption and K^+ secretion by the principal cells of the late distal tubule and collecting duct. Thus in the presence of an aldosterone antagonist, these effects are inhibited and both Na^+ reabsorption and K^+ secretion are reduced.

The ability of the Na^+ channel blockers amiloride and triamterene to inhibit Na^+ reabsorption and K^+ secretion is similar to that of spironolactone, but the cellular mechanism is different. Amiloride and triamterene block the entry of Na^+ into the principal cell by directly inhibiting the Na^+ channel (ENaC) in the apical membrane. With decreased Na^+ entry, reduced Na^+ extrusion occurs across the basolateral membrane through Na^+-K^+–adenosine triphosphatase (ATPase). This effect in turn reduces cellular K^+ uptake and ultimately its secretion into the tubular fluid. Inhibition of apical membrane Na^+ channels also alters the electrical profile across the luminal membrane, with the voltage across this membrane increasing in magnitude. Because of this voltage change, the electrochemical gradient for K^+ movement out of the cell is reduced.

This membrane voltage effect also contributes to the inhibition of K^+ secretion.

IN THE CLINIC

Trimethoprim is an antibiotic used to treat *Pneumocystis jerovecii* infections. *P. jerovecii* infections are commonly seen in persons whose immune systems are compromised (e.g., persons with acquired immunodeficiency syndrome). Hyperkalemia may occur in persons treated with trimethoprim as a result of reduced renal K^+ excretion. K^+ excretion is reduced because trimethoprim inhibits K^+ secretion by the principal cells of the late distal tubule and cortical collecting duct. The mechanism for this inhibition of K^+ secretion is similar to that of amiloride and triamterene (i.e., direct inhibition of the Na^+ channel [ENaC] in the apical membrane of the cell).

Aquaretics

In recent years, drugs that are antagonists of the AVP receptor (V_2) have been developed (e.g., tolvaptan and lixivaptan). These drugs act on the late portion of the distal tubule and the collecting duct to block the action of AVP. As a result of their action, the urine cannot be concentrated and dilute urine is excreted, reflecting the fact that tubular fluid reaching these AVP-sensitive segments of the nephron is hypoosmotic to the ECF (see Chapter 5). These drugs are particularly helpful in treating patients whose ECF is hypoosmotic as a result of the failure of the kidneys to excrete solute-free water because AVP levels are elevated by nonosmotic and nonhemodynamic mechanisms (e.g., syndrome of inappropriate AVP secretion [SIADH]*).

EFFECT OF DIURETICS ON THE EXCRETION OF WATER AND SOLUTES

Through their effects on Na^+ handling along the nephron, diuretics also influence the handling of water and solutes. Table 10-1 summarizes the effects of the

---

*Note that AVP is also called *antidiuretic hormone* (ADH); thus, the syndrome of inappropriate ADH secretion (SIADH, the term used in the clinical setting) also could be called SIAVP.

various diuretics on the handling of some of these solutes and the ability of the kidneys to excrete (C_{H_2O}) and reabsorb ($T^C_{H_2O}$) solute-free water.

Solute-Free Water

As discussed in Chapter 5, the ability of the kidneys to excrete or reabsorb solute-free water depends on several factors. With regard to the action of diuretic agents, the factors of concern are as follows:

1. The normal function of the nephron segments (particularly the thick ascending limb)
2. The delivery of adequate solute to Henle's loop
3. The maintenance of a hyperosmotic medullary interstitium (selective reabsorption of solute-free water)

The thick ascending limb of Henle's loop is the most important site for the separation of solute and water. As noted, this separation not only dilutes the tubular fluid but also, by establishing a hyperosmotic medullary interstitium, allows water reabsorption from the collecting duct and thus concentration of the urine. Inhibition of thick ascending limb Na^+ reabsorption by loop diuretics therefore results in inhibition of both solute-free water excretion (C_{H_2O}) and solute-free water reabsorption ($T^C_{H_2O}$).

The early portion of the distal tubule is also a site of solute and water separation and thus tubular fluid dilution. Accordingly, inhibition of Na^+ reabsorption by the thiazide diuretics impairs dilution of the urine. However, thiazide diuretics impair urine dilution to a lesser degree than do loop diuretics, reflecting the difference in the NaCl reabsorptive capacity between the distal tubule (5% of the filtered Na^+) and the thick ascending limb (25% of the filtered Na^+). In contrast to the loop diuretics, thiazide diuretics do not significantly impair the ability of the kidneys to concentrate the urine. As already noted, concentration of the urine requires a hyperosmotic medullary interstitium so that water can be reabsorbed from the collecting duct in the presence of AVP. Because thiazide diuretics act on distal tubules that are located in the cortex, their action at this site does not appreciably alter the medullary interstitial osmotic gradient. Consequently, urine-concentrating ability is unaffected by thiazide diuretics.

The action of diuretics in the proximal tubule (osmotic diuretics and carbonic anhydrase inhibitors) results in an increase in the delivery of NaCl and water to Henle's loop. In view of the ability of the thick ascending limb to increase its transport rate in response to an increased delivered load of NaCl, the separation of solute and water increases. As a result, these diuretic agents increase the ability of the kidneys to excrete solute-free water and reabsorb solute-free water. Thus diuretics that act on the proximal tubule enhance the ability to concentrate and dilute the urine.

Although the late portion of the distal tubule and the collecting duct are able to dilute the luminal fluid in the absence of AVP, Na^+ transport in these segments is not of sufficient magnitude to contribute significantly to the excretion of solute-free water. Consequently, the K^+-sparing diuretics do not appreciably alter free-water excretion. Like thiazide diuretics, K^+-sparing diuretics do not alter solute-free water reabsorption because the nephron sites of action are located in the cortex. Aquaretics, because they act directly on the medullary portion of the collecting duct, increase solute-free water excretion and impair solute-free water reabsorption.

K^+ Excretion

One of the major consequences of diuretic use (excluding the K^+-sparing diuretics) is increased excretion of K^+, which can be of sufficient magnitude to result in hypokalemia. The basis for this diuretic-induced increase in renal K^+ excretion lies in the fact that when a diuretic inhibits Na^+ and water reabsorption in segments upstream from the late portion of the distal tubule and cortical collecting duct (K^+ secretory site of the nephron), tubular fluid flow rate increases. The increased tubular fluid flow rate stimulates K^+ secretion at this site (see Chapter 7 for details). In addition, by their action on Na^+ balance, diuretics decrease the ECF volume. This mechanism, in turn, leads to increased secretion of aldosterone by the adrenal cortex (see Chapter 6), which acts at this site to stimulate K^+ secretion.

The decrease in ECF volume also stimulates AVP secretion. As described in Chapter 7, AVP stimulates K^+ secretion by the principal cells of the late distal tubule and collecting duct. This stimulatory effect normally is offset by the inhibitory effect of the reduced tubular flow rate, which also is induced by AVP. As a result, AVP does not normally alter renal K^+ excretion. However, in the presence of a diuretic that is acting upstream to the late portion of the distal tubule and the collecting duct, AVP does increase renal K^+ excretion because in this setting tubular fluid flow is elevated by the action of the diuretics.

Because K^+-sparing diuretics prevent the increase in K^+ excretion caused by the other diuretics, they usually are given in combination with these other diuretics to prevent or at least minimize the development of hypokalemia.

HCO_3^- Excretion

By inhibiting H^+ secretion in the proximal tubule and thereby increasing HCO_3^- excretion, carbonic anhydrase inhibitors can result in the development of a metabolic acidosis.

Although only carbonic anhydrase inhibitors directly alter H^+ secretion by the nephron, all diuretics can affect systemic acid-base balance secondarily. Both loop and thiazide diuretics can induce a metabolic alkalosis, which is a consequence of the decrease in ECF volume that accompanies their use. With a decrease in the ECF volume, Na^+ is more avidly reabsorbed by the nephron. In the proximal tubule, this enhanced Na^+ reabsorption results in enhanced H^+ secretion through the Na^+-H^+ antiporter. Thus a greater fraction of the filtered HCO_3^- is reabsorbed. In addition, the reduction in ECF volume stimulates aldosterone secretion by the adrenal cortex. As discussed in Chapter 8, aldosterone stimulates H^+ secretion by intercalated cells of the distal tubule and collecting duct. Because, as noted, proximal tubule HCO_3^- reabsorption is increased, virtually none of the filtered HCO_3^- reaches the distal tubule. Therefore the increased H^+ secretion that occurs in the distal tubule and collecting duct results in the production of new HCO_3^- as the H^+ is excreted with non-HCO_3^- urinary buffers (i.e., titratable acid). The increased secretion of H^+ in the distal tubule and collecting duct also enhances the excretion of NH_4^+, which results in the addition of new HCO_3^- to the ECF. As a result, net acid excretion by the kidneys is increased and metabolic alkalosis develops.

By inhibiting Na^+ reabsorption in the late portion of the distal tubule and cortical collecting duct, K^+-sparing

diuretics secondarily inhibit H^+ secretion and thus can lead to the development of a metabolic acidosis. H^+ secretion by these nephron segments is facilitated by the lumen-negative transepithelial voltage. Normally, Na^+ reabsorption in these nephron segments results in the generation of such a voltage. By inhibiting Na^+ reabsorption and thus the negative luminal voltage, K^+-sparing diuretics reduce H^+ secretion. With reduced H^+ secretion, insufficient quantities of net acid are excreted and a metabolic acidosis ensues.

Ca^{++} and P_i Excretion

With the exception of K^+-sparing diuretics, all the diuretics can significantly alter Ca^{++} excretion by the kidney. With inhibition of proximal tubule solute and water reabsorption (osmotic diuretics and carbonic anhydrase inhibitors), reduced reabsorption of Ca^{++} and thus increased excretion occurs. The amount of Ca^{++} excreted is less than expected from inhibition of proximal tubule transport. This situation again reflects the ability of the downstream segments (particularly the thick ascending limb of Henle's loop) to increase reabsorption after an increased delivery of Ca^{++}. The mechanism by which these diuretics inhibit proximal tubule Ca^{++} reabsorption is related to their ability to reduce solvent drag (see Chapter 9). With the use of carbonic anhydrase inhibitors, increased Ca^{++} excretion occurs in the setting of an alkaline urine (increased urinary $[HCO_3^-]$). Because Ca^{++} is less soluble in alkaline urine, the potential exists for the formation of renal stones that contain Ca^{++}.

Loop diuretics also increase Ca^{++} excretion, an action explained by the effect of these diuretics on the transepithelial voltage of the thick ascending limb of Henle's loop. Normally, the transepithelial voltage of this segment is oriented lumen positive (see Chapter 4), providing a driving force for the movement of Ca^{++} from the lumen to blood through the paracellular pathway (see Chapter 9). When transport of NaCl by Henle's loop is blocked by loop diuretics, this lumen-positive voltage is abolished, and thus the driving force for Ca^{++} reabsorption is reduced. Normally, Henle's loop reabsorbs about 15% of the filtered Ca^{++} (see Chapter 9). Inhibition of Ca^{++} reabsorption by loop diuretics therefore can have a significant effect on Ca^{++} excretion. For this reason, loop diuretics often are used to treat hypercalcemia. Despite this action of loop diuretics, hypercalcemia can occur with their long-term use. The mechanism responsible for this effect is related to the diuretic-induced decrease in the ECF volume. When the ECF volume is decreased, proximal tubule reabsorption is enhanced, which increases Ca^{++} reabsorption at this site and therefore decreases urinary Ca^{++} excretion.

Thiazide diuretics stimulate Ca^{++} reabsorption by the cells of the distal tubule and thus reduce Ca^{++} excretion. The distal tubule normally reabsorbs approximately 10% to 15% of the filtered Ca^{++} (see Chapter 9). The reabsorption of Ca^{++} at this site is an active, transcellular process involving entry of Ca^{++} into the cell through channels in the apical membrane and extrusion from the cell across the basolateral membrane by the Ca^{++}-ATPase and $3Na^+$-Ca^{++} antiporter. Thiazide diuretics, by inhibiting the entry of NaCl into the cell, cause the membrane potential to hyperpolarize (i.e., the cell interior becomes more electrically negative).* This hyperpolarization in turn activates the Ca^{++} channel (TRPV5) in the apical

---

*Hyperpolarization of the membrane potential occurs as a result of a decrease in the intracellular $[Cl^-]$. The basolateral membrane of the distal tubule cell contains Cl^- channels; thus the membrane potential is determined in part by the Cl^- equilibrium potential. A decrease in the intracellular $[Cl^-]$ therefore increases the magnitude of this equilibrium potential (i.e., it becomes more negative).

membrane of the cell and increases the electrochemical gradient for Ca^{++} entry into the cell. The increased entry of Ca^{++} into the cell is matched by increased extrusion across the basolateral membrane by the Ca^{++}-ATPase and $3Na^+$-Ca^{++} antiporter (extrusion of Ca^{++} via the $3Na^+$-Ca^{++} antiporter is stimulated because the intracellular concentration of Na^+ is decreased as a result of the diuretic blocking Na^+ entry into the cell across the apical membrane). The net effect is an increase in Ca^{++} reabsorption. With long-term use of thiazide diuretics, the associated decrease in ECF volume stimulates proximal tubule reabsorption (see Chapter 6), including that of Ca^{++}. Because thiazides reduce urinary Ca^{++} excretion, they sometimes are used to lower the incidence of the formation of stones containing Ca^{++} in persons who normally excrete high levels of Ca^{++} in their urine.

With the exception of the K^+-sparing diuretics, all diuretics acutely increase Pi excretion. However, the cellular mechanisms for this effect are not completely understood. The effect is modified, however, with long-term diuretic therapy. With the decrease in ECF volume that accompanies long-term diuretic use, proximal tubule Na^+ reabsorption is stimulated. Because the proximal tubule reabsorbs the largest portion of the filtered Pi and because this reabsorptive process is coupled with Na^+ (see Chapters 4 and 9), P_i excretion is reduced in this setting.

S U M M A R Y

1. Diuretics inhibit solute (primarily NaCl) transport at various sites along the nephron. As a result of their action, the net excretion of solute and water by the kidneys increases.

2. By increasing the excretion of NaCl by the kidneys, diuretics cause a decrease in the volume of the ECF. This decreased ECF volume results in a loss of body weight because 1 L of ECF fluid weighs 1 kg.

3. The ability of a particular diuretic to increase solute and water excretion depends on several factors, including the nephron segment(s) where the

diuretic acts, the ability of other nephron segments not directly affected by the diuretic to increase their reabsorption of solute and water, the delivery of sufficient quantities of the diuretic to its site of action, and diuretic-induced changes in ECF volume that may affect renal solute and water transport.

4. Osmotic diuretics inhibit solute and water reabsorption in the proximal tubule and descending thin limb of Henle's loop. Quantitatively, the proximal tubule is the most important site of action.

5. Carbonic anhydrase inhibitors act primarily in the proximal tubule to inhibit Na^+, HCO_3^-, and water reabsorption.

6. Loop diuretics inhibit NaCl reabsorption by the thick ascending limb of Henle's loop. They are the most potent diuretic and can increase Na^+ excretion to as much as 25% of the filtered NaCl.

7. Thiazide diuretics inhibit NaCl reabsorption in the early portion of the distal tubule.

8. K^+-sparing diuretics act at the late portion of the distal tubule and the cortical collecting duct. They inhibit Na^+ reabsorption and in doing so inhibit K^+ secretion. Their most important use is related to their ability to reduce renal K^+ excretion.

9. Aquaretics block the AVP receptor (V_2) in the late portion of the distal tubule and the collecting duct. They impair the ability of the kidneys to concentrate the urine, leading to the excretion of solute-free water.

10. Osmotic diuretics and carbonic anhydrase inhibitors increase the kidneys' ability to excrete and reabsorb solute-free water (i.e. both urinary diluting and concentrating mechanisms, respectively). The loop diuretics impair both solute-free water reabsorption (i.e., the ability to produce concentrated urine) and excretion (i.e., the ability to produce dilute urine), whereas the thiazide diuretics impair only solute-free water excretion (i.e., the ability to produce dilute urine). The K^+-sparing diuretics do not have a significant effect on solute-free water excretion. Aquaretics increase solute-free water excretion and impair solute-free water reabsorption.

11. All diuretics, with the exception of the K^+-sparing diuretics, increase the renal excretion of K^+. This effect is in response to increased delivery of tubular fluid to the K^+ secretory portion of the nephron (distal tubule and cortical collecting duct) and increased aldosterone and AVP levels secondary to the diuretic-induced decrease in ECF volume.

12. The carbonic anhydrase inhibitors and K^+-sparing diuretics can induce a metabolic acidosis. The loop diuretics and thiazide diuretics can cause a metabolic alkalosis.

13. Acutely, loop diuretics increase Ca^{++} excretion. By reducing the ECF volume, chronic administration of loop diuretics can secondarily enhance proximal Ca^{++} reabsorption and limit net Ca^{++} excretion. Thiazide diuretics decrease Ca^{++} excretion.

14. With the exception of K^+-sparing diuretics, all diuretics acutely increase P_i excretion. When the ECF volume is decreased by chronic diuretic use, P_i excretion is reduced.

KEY WORDS AND CONCEPTS

- Organic anion secretory system
- Organic cation secretory system
- Steady state
- Diuretic braking phenomenon
- Osmotic diuretics
- Syndrome of inappropriate ADH/AVP secretion (SIADH/SIAVP)
- Carbonic anhydrase inhibitors
- Loop diuretics
- Thiazide diuretics
- K^+-sparing diuretics
- Aquaretics

SELF-STUDY PROBLEMS

1. Patients with nephrogenic diabetes insipidus can obtain symptomatic relief from their polyuria with long-term use of a thiazide diuretic. What are the mechanisms by which long-term thiazide therapy produces a decrease in urine volume in these patients?

2. An individual takes a thiazide diuretic as partial therapy for hypertension. Before therapy, plasma $[K^+]$ is 4 mEq/L. After several months of therapy, the individual's blood pressure is reduced and plasma $[K^+]$ is 3 mEq/L.

   a. By what mechanism could the diuretic lead to a decrease in blood pressure?

   b. By what mechanism did the plasma $[K^+]$ decrease? What other classes of diuretics would produce this effect?

   c. What can be done to increase the plasma $[K^+]$ to the level it was at before diuretic therapy was initiated?

3. The antibiotic penicillin is secreted into the urine by the organic anion secretory system of the proximal tubule. If an infection requiring penicillin develops in a person taking a thiazide diuretic for hypertension, what effect, if any, could this have on the action of the diuretic?

4. A diuretic is administered to two individuals for several weeks. Individual A receives a loop diuretic and individual B receives a thiazide diuretic. Both ingest a diet that contains 100 mEq/day of Na^+. After these persons have taken their respective diuretics for 2 weeks, consider the following questions:

   a. How much Na^+ does each person excrete in a day, and why?

   b. Both individuals are deprived of water. Individual A is able to concentrate the urine to 400 mOsm/kg H_2O. Individual B is able to concentrate the urine to 1000 mOsm/kg H_2O. How do you explain the difference in response of these two individuals to water deprivation?

   c. Both individuals are water loaded. Individual A is able to dilute his urine to 300 mOsm/kg H_2O. Individual B is able to dilute his urine to 250 mOsm/kg H_2O. How do you explain the inability of these individuals to dilute their urine maximally?

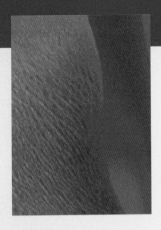

ADDITIONAL READING

The following resources are offered as suggestions for students who wish to learn more about the kidney and the urinary tract and build on the foundation laid out in this book.

Alpern RJ, Hebert SC, editors: *Seldin and Giebisch's The kidney: physiology and pathophysiology*, ed 4. Philadelphia, 2008, Elsevier. (A two-volume, comprehensive text on the kidney, similar in many ways to the Brenner text. Includes sections on normal physiology, pathophysiology, and clinical nephrology. Each chapter is written by experts in the field and includes an extensive list of references.)

Taal M, et al, editors: Brenner and Rector's *The kidney*, ed 9. Philadelphia, 2012, Saunders Elsevier. (A two-volume, comprehensive text on the kidney. Includes sections on normal physiology, pathophysiology, and clinical nephrology. Each chapter is written by experts in the field and includes an extensive list of references.)

Costanzo LS. *Physiology, BRS Board Review Series*, ed 5. Philadelphia, 2011, Wolters Kluwer, Lippincott Williams & Wilkins. (This book reviews physiological principles and includes clinical correlations and 350 USMLE-style questions with answers.)

Floege J, Johnson RJ, Freehally J, editors: *Comprehensive clinical nephrology*, ed 4. Philadelphia, 2011, Mosby Elsevier. (A clinically oriented textbook of nephrology, which has overviews of normal physiology and pathophysiology.)

Schrier RW, editor: *Diseases of the kidney and urinary tract*, ed 8. Philadelphia, 2007, Lippincott Williams & Wilkins. (A three-volume, comprehensive text on pathophysiology and clinical nephrology. Each chapter is written by experts in the field and includes an extensive list of references.)

UpToDate is a website for clinicans and patients that answers clinical questions. For clinical questions on nephrology go to http://www.uptodate.com/home/clinicians/specialties/nephrology.html.

APPENDIX A

INTEGRATIVE CASE STUDIES

CASE 1

A 65-year-old man has congestive heart failure. He is seen by his physician because he has run out of his medications. He presents with easy fatigability, shortness of breath, and swelling of his ankles. On physical examination he is found to have distended neck veins and pitting edema of the ankles. His breathing is rapid (20 breaths/min), and rales (i.e., fluid in the lungs) are heard bilaterally at the bases of the lungs. He is afebrile, with a pulse rate of 110 beats/min and a blood pressure of 110/70 mm Hg. A blood sample is obtained, and the following abnormalities are noted:

Serum $[Na^+]$ = 130 mEq/L

Serum $[K^+]$ = 3.0 mEq/L

Serum [creatinine] = 1.4 mg/dL

Questions

1a. Is the extracellular fluid (ECF) volume in this man increased or decreased from normal? What evidence in the physical examination supports your conclusion?

1b. Is the effective circulating volume (ECV) in this man increased or decreased from normal?

1c. What would you predict to be the levels (activities) of atrial natriuretic peptide, brain natriuretic peptide, arginine vasopressin, renin-angiotensin-aldosterone, and the sympathetic nervous system in this man, and why?

1d. How would you characterize renal Na^+ handling in this man? What evidence in the physical examination supports this conclusion?

1e. What is the mechanism for the development of hyponatremia in this man?

1f. What is the mechanism for the development of hypokalemia in this man?

1g. The physician treating this man prescribes a loop diuretic to reduce Na^+ retention and reduce his edema. It is known that patients with congestive heart failure do not respond as well to loop diuretics as healthy patients would (i.e., the degree of natriuresis is less). What explains the decreased effect of the loop diuretic in a patient with congestive heart failure?

1h. What effect will the loop diuretic have on this man's ECF volume and ECV?

1i. While he is taking the loop diuretic, the serum $[K^+]$ of this man decreases from 3.0 to 2.5 mEq/L. What is the mechanism for this diuretic-induced hypokalemia?

1j. After administration of the diuretic, the serum [creatinine] increases from 1.4 to 1.8 mg/dL. Why was the serum [creatinine] elevated, and why did it increase further after treatment with the loop diuretic?

CASE 2

A 49-year-old woman sees her physician because of weakness, easy fatigability, and loss of appetite. During the past month she has lost 7 kg (15 lb). On physical examination she is found to have hyperpigmentation, especially of the oral mucosa and gums. She is hypotensive, and her blood pressure (BP) falls when she assumes an upright posture (BP = 100/60 mm Hg supine and 80/50 mm Hg erect). The following laboratory data are obtained:

Serum $[Na^+]$ = 132 mEq/L

Serum $[K^+]$ = 6.5 mEq/L

Serum $[HCO_3^-]$ = 20 mEq/L

Urine $[Na^+]$ = 20 mEq/L

Questions

2a. The plasma level of what hormone(s) would be expected to be below normal in this woman?

2b. How do you explain the urine $[Na^+]$ of 20 mEq/L in this woman? What would you expect the urine $[Na^+]$ to be in an individual who is volume depleted? What relationship does this have to the hypotension in this woman?

2c. What is the mechanism for development of hyponatremia in this woman?

2d. Why does this woman have hyperkalemia?

2e. What is the acid-base disturbance in this woman, and what is its cause?

CASE 3

A 70-year-old man with lung cancer develops the syndrome of inappropriate antidiuretic hormone secretion (SIADH). He is admitted to the hospital, and the following data are obtained. His vital signs are normal, as is the physical examination. There is no evidence of ECF volume contraction or ECF volume expansion.

Body weight = 70 kg

Serum $[Na^+]$ = 120 mEq/L (normal = 135-147 mEq/L)

Urine osmolality = 600 mOsm/kg H_2O

Urine $[Na^+]$ excretion = 80 mEq/day

Questions

3a. What determines the amount of Na^+ that is excreted in the urine, and is Na^+ excretion in this patient normal (assume that he ingests approximately 80 mEq/day of Na^+)?

3b. 1 L of isotonic saline is administered intravenously with the goal of raising the serum $[Na^+]$. How much of the infused NaCl will be excreted in the urine (for simplicity, assume that 1 L of isotonic saline contains 150 mmol/L of NaCl)? What effect will this infusion have on the plasma $[Na^+]$?

3c. What effect would the administration of 1 L of hypertonic saline (3% NaCl solution) have on the plasma $[Na^+]$?

3d. What other therapies could be used to treat this man's hyponatremia?

CASE 4

An 18-year-old man with insulin-dependent (type 1) diabetes mellitus is seen in the emergency department. He reports not taking his insulin during the previous 24 hours because he did not feel well and was not eating. He now has weakness, nausea, thirst, and frequent urination. His blood pressure is 100/60 mm Hg supine and 80/50 mm Hg erect. His pulse rate increases from 100 beats/min supine to 110 beats/min when erect. On physical examination he is found to have deep and rapid respiration (Kussmaul's respiration). At 1:00 AM the following laboratory data are obtained:

Plasma $[Na^+]$ = 140 mEq/L

Serum $[Cl^-]$ = 95 mEq/L

Plasma $[K^+]$ = 6.5 mEq/L

Plasma $[HCO_3^-]$ = 7 mEq/L

Blood pH = 6.99

Arterial P_{CO_2} = 18 mm Hg

Plasma [glucose] = 600 mg/dL

Urine contains glucose and ketones

The diagnosis of diabetic ketoacidosis is made, and the man is admitted to the hospital. Saline is administered intravenously and insulin therapy begun. The results of therapy are illustrated in the following table.

TIME	SERUM $[K^+]$ (mEq/L)	PLASMA pH	SERUM $[HCO_3^-]$ (mEq/L)	SERUM [GLUCOSE] (mg/dL)
1:00 AM	6.5	6.99	7	600
3:00 AM	4.5	7.10	12	400
4:00 AM	4.0	7.16	14	300
5:00 AM	3.5	7.20	16	250
7:00 AM	3.2	7.24	18	200

Questions

4a. What type of acid-base disorder does this man have? What is the plasma anion gap, and what is its significance?

4b. What can you conclude about K^+ balance in this man?

4c. Explain why the serum $[K^+]$ fell during the first hour of treatment.

CASE 5

A previously healthy 28-year-old man is seen in the emergency department with right side flank pain. Shortly after arrival, he passes a small kidney stone. He denies any significant previous renal or gastrointestinal problems. There is a family history of kidney stones. The results of laboratory tests done in the emergency department include the following:

Serum $[Na^+]$ = 137 mEq/L

Serum $[K^+]$ = 3.1 mEq/L

Serum $[Cl^-]$ = 111 mEq/L

Serum $[HCO_3^-]$ = 13 mEq/L

Arterial pH = 7.28

Arterial $P{CO_2}$ = 28 mm Hg

Urine pH = 6.4

Questions

5a. What is the acid-base disorder? What is the anion gap, and what does it tell you about this man's acid-base disorder?

5b. How do you explain the urine pH of 6.4 when his plasma $[HCO_3^-]$ is 13 mEq/L and the plasma pH is 7.28?

5c. The man's "urinary net charge" is calculated, and a value of +13 is obtained. What information does this give you regarding renal acid-base transport, and how does this help you to determine the cause of his acid-base disorder?

CASE 6

Paramedics bring a 16-year-old asthmatic patient to the emergency department. History obtained from the parents indicates that she has had asthma for 4 years, which is induced by exercise and is exacerbated during upper respiratory infections. She currently uses an inhaler (β-adrenergic agonist) before exercise. Four days ago she developed symptoms of an upper respiratory infection, and she increased the use of her inhaler. This morning she had acute shortness of breath and her parents called 911. When the paramedics arrived she was cyanotic, and epinephrine was administered with some improvement.

On physical examination she appears anxious and in moderate distress. On auscultation of the chest, wheezes are heard throughout both lung fields. The following laboratory data are obtained:

Serum $[Na^+]$ = 140 mEq/L

Serum $[K^+]$ = 3.3 mEq/L

Serum $[Cl^-]$ = 105 mEq/L

Serum $[HCO_3^-]$ = 15 mEq/L

Serum [creatinine] = 1.0 mg/dL

Arterial pH = 7.0

Arterial $P{CO_2}$ = 60 mm Hg

Arterial $P{O_2}$ = 40 mmHg

Questions

6a. What is the acid-base disorder in this girl?

6b. What is the most likely cause of her hypokalemia?

CASE 7

A child (body weight = 30 kg) develops gastroenteritis with vomiting and diarrhea. Over a 2-day period he loses 2 kg of weight. His plasma $[Na^+]$ was initially 140 mEq/L, and is unchanged. Calculate the following:

	INITIAL	AFTER DAY 2
Total body water (L)		
ECF volume (L)		
ICF volume (L)		
Total body osmoles (mOsm)		
ECF osmoles (mOsm)		
ICF osmoles (mOsm)		

CASE 8

Another child (body weight = 30 kg) also develops gastroenteritis with vomiting and diarrhea. Over a 2-day period he also loses 2 kg of weight. However, his plasma [Na⁺], which was initially 140 mEq/L, is now 120 mEq/L. Calculate the following:

	INITIAL	AFTER DAY 2
Total body water (L)		
ECF volume (L)		
ICF volume (L)		
Total body osmoles (mOsm)		
ECF osmoles (mOsm)		
ICF osmoles (mOsm)		

CASE 9

Another child (body weight = 30 kg) also develops gastroenteritis with vomiting and diarrhea. Over a 2-day period he also loses 2 kg of weight. However, his plasma [Na⁺], which was initially 140 mEq/L, is now 160 mEq/L. Calculate the following:

	INITIAL	AFTER DAY 2
Total body water (L)		
ECF volume (L)		
ICF volume (L)		
Total body osmoles (mOsm)		
ECF osmoles (mOsm)		
ICF osmoles (mOsm)		

Compare the fluid and electrolyte treatment strategies that would be used to restore the volume and composition of the body fluids in the children in cases 7 to 9.

CASE 10

A 12-year-old girl presents to the emergency department with an acute asthmatic attack. Her respiratory rate is increased (tachypnea). Initial arterial blood gas values on room air are:

Serum $[HCO_3^-]$ = 22 mEq/L

Arterial pH = 7.55

Arterial P_{CO_2} = 28 mm Hg

Arterial P_{O_2} (room air) = 60 mm Hg

10a. What was the acid-base disorder?

Five hours later, after receiving therapy (including 40% O_2 by mask), she is tired and has quiet breath sounds on auscultation. Repeat arterial blood gases are obtained:

Serum $[HCO_3^-]$ = 22.4 mEq/L

Arterial pH = 7.32

Arterial P_{CO_2} = 45 mm Hg

Arterial P_{O_2} (room air) = 60 mm Hg

10b. What is the acid-base disorder after therapy?

10c. How do you account for the change in the patient's condition after therapy?

APPENDIX B

NORMAL LABORATORY VALUES

	TRADITIONAL UNITS	SI UNITS
Arterial Blood Gases		
P_{CO_2}	33-44 mm Hg	4.4-5.9 kPa
P_{CO_2}	75-105 mm Hg	10.0-14.0 kPa
pH	7.35-7.45	$[H^+]$ 36-44 nmol/L
Serum Electrolytes*		
Na^+	135-147 mEq/L	135-147 mmol/L
Cl^-	95-105 mEq/L	95-105 mmol/L
K^+	3.5-5.0 mEq/L	3.5-5.0 mmol/L
HCO_3^-	22-28 mEq/L	22-28 mmol/L
Ca^{++}	8.4-10.0 mg/dL	2.1-2.8 mmol/L
P_i	3.0-4.5 mg/dL	1.0-1.5 mmol/L
Anion gap	8-16 mEq/L	8-16 mmol/L
Serum Proteins		
Total	6.0-7.8 g/dL	60-78 g/L
Albumin	3.5-5.5 g/dL	35-55 g/L
Globulin	2.3-3.5 g/dL	23-35 g/L
Other Serum Constituents		
Creatinine	0.6-1.2 mg/dL	53-106 mmol/L
Glucose (fasting)	70-110 mg/dL	3.8-6.1 mmol/L
Urea nitrogen (BUN)	7-18 mg/dL	1.2-3.0 mmol/L
Serum osmolality	285-295 mOsm/kg H_2O	285-295 mOsm/kg H_2O
Creatinine Clearance		
Male	90-140 mL/min	90-140 mL/min
	130-200 L/day	130-200 L/day
Female	80-125 mL/min	80-125 mL/min
	115-180 L/day	115-180 L/day

*Serum is derived from clotted blood (devoid of clotting factors), whereas plasma is derived from unclotted blood (contains clotting factors). However, concentrations of most substances are the same whether determined on a sample of plasma or serum. Most clinical chemistry laboratories determine concentrations of serum samples.
BUN, blood urea nitrogen.

APPENDIX C

NEPHRON FUNCTION

SUMMARY BY TRANSPORT PROCESS

TABLE C-1		
Na$^+$ and Cl$^-$ Reabsorption		
NEPHRON SEGMENT	**MECHANISM**	**REGULATION**
Proximal tubule	Na$^+$-H$^+$ antiport Na$^+$-solute symport Cl$^-$ anion exhange Paracellular	↓ ECF volume (+) ↑ ECF volume (−) Angiotensin II (+) Sympathetic nerves (+) Epinephrine (+) Dopamine (−) Starling forces (+)

Henle's loop
   Thin descending limb
   Thin ascending limb
   Thick ascending limb
	
	None
	Paracellular
	Na$^+$-K$^+$-2Cl$^-$ symport
		
		Aldosterone (+)
		Sympathetic nerves (+)

Early distal tubule	Paracellular Na$^+$-Cl$^-$ symport	 Aldosterone (+) Sympathetic nerves (+) Angiotensin II (+)
Late distal tubule and collecting duct	Na$^+$ channel (ENaC)	Aldosterone (+) Sympathetic nerves (+) Angiotensin II (+) ANP, BNP, urodilation (−) Uroguanylin, guanylin (−)

ANP, atrial natriuretic peptide; *BNP*, brain natriuretic peptide; *ECF*, extracellular fluid; (+), stimulation; (−), inhibition.

TABLE C-2
K⁺ Reabsorption

NEPHRON SEGMENT	MECHANISM	REGULATION
Proximal tubule	Paracellular	↓ ECF volume (+)
		↑ ECF volume (−)
Henle's loop		
Thin descending limb	None	
Thin ascending limb	None	
Thick ascending limb	Na^+-K^+-$2Cl^-$ symport	Aldosterone (+)
	Paracellular	
Early distal tubule	None	
Late distal tubule and collecting duct	H^+-K^+-ATPase	Dietary K^+ depeltion (+)

ECF, extracellular fluid; (+), stimulation; (−), inhibition.

TABLE C-3
K⁺ Secretion

NEPHRON SEGMENT	MECHANISM	REGULATION
Promixmal tubule	None	
Henle's loop		
Thin descending limb	None	
Thin ascending limb	None	
Thick ascending limb	None	
Early distal tubule	None	
Late distal tubule and collecting duct	K^+ channel	Plasma [K+] (+)
		Aldosterone (+)
		AVP (+)
		Flow rate (+)
		Acid-base balance (+/−)
		Glucocortiocoids (+)

AVP, arginine vasopressin; (+), stimulation; (−), inhibition.

TABLE C-4
H⁺ Secretion (HCO₃⁻ Reabsorption)

NEPHRON SEGMENT	MECHANISM	REGULATION
Promixmal tubule	Na^+-H^+ antiport	↑ Filtered load of HCO_3^- (+)
	H^+-ATPase	↓ ECF volume (+)
		↑ P_{CO_2} (+)
		↓ Plasma [HCO_3^-] (+)
		Endothelin (+)
		Glucocorticoid (+)
		Acute PTH (−)
Henle's loop		
Thin descending limb	None	
Thin ascending limb	None	
Thick ascending limb	Na^+-H^+ antiport	↑ P_{CO_2} (+)
	H^+-ATPase	↓ Plasma [HCO_3^-] (+)
		Chronic PTH (+)
Early distal tubule	Na^+-H^+ antiport	↑ P_{CO_2} (+)
	H^+-ATPase	↓ Plasma [HCO_3^-] (+)
Late distal tubule and collecting duct	H^+-ATPase	↑ P_{CO_2} (+)
	H^+-K^+-ATPase	↓ Plasma [HCO_3^-] (+)
		Aldosterone (+)

ATPase, adenosine triphosphatase; *ECF*, extracellular fluid; *PTH*, parathyroid hormone; (+), stimulation; (−), inhibition.

TABLE C-5
HCO₃⁻ Secretion

NEPHRON SEGMENT	MECHANISM	REGULATION
Promixmal tubule	None	
Henle's loop		
Thin descending limb	None	
Thin ascending limb	None	
Thick ascending limb	None	
Early distal tubule	None	
Late distal tubule and collecting duct	H^+– ATPase Cl⁻–HCO₃⁻ antiport	Metabolic alkalosis (+)

ATPase, adenosine triphosphatase; (+), stimulation; (−), inhibition.

TABLE C-6
Water Reabsorption

NEPHRON SEGMENT	MECHANISM	REGULATION
Promixmal tubule	AQP water channel	Starling forces
Henle's loop		
Thin descending limb	AQP water channel	
Thin ascending limb	None	
Thick ascending limb	None	
Early distal tubule	None	
Late distal tubule and collecting duct	AQP water channel	AVP (+) ANP, BNP, urodilation, uroguanylin, guanylin (−)

ANP, atrial natriuretic peptide; *AQP*, aquaporin; *AVP*, arginine vasopressin; *BNP*, brain natriuretic peptide; (+), stimulation; (−), inhibition.

Table C-7
Pᵢ Reabsorption

NEPHRON SEGMENT	MECHANISM	REGULATION
Promixmal tubule	$3Na^+$-P_i symport $2Na^+$-P_i symport	PTH P_i depletion (+) ↓ ECF volume (+) Acidosis (−) Glucocorticoids (−) FGF-23 (−)
Henle's loop		
Thin descending limb	None	
Thin ascending limb	None	
Thick ascending limb	None	
Early distal tubule	None	
Late distal tubule and collecting duct	None	

ECF, extracellular fluid; *FGF*, fibroblast growth factor; *PTH*, parathyroid hormone; (+), stimulation; (−), inhibition.

TABLE C-8
Ca⁺⁺ Reabsorption

NEPHRON SEGMENT	MECHANISM	REGULATION
Proximal tubule	Ca^{++} channel Paracellular	PTH (−) ↓ ECF volume (+) ↓ Plasma [P_i] (+)
Henle's loop		
Thin descending limb	None	
Thin ascending limb	None	
Thick ascending limb	Paracellular	PTH (+) ↓ Plasma [P_i] (+) CaSR (−)
Early distal tubule	Ca^{++} channel	PTH (+) Calcitriol (+) ↓ Plasma [P_i] (+) Acidosis (−) CaSR (−)
Late distal tubule and collecting duct	None	

CaSR, calcium-sensing receptor; *ECF*, extracellular fluid; *PTH*, parathyroid hormone; (+), stimulation; (−), inhibition.

SUMMARY BY NEPHRON SEGMENT

Proximal Tubule

Reabsorption

Water	67% of the filtered load
NaCl	67% of the filtered load
K^+	67% of the filtered load
Ca^{++}	70% of the filtered load
P_i	80% of the filtered load
HCO_3^-	80% of the filtered load
Protein	100% of the filtered load
Urea	67% of the filtered load

Secretion

NH_4^+	Variable
Organic anions	Variable
Organic cations	Varaible

Henle's Loop (Thick Ascending Limb)

Reabsorption

Water	15% of the filtered load (thin descending limb only)
NaCl	25% of the filtered load
Ca^{++}	20% of the filtered load
HCO_3^-	10% of the filtered load
NH_4^+	Variable

Secretion
Urea (thin descending limb only)

Distal Tubule

Reabsorption

NaCl	5% of the filtered load
Ca^{++}	9% of the filtered load
HCO_3^-	6% of the filtered load
P_i	10% of the filtered load
Water	Variable in the late portion depending on AVP, ANP, BNP, uroguanylin, and guanylin levels

Collecting Duct

Reabsorption

Water	Variable depending on AVP, ANP, BNP, uroguanylin and guanylin levels
NaCl	3% of the filtered load
K^+	Normally zero
HCO_3^-	4% of the filtered load
Urea	Variable in medullary collecting duct depending on AVP levels

Secretion

K^+	0%-70% of the filtered load
NH_4^+	Variable
Urea	Variable (medullary portion only)

APPENDIX D

ANSWERS TO SELF-STUDY PROBLEMS

CHAPTER 1

1.

		MOLARITY (mmol/L)	OSMOLALITY (mOsm/kg H$_2$O)
9 g	NaCl	154	308
72 g	Glucose	400	400
22.2 g	CaCl$_2$	200	600
3 g	Urea	50	50
8.4 g	NaHCO$_3$	100	200

2. The cell will swell when placed in the solution because the solute is only a partially effective osmole (i.e., this is a hypotonic solution). Because the reflection coefficient (σ) is 0.5, the effective osmolality of the solution is only 150 mOsm/kg H$_2$O. The solution would have to contain 600 mmol/L of this solute to be isotonic.

3. Na$^+$, with its anions Cl$^-$ and HCO$_3^-$, constitutes the majority of particles in the ECF and is therefore the major determinant of plasma osmolality. Consequently, plasma osmolality can be estimated by simply doubling the plasma [Na$^+$]. Thus the estimated plasma osmolality in this individual is as follows:

$$P_{osm} = 2(130) = 260 \text{ mOsm/kg H}_2\text{O}$$

This value is well below the normal range of 285 to 295 mOsm/kg H$_2$O and will result in movement of water from the ECF into the ICF. Because ions move freely across the capillary wall, the [Na$^+$] (and osmolality) of the plasma and interstitial fluid will be the same. Therefore, water movement across the capillary endothelium will not be affected.

4. The increase in venous pressure causes increased movement of fluid out of the capillary. As a result, fluid accumulates in the interstitial space. Some of this fluid will be taken up by the lymphatics, and lymphatic flow will increase. However, when the capacity of the lymphatics to remove this fluid is exceeded, the volume of the interstitial space increases, and edema forms (see also Chapter 6).

5. This is an isotonic solution and will therefore remain confined initially to the ECF. The ECF volume will increase by 1 L, and ICF volume will be unchanged (initial volumes being 10 L [ECF] and 20 L [ICF], respectively). Plasma [Na$^+$] will decrease because of the addition of 1 L of Na$^+$-free solution to the ECF. The new plasma [Na$^+$] is calculated by:

Initial ECF Na$^+$ content	= 145 mEq/L $\times$ 10 L
	= 1450 mEq
New [Na$^+$]	= 1450 mEq/11 L
	= 132 mEq/L

Therefore the immediate effect is:

ECF volume	11 L
ICF volume	20 L
Plasma [Na$^+$]	132 mEq/L

In the long term, the dextrose will be metabolized to CO$_2$ and H$_2$O. Thus infusion of a dextrose solution is equivalent to infusion of solute-free water. After metabolism of dextrose (several hours) and equilibration, the 1 L of infused H$_2$O will distribute into both the ICF and ECF in proportion to the ratio of their volumes (two thirds into the ICF and one third into the ECF):

ICF volume	= 20 L + 0.67 L	= 20.67 L
ECF volume	= 10 L + 0.33 L	= 10.33 L
New [Na$^+$]	= 1450 mEq/10.33 L	= 141 mEq/L

Therefore the long-term effect is:

ECF volume	10.3 L
ICF volume	20.7 L
Plasma [Na$^+$]	141 mEq/L

As noted previously, a dextrose solution is equivalent to solute-free water. Therefore, these solutions would be used when the patient had lost solute-free water and body fluid osmolality is elevated (i.e., hypernatremia).

6. A 0.9% NaCl solution is isotonic saline. Therefore, the entire infused volume will remain in the ECF. In this example, the ECF will increase by 1 L and the ICF will not change. One approach to this problem is to calculate the amount of Na$^+$ in the infused volume and then determine the effect on the plasma [Na$^+$]. For example:

0.9% NaCl	= 154 mEq/L
Amount of infused Na$^+$	= 1 L × 154 mEq/L
	= 154 mEq
New ECF Na$^+$ content	= 1450 mEq + 154 mEq
	= 1604 mEq
New plasma [Na$^+$]	= 1604 mEq/11 L
	= 146 mEq/L

Therefore the immediate effect is:

ECF volume	11 L
ICF volume	20 L
Plasma [Na$^+$]	146 mEq/L

The long-term effect of this infusion is identical to that seen immediately. Thus the long-term effect is:

ECF volume	11 L
ICF volume	20 L
Plasma [Na$^+$]	146 mEq/L

From this it is apparent that infusion of isotonic saline into an individual with a normal serum [Na$^+$] will result in an increase in the volume of the ECF, equal to the entire infused volume, with no appreciable change in the serum [Na$^+$].

7. The initial volumes of the body fluid compartments and the osmoles in these compartments are calculated as follows (osmolality is estimated as 2 × [Na$^+$] = 280 mOsm/kg H$_2$O):

Initial total body water	= 0.6(60 kg) = 36 L
Initial ICF volume	= 0.4(60 kg) = 24 L
Initial ECF volume	= 0.2(60 kg) = 12 L
Initial total body osmoles	= (total body water)(body fluid osmolality)
	= (36 L)(280 mOsm/kg H$_2$O)
	= 10,080 mOsm
Initial ICF osmoles	= (ICF volume)(body fluid osmolality)
	= (24 L)(280 mOsm/kg H$_2$O)
	= 6720 mOsm
Initial ECF osmoles	= Total body osmoles − ICF osmoles
	= 10,080 mOsm = 6720 mOsm
	= 3360 mOsm

Four kilograms of body weight are lost. It is assumed that this entire weight reduction reflects fluids lost through vomiting and diarrhea. Thus 4 L of fluid are lost. Because the plasma [Na$^+$] is unchanged, a proportional amount of solute was also lost (isotonic loss of fluid). No fluid shifts occur between the ECF and ICF because of the absence of an osmotic gradient between these compartments. Therefore the ECF loses 4 L of volume, and 4 × 280 = 1120 mOsm of solute.

New total body water	= 36 L − 4 L = 32 L
New ICF volume	= 24 L (unchanged)
New ECF volume	= 12 L − 4 L = 8 L
New total body osmoles	= 10,080 mOsm − 1120 mOsm
	= 8960 mOsm
New ICF osmoles	= 6720 mOsm (unchanged)
New ECF osmoles	= 3360 mOsm − 1120 mOsm
	= 2240 mOsm

8. The initial volumes of the body fluid compartments and the osmoles in these compartments are calculated as in problem 7:

Initial total body water	= 0.6(50 kg) = 30 L
Initial ICF volume	= 0.4(50 kg) = 20 L
Initial ECF volume	= 0.2(50 kg) = 10 L
Initial total body osmoles	= (total body water) × (body fluid osmolality)
	=(30 L)(290 mOsm/kg H$_2$O)
	= 8700 mOsm
Initial ICF osmoles	= (ICF volume)(body fluid osmolality)
	= (20 L)(290 mOsm/kg H$_2$O)
	= 5800 mOsm

Initial ECF osmoles = Total body osmoles − ICF osmoles
= 8700 mOsm − 5800 mOsm
= 2900 mOsm

The total amount of mannitol added to the ECF must be calculated to determine its effect on body fluids. At 5 g/kg, a total of 250 g was added to the ECF (1.374 moles of mannitol). Because mannitol is a single particle in solution, this adds 1374 mOsm to the ECF. The mannitol will raise ECF osmolality and result in the shift of fluid from the ICF into the ECF.

New total body water = 30 L (unchanged)
New total body osmoles = 8700 mOsm + 1374 mOsm
= 10,074 mOsm
New ICF osmoles = 5800 mOsm (unchanged)
New ECF osmoles = 2900 mOsm + 1374 mOsm
= 4274 mOsm
New plasma osmolality = New total osmoles/Total body water
= 10,074 mOsm/30L
= 336 mOsm/kg H_2O
New ICF volume = ICF osmols/New P_{osm}
= 5800 mOsm/336 mOsm/kg H_2O
= 17.3 L
New ECF volume = Total body water − ICF volume
= 30 L − 17.3 L = 12.7 L

Because mannitol increases the osmolality of the ECF, 2.7 L of fluid shifts from the ICF into the ECF. To calculate the new plasma [Na^+], assume that the amount of Na^+ in the ECF is unchanged after mannitol infusion. Originally, there were 2900 mOsm attributable to Na^+ ($2 \times$ [Na^+] = ECF volume) in the ECF. Because the Na^+ osmoles are unchanged but are now present in a larger volume, the new plasma [Na^+] is calculated as follows:

New plasma Na^+ osmoles = 2900 mOsm from Na^+/12.7L
= 228 mOsm/L
New plasma [Na^+] = Na^+ Osm/2
= 228 mOsm/L
= 114 mEq/L

9. Both individuals start out with the same total body water (36 L) and total body osmoles (10,440 mOsm) assuming a plasma [Na^+] of 145 mEq/L and a plasma osmolality of 290 mOsm/kg H_2O. Subject A loses 1 L of total body water and 1000 osmoles of total body solute, resulting in a new plasma osmolality of:

$$P_{osm} = (10,440 \text{ mOsm} − 1000 \text{ mOsm})/35 \text{ L}$$
$$= 270 \text{ mOsm/kg } H_2O$$

Subject B loses 4 L of total body water and 1600 mOsm of total body solute, resulting in a new plasma osmolality of:

$$P_{osm} = (10,440 \text{ mOsm} − 1600 \text{ mOsm})/32 \text{ L}$$
$$= 276 \text{ mOsm/kg } H_2O$$

CHAPTER 2

1. The gross anatomic features of the kidney include the cortex, medulla, nephrons, blood vessels, lymphatics, nerves, renal pyramids, papilla, minor calyx, major calyces, and pelvis.

2. The nephron consists of a renal corpuscle, proximal tubule, loop of Henle, distal tubule, and collecting duct system.

3. The renal artery branches progressively to form the interlobar artery, the arcuate artery, the interlobular artery, and the afferent arteriole, which leads into the glomerular capillaries (i.e., glomerulus). The glomerular capillaries come together to form the efferent arteriole, which leads into a second capillary network, the peritubular capillaries, which supply blood to the nephron. The vessels of the venous system run parallel to the arterial vessels and progressively form the interlobular vein, arcuate vein, interlobar vein, and renal vein, which courses beside the ureter.

4. The renal corpuscle is the first part of the nephron and is composed of glomerular capillaries and Bowman's capsule.

5. The glomerular capillary endothelium, basement membrane, and foot processes of podocytes form the so-called *filtration barrier*. Proteins are filtered on the basis of size.

6. Structures that compose the juxtaglomerular apparatus include the macula densa of the thick ascending limb, extraglomerular mesangial cells, and the renin-producing granular cells of the afferent arterioles.

7. The juxtaglomerular apparatus is one component of a feedback mechanism (i.e., tubuloglomerular feedback) that regulates renal blood flow and glomerular filtration rate. It also regulates renin secretion by the granular cells of the afferent arteriole.

8. The mesangium consists of mesangial cells and the mesangial matrix. Mesangial cells, which possess many properties of smooth muscles cells, surround the glomerular capillaries, provide structural support for the glomerular capillaries, secrete the extracellular matrix, exhibit phagocytic activity that removes macromolecules from the mesangium, and secrete prostaglandins and proinflammatory cytokines. Because they also contract and are adjacent to glomerular capillaries, mesangial cells may influence the GFR by regulating blood flow through the glomerular capillaries or by altering the capillary surface area. Mesangial cells located outside the glomerulus (between the afferent and efferent arterioles) are called extraglomerular mesangial cells.

9. Renal nerves regulate renal blood flow, glomerular filtration rate, and salt and water reabsorption by the nephron. The nerve supply to the kidneys consists of sympathetic nerve fibers that originate in the celiac plexus. There is no parasympathetic innervation. Adrenergic fibers that innervate the kidneys release norepinephrine. The adrenergic fibers lie adjacent to the smooth muscle cells of the major branches of the renal artery (interlobar, arcuate, and interlobular arteries) and the afferent and efferent arterioles. Moreover, sympathetic nerves innervate the renin-producing granular cells of the afferent arterioles. Renin secretion is stimulated by increased sympathetic activity. Nerve fibers also innervate the proximal tubule, loop of Henle, distal tubule, and collecting duct; activation of these nerves enhances Na^+ reabsorption by these nephron segments.

CHAPTER 3

1. Before phlorhizin administration:

Serum [inulin]	1 mg/mL
Serum [glucose]	1 mg/mL
Inulin excretion rate	100 mg/min
Glucose excretion rate	0 mg/min

Inulin clearance	100 mL/min
Glucose clearance	0 mL/min

After phlorhizin administration:

Serum [inulin]	1 mg/mL
Serum [glucose]	1 mg/mL
Inulin excretion rate	100 mg/min
Glucose excretion rate	100 mg/min
Inulin clearance	100 mL/min
Glucose clearance	100 mL/min

Before treatment with phlorhizin, the filtered load of glucose (GFR × serum [glucose]) is 100 mg/min (GFR calculated from inulin clearance). With this filtered load of glucose, all the glucose is reabsorbed and none is excreted. Thus, the clearance of glucose is zero. After phlorhizin the filtered load is unchanged, but there is no glucose reabsorption. Therefore, all the glucose that is filtered is excreted, and the clearance of glucose equals that of inulin.

2. a. Although the appearance of red cells in the urine can result from damage to the glomerular filtration barrier, red cells can also appear in the urine for other reasons. For example, they can appear as a result of bleeding in any part of the lower urinary tract. Such bleeding is seen with kidney stones and occasionally as a result of a bacterial infection of the lower urinary tract, which causes bleeding. Thus, the appearance of blood in the urine does not necessarily mean the glomerular filtration barrier is damaged.

   b. Because glucose is filtered and completely reabsorbed by the proximal tubule, it is not normally found in the urine. Its presence in the urine indicates an elevated serum glucose level such that the filtered load (i.e., GFR × serum [glucose]) is greater than the ability of the proximal tubule to reabsorb glucose. Because glucose is freely filtered by the normal glomerulus, damage to the ultrafiltration barrier would not increase its filtration.

   c. In healthy individuals, Na^+ normally appears in the urine. Like glucose, Na^+ is freely filtered by the normal glomerulus. Therefore damage to the filtration barrier does not increase the rate of Na^+ excretion.

d. This is the correct answer. Normally, the urine contains essentially no protein. The glomerulus prevents the filtration of plasma proteins. However, when the glomerulus is damaged, large amounts of plasma proteins are filtered. If the amount filtered overwhelms the reabsorptive capacity of the proximal tubule, protein appears in the urine (proteinuria).

3. The equation for blood flow through an organ is $Q = \Delta P/R$. Sympathetic agonists, angiotensin II, and prostaglandins change blood flow by altering the resistance (R). Whereas sympathetic agonists and angiotensin II increase R and thereby decrease renal blood flow (RBF), prostaglandins decrease R and thereby increase RBF.

4. Normally, renal prostaglandin production is low, and nonsteroidal antiinflammatory drugs (NSAIDs) do not have an appreciable effect on prostaglandin production. However, during reductions in GFR and RBF, elevated prostaglandin levels cause vasodilation of the afferent and efferent arterioles. This effect prevents excessive decreases in RBF and GFR. Administration of NSAIDs to patients with low GFR and RBF inhibits prostaglandin production and further reduces GFR and RBF.

CHAPTER 4

1. The glomeruli filter 25,200 mEq of Na^+ and 18,000 mEq of Cl^- each day (assuming GFR = 180 L/day), and 99% is reabsorbed by the nephrons, with less than 1% appearing in the urine. Although Na^+ and Cl^- uptake into cells across the apical membrane and NaCl reabsorption across the paracellular pathway are passive processes (i.e., they do not require the direct input of adenosine triphosphate [ATP]), they ultimately depend on the operation of the Na^+-K^+-ATPase. Accordingly, reabsorption of NaCl requires a considerable quantity of ATP, the synthesis of which by kidney cells requires large amounts of oxygen and, hence, high blood flow.

2. "Normal" or "average" urine composition does not actually exist because of the variability in the volume of urine excreted, as well as variations in the intake of solutes in the diet (Table D-1). Urine was

Table D-1
Urine Flow Rate

	0.5 L/DAY	1 L/DAY	2 L/DAY
Na^+ (mEq/L)	300	150	75
K^+ (mEq/L)	200	100	50
Cl^- (mEq/L)	300	150	75
HCO_3^- (mEq/L)	4	2	1
Ca^{++} (mg/dL)	40	20	10
NH_4^+ (mEq/L)	100	50	25
Creatinine (mg/L)	2000	1000	500
Glucose (mmol/L)	1.0	0.5	0.25
Urea (mmol/L)	600	300	150
Urea (mg/L)	14000	7000	3500
pH	5.0	to	7.0
Osmolality (mOsm/kg H_2O)	1600	800	400

Modified from Valtin HV: *Renal function*, ed 2, Boston, 1983, Little, Brown. Lab values from DMS, 1989.

Table D-2

SOLUTE	SOLUTE EXCRETION/DAY
Na^+ (mEq)	150
K^+ (mEq)	100
Cl^- (mEq)	150
HCO_3^- (mEq)	2
Ca^{++} (mg)	200
NH_4^+ (mEq)	50
Creatinine (mg)	1000
Glucose (mmol)	0.5
Urea (mmol)	300
Urea (mg/L)	7000
Osmolytes (mOsm)	800

collected on three different days from a subject who ate a consistent diet but ingested different amounts of water each day. Although the amount of each solute excreted was similar each day (Table D-2), the concentration of each solute in the urine was different because the volume of urine varied each day. This question demonstrates that the amount (or rate) of a solute excreted, not the concentration of the solute in the urine, is important in the clinical evaluation of urine.

3. Passive transport always occurs down an electrochemical gradient. For coupled transporters

(antiport and symport), the movement of one molecule down its electrochemical gradient can drive uphill movement of the coupled molecule. When this occurs, the uphill movement is termed secondary active transport because the transporter is not coupled directly to the hydrolysis of ATP. Active transport occurs against an electrochemical gradient and requires the direct input of energy (i.e., ATP). Some authors refer to such transport as primary active to emphasize the direct coupling to ATP.

4. Because the Na^+-K^+-ATPase is ultimately responsible for the reabsorption and secretion of all solutes (except H^+) and water by the nephron, complete inhibition of this transport protein would block all solute and water transport (both cellular and paracellular). Hence, in this hypothetical example, each day the kidneys would excrete 180 L of fluid (assuming GFR = 180 L/day) that would be similar in composition to the glomerular ultrafiltrate.

5. The reabsorption of Na^+ in the first half of the proximal tubule is coupled to that of HCO_3^- and a number of organic molecules, and this generates a negative transepithelial voltage across the proximal tubule that provides the driving force for the paracellular reabsorption of Cl^-. The reabsorption of many organic molecules is so avid that they are almost completely removed from the tubular fluid in the first half of the proximal tubule. The reabsorption of $NaHCO_3$ and Na^+ organic solutes across the proximal tubule establishes a transtubular osmotic gradient that provides the driving force for the passive reabsorption of water by osmosis. Because more water than Cl^- is reabsorbed in the first half of the proximal tubule, the Cl^- concentration in tubular fluid rises along the length of the proximal tubule. In the second half of the proximal tubule, Na^+ is mainly reabsorbed with Cl^- across the transcellular pathway. Na^+ is primarily reabsorbed with Cl^- rather than organic solutes or HCO_3^- as the accompanying anion because the Na^+ transport mechanisms in the second half of the proximal tubule differs from those in the first half. Furthermore, the tubular fluid that enters the second half contains very little glucose and amino acids, but the high concentration of Cl^- (140 mEq/L) in tubule fluid exceeds that in the first half (105 mEq/L). The high Cl^- concentration is due to the preferential reabsorption of Na^+ with HCO_3^- and organic solutes in the first half of the proximal tubule. In the second half of the proximal tubule Na^+ enters the cell across the luminal membrane primarily through the parallel operation of a Na^+-H^+ antiporter and one or more Cl^--base antiporters. Because the secreted H^+ and base combine in the tubular fluid and reenter the cell, the operation of the Na^+-H^+ and Cl^--anion antiporters is equivalent to NaCl uptake from tubular fluid into the cell. Na^+ leaves the cell through Na^+-K^+-ATPase, and Cl^- leaves the cell and enters the blood through a K^+-Cl^- symporter and a Cl^- channel in the basolateral membrane. Some NaCl is also reabsorbed across the second half of the proximal tubule by a paracellular route. The transport of solutes (NaCl) across the cellular and paracellular pathways lowers the osmolality of the tubular fluid and increases the osmolality of the interstitial fluid, which establishes a driving force for water reabsorption across the proximal tubule. Some solutes are reabsorbed with this water by the process of solvent drag. Starling forces across the wall of the peritubular capillary are important for the uptake of this interstitial fluid and can regulate the rate of solute and water back-flux across the tight junctions and thereby modulate net solute and water reabsorption.

6. NaCl is reabsorbed across the thick ascending limb by two mechanisms. First, transcellular transport involves Na^+ and Cl^- entry into the cell across the apical membrane by the Na^+-K^+-$2Cl^-$ symporter (some Na^+ is also reabsorbed by the apical membrane Na^+-H^+ antiporter) and exit across the basolateral membrane by the Na^+-K^+-ATPase (for Na^+) and a K^+-Cl^- symporter and Cl^- channel (for Cl^-). Second, Na^+ is also reabsorbed across the paracellular pathway, owing to the lumen-positive transepithelial voltage. Furosemide would have no effect on water reabsorption in the thick ascending limb because this segment of the nephron is relatively impermeable to water and water is not reabsorbed even when NaCl reabsorptive rates are high. Furosemide increases water excretion by reducing the osmolality of the medullary interstitial fluid, which

in turn reduces water reabsorption from the descending thin limb of Henle's loop and medullary collecting duct.

7. Glomerulotubular balance describes the phenomenon whereby an increase in the filtered load of water and NaCl is accompanied by a parallel increase in water and NaCl reabsorption by the proximal tubule. If a constant amount of NaCl and water was reabsorbed by the proximal tubule, increases in GFR and the filtered load of NaCl and water would result in an increased delivery to more distal segments. If these segments were not able to reabsorb the excess NaCl and water, large amounts could be lost in the urine. If such an increase in excretion were not accompanied by a corresponding rise in dietary intake, the organism would develop negative NaCl and water balance. Hence, glomerulotubular balance helps maintain NaCl and water homeostasis despite changes in GFR and the filtered load of water and NaCl.

8. See Table 4-6.

CHAPTER 5

1. This problem illustrates the importance of effective versus ineffective osmoles in regulating AVP secretion. Although plasma osmolality is elevated, the increased osmolality is due to urea. Because urea is an ineffective osmole with regard to AVP secretion, it is necessary to estimate the osmolality of plasma that is due to effective osmoles (Na^+ and its anions). The effective osmolality of the plasma is estimated by doubling the plasma [Na^+], which yields a value of 270 mOsm/kg H_2O (see Chapter 1). Because the effective osmolality is reduced, AVP secretion is suppressed and plasma levels are reduced.

2. Osmolality of tubular fluid

Nephron Site	0- AVP	Max. AVP
Proximal tubule	300	300
Beginning of descending thin limb	300	300
Beginning of ascending thin limb	1200	1200
End of thick ascending limb	=150	=150
End of cortical collecting duct	<100	300
Urine	=50	1200

Regardless of the presence or absence of AVP, tubular fluid osmolality is the same in all segments except the late portion of the distal tubule and collecting duct. When AVP is present, the tubular fluid within the lumen of these segments comes to osmotic equilibrium with the surrounding interstitial fluid (300 mOsm/kg H_2O in the cortex and 1200 mOsm/kg H_2O in the papilla). In the absence of AVP, solute reabsorption by these segments leads to further dilution of the tubular fluid.

3. a. Decreased renal perfusion: With a decrease in renal perfusion, as would occur with contraction of the extracellular fluid volume, delivery of solute and water to Henle's loop is reduced (GFR is decreased, and therefore filtered load is decreased and proximal tubule fractional reabsorption is enhanced [see Chapter 6]). As a result, there will be less separation of solute and water and a reduction in $T^c_{H_2O}$. Urine osmolality will be maximal, but the total volume of solute-free water reabsorbed by the nephron (i.e., $T^c_{H_2O}$) will be reduced.

b. Inhibition of thick ascending limb transport: Inhibition of thick ascending limb NaCl transport decreases the separation of solute and water that occurs at this site. Because transport by the thick ascending limb is necessary for the generation of the medullary interstitial osmotic gradient, the osmolality of the interstitium falls. This impairs the reabsorption of water from the medullary collecting duct. As a result, $T^c_{H_2O}$ is reduced. The urine osmolality will approach 300 mOsm/kg H_2O, reflecting the fact that fluid entering Henle's loop from the proximal tubule has an osmolality of this value, and separation of solute and water is impaired.

c. Nephrogenic diabetes insipidus: In nephrogenic diabetes insipidus, the collecting duct does not respond to AVP. As a result, water cannot be absorbed. This impairs the ability of the kidneys to concentrate the urine and reabsorb solute-free water ($T^c_{H_2O}$). Dilute urine will be excreted.

d. Defect in the urea transporter in the vasa recta: The urea transporter in the vasa recta (UT-B) helps to trap urea in the inner interstitium of the medulla by the process of countercurrent exchange. In the absence of this transporter, trapping of urea is impaired. As a result, the osmolality of the inner medullary interstitium is reduced and the urine cannot be maximally concentrated.

4. If daily solute excretion is 800 mOsm and the individual can produce concentrated urine that has an osmolality of only 400 mOsm/kg H_2O, the minimum volume of urine required for this solute excretion is:

$$\frac{800 \text{ mOsm}}{400 \text{ mOsm/kg } H_2O} = 2 \text{ L}$$

If insensible loss is 1 L, this individual must drink at least 3 L of water (or other dilute beverage) in that 24-hour period to prevent the development of hyperosmolality. This is slightly more than the average daily intake of most individuals. For the second individual, the daily water requirement is much less because of the ability to excrete a more concentrated urine. The minimum urine volume required in this individual:

$$\frac{800 \text{ mOsm}}{1200 \text{ mOsm/kg } H_2O} = 0.67 \text{ L}$$

With insensible loss of 1 L, daily water intake could be less than 2 L, and body fluid osmolality would be maintained. A corollary to these examples is that solute excretion also places constraints on the maximum volume of water that can be ingested. For example, if an individual who can dilute urine to 100 mOsm/kg H_2O excretes 800 mOsm of solute, this person could drink as much as 8 L of water without reducing body fluid osmolality. If, however, the individual excretes more solute (e.g., 1200 mOsm), 12 L of water could be ingested. Indeed, a decline in body fluid osmolality can be seen in individuals who drink large quantities of water without sufficient solute intake.

5. Osmolar clearance and free water clearance are calculated as:

$$C_{osm} = \frac{200 \text{ mOsm/kg } H_2O \times 6 \text{ L/day}}{280 \text{ mOsm/kg } H_2O} = 4.3 \text{ L}$$

and

$$C_{H2O} = 6 \text{ L/day} - 4.3 \text{ L/day} = 1.7 \text{ L/day}$$

CHAPTER 6

1. It is assumed that the 3-kg weight loss reflects only the loss of ECF. Because the plasma $[Na^+]$ is unchanged, this represents a loss of isotonic fluid (3 L) from the ECF.

   Plasma osmolality: Because the plasma $[Na^+]$ is unchanged, the plasma osmolality is unchanged.

   ECF volume: The ECF volume has been decreased by 3 L.

   Effective circulating volume (ECV): The loss of fluid from the ECF will be detected by the vascular volume sensors as a decrease in the ECV.

   Plasma AVP levels: The vascular volume sensors will detect the decreased ECV and cause increased AVP secretion (see Chapter 5).

   Urine osmolality: The increased levels of AVP lead to water conservation by the kidneys and excretion of a concentrated urine (see Chapter 5).

   Sensation of thirst: Again, the detection of a decrease in ECV by the vascular volume sensors leads to an enhanced sensation of thirst. The elevated levels of angiotensin II, which would also exist in this situation, will also stimulate the thirst center in the hypothalamus (see Chapter 5).

2. The individual is euvolemic. To maintain Na^+ balance, the amount of Na^+ ingested in the diet must equal the amount excreted from the body. Because the kidneys are the primary route for Na^+ excretion, the amount of Na^+ excreted daily is very nearly equal to the amount ingested in the diet (small amounts of Na^+ are lost in perspiration and feces). Therefore, the Na^+ excretion rate in this individual is approximately 100 mEq/day.

3.

	Volume Expansion	Volume Contraction
Renal sympathetic nerve activity	Decreased	Increased
ANP and BNP levels	Increased	Decreased
Angiotensin II levels	Decreased	Increased
Aldosterone levels	Decreased	Increased
Vasopressin levels	Decreased	Increased

4. Volume of accumulated edema fluid   = 4 L
   Amount of Na^+ retained by the kidneys = 580 mEq

   The man has gained 4 kg. This represents an increase in the volume of his ECF of 4 L of fluid (1 kg = 1 L). A portion of this will accumulate in the interstitial fluid compartment as edema because of the altered Starling forces across his capillary walls. The composition of this fluid is the same as that of serum and therefore has a $[Na^+]$ of 145 mEq/L. Because the accumulation of the fluid requires NaCl and water retention by the kidneys, the amount of Na^+ retained by the kidneys must be equal to the amount contained in 4 L of fluid having an $[Na^+]$ of 145 mEq/L or 580 mEq of Na^+.

5. Aldosterone stimulates Na^+ reabsorption primarily in the late distal tubule and collecting duct, which explains the reduction in Na^+ excretion seen during the beginning of aldosterone treatment. As a result of the positive Na^+ balance, the ECF volume is increased. This in turn increases the GFR (i.e., increases the filtered load of Na^+), reduces proximal tubule reabsorption, and thereby enhances delivery of Na^+ to the distal tubule and collecting duct. In addition, natriuretic peptides (ANP and BNP) and urodilatin levels are increased, and their action on the collecting duct to inhibit Na^+ reabsorption, together with increased Na^+ delivery to this site, results in the return of Na^+ excretion to its previous level. A new steady state is reached (Na^+ intake = Na^+ excretion) but at an expanded ECF volume. Body weight is increased, reflecting the increased ECF volume. With cessation of aldosterone treatment, the Na^+ reabsorptive rate of the late distal tubule and collecting duct decreases. Because of the increased ECF volume and, therefore, enhanced Na^+ delivery to the distal tubule, the reabsorptive capacity of the distal tubule and collecting duct is overwhelmed, and Na^+ excretion increases. After a period of negative Na^+ balance, the ECF volume decreases back to normal. A new steady state is reached (Na^+ intake = Na^+ excretion), and the body weight returns to its original value as the ECF volume decreases.

6. ECF volume: With decreased cardiac performance there is NaCl and water retention (see Figure 6-6). This will increase ECF volume, blood volume, and interstitial fluid volume. The increased interstitial fluid volume is manifested as edema.

   ECV: Because of the poor cardiac performance (decreased blood pressure and cardiac output), the vascular volume receptors, especially those in the high-pressure side of the circulation, will detect a decreased ECV.

   Plasma osmolality: Because the plasma $[Na^+]$ is unchanged, the plasma osmolality is unchanged.

   Fractional Na^+ excretion: Because the ECV is decreased, renal sympathetic nerve activity is increased, and the renin-angiotensin-aldosterone system is activated. This results in a decrease in the filtered load of Na^+ and also an increase in the reabsorption of Na^+ by the nephron. This increase in Na^+ reabsorption eliminates almost all the Na^+ from the urine. Therefore, the fractional Na^+ excretion decreases.

   Renal sympathetic nerve activity: The vascular volume sensors will detect the decreased ECV and increase the activity of the sympathetic fibers innervating the kidney.

   ANP and BNP levels: Because of the increased blood and venous volumes, the heart will be dilated. This will stimulate ANP and BNP secretion, and their levels in the blood will be increased.

   Angiotensin II levels: The vascular volume sensors will detect the decreased ECV and activate the renin-angiotensin-aldosterone system.

   Aldosterone levels: The vascular volume sensors will detect the decreased ECV and activate the renin-angiotensin-aldosterone system.

   Plasma AVP levels: The vascular volume sensors will detect the decreased ECV and cause increased AVP secretion (see Chapter 5).

CHAPTER 7

1. Intravenous infusion of K^+ into a subject with a combination of sympathetic blockade (i.e., no catecholamine release) and insulin deficiency

would result in significant hyperkalemia compared with a similar infusion of K^+ in a normal subject. Although aldosterone secretion would be stimulated by the hyperkalemia, this hormone stimulates cell K^+ uptake after a 1-hour lag period. In the first hour following K^+ infusion, less than 50% of the infused K^+ is excreted by the kidneys, and because sympathetic activity and insulin release are suppressed, most of the K^+ remaining in the body is retained in the ECF.

2. Aldosterone deficiency would initially reduce urinary potassium excretion, and K^+ would be retained in the body (i.e., dietary intake would exceed excretion). This would lead to hyperkalemia, which is a potent stimulus of K^+ excretion. Because the individual is initially in positive K^+ balance, plasma K^+ rises until urinary K^+ excretion becomes equal to dietary K^+ intake. In the new steady state, K^+ intake would equal K^+ excretion; however, the subject has hyperkalemia. Thus, it is possible to match dietary K^+ intake with excretion in the absence of aldosterone, although this occurs at an elevated plasma $[K^+]$.

3. In the first hour after a meal, the rise in plasma $[K^+]$ is blunted by the rapid (minutes) uptake of K^+ into skeletal muscle, liver, bone, and red blood cells. Some K^+ is excreted by the kidneys, but in the first hour after the meal, most K^+ is sequestered in the intracellular fluid. In the ensuing hours, K^+ slowly leaves the cells and is excreted by the kidneys, thereby maintaining K^+ balance and plasma $[K^+]$.

4. Normally, K^+ excretion is determined primarily by the rate of K^+ secretion by the late distal tubule and collecting duct and is largely independent of the GFR and the filtered load of K^+. When 50% of the nephrons are lost, the late distal tubules and collecting ducts in the remaining functioning nephrons secrete more K^+ so that K^+ excretion and plasma $[K^+]$ are maintained at normal levels. However, if 80% to 85% of the nephrons are lost and GFR falls below 15% to 20% of normal, K^+ secretion by the distal tubule and collecting duct cannot increase enough to maintain constant urinary K^+ excretion, and hyperkalemia ensues.

CHAPTER 8

If urinary buffers were not available, the 70 mEq of acid needed to be excreted by the kidneys to maintain acid-base balance (net acid excretion = nonvolatile acid production) would have to be excreted as free H^+. If the minimum urine pH equals 4.0, this represents only 0.1 mEq/L of H^+. Thus, for 70 mEq of H^+ to be excreted, the daily urine output would need to be:

$$\frac{70 \text{ mEq/day}}{0.1 \text{ mEq/L}} = 700 \text{ L/day}$$

This exceeds the daily GFR (180 L/day). Thus, the urinary buffers are essential for the kidneys' ability to excrete sufficient quantities of H^+ and maintain acid-base balance.

2.

pH	$[HCO_3^-]$ (mEq/L)	P_{CO_2} mm Hg	Disorder
7.23	10	25	Metabolic acidosis
7.46	30	44	Metabolic alkalosis
7.37	28	50	Chronic respiratory acidosis
7.66	22	20	Acute respiratory alkalosis
7.34	26	50	Acute respiratory acidosis
7.54	18	22	Chronic respiratory alkalosis

3. The initial set of laboratory data indicates the presence of a metabolic alkalosis with appropriate respiratory compensation. Given the individual's history, the most likely cause of this simple acid-base disorder is the loss of gastric acid by vomiting. The second set of laboratory data continues to show the presence of metabolic alkalosis with respiratory compensation. In addition, there is evidence of fluid loss (decrease in body weight by 2 kg) and a resultant decrease in ECF volume (decrease in blood pressure). Given the worsening of this individual's metabolic alkalosis, it is somewhat surprising that the urine pH is so acidic. The appropriate renal response

should be an increase in HCO_3^- excretion (i.e., decreased net acid excretion) to correct the alkalosis. However, the kidneys' response to the ECF volume contraction prevents this from occurring (see Chapter 6). Thus, the filtered load of HCO_3^- is decreased because of a reduction in GFR, and proximal tubule HCO_3^- reabsorption is enhanced because of the need to conserve Na^+ (i.e., H^+ secretion is stimulated because of the increased activity of the Na^+-H^+ antiporter). In addition, the ECF volume contraction stimulates aldosterone secretion, which increases H^+ secretion by α-intercalated cells of the late distal tubule and collecting duct. Therefore, the urine is more acidic than expected for the degree of alkalosis. The ECF volume must be restored to its normal value to correct this situation. Infusion of isotonic NaCl would accomplish this and also allow the kidneys to excrete the excess HCO_3^-, thereby restoring acid-base balance.

4. Carbonic anhydrase plays an important role in the secretion of H^+ (reabsorption of HCO_3^-) by the cells of the proximal tubule, thick ascending limb of Henle's loop, and α-intercalated cells of the late distal tubule and collecting duct. Inhibition of this enzyme would therefore inhibit the secretion of H^+ by these nephron segments. Because the proximal tubule reabsorbs the largest fraction of the filtered load of HCO_3^- (80%), the effect of carbonic anhydrase inhibitors at this site is quantitatively the most important. With decreased reabsorption, more HCO_3^- would be excreted in the urine, and urine pH would become alkaline. This loss of HCO_3^- from the body would result in the development of metabolic acidosis.

5. This man has a metabolic acidosis with respiratory compensation. The plasma anion gap is calculated from the serum concentrations of Na^+, Cl^-, and HCO_3^-, and is:

$$Anion\ gap = [Na^+] - ([Cl^-] + [HCO_3^-])$$

$$13\ mEq/L = 137\ mEq/L - (111\ mEq/L + 13\ mEq/L)$$

Thus, this is a normal anion gap metabolic acidosis, which may be seen either in patients who lose alkali in the feces secondary to diarrhea or in patients with renal tubular acidosis. Because his urine is more alkaline than expected for someone with his degree of acidosis (a urine pH of at least 5.5 would be expected), it is most probable that he has renal tubular acidosis. This would predispose him to the formation of kidney stones. Because of his acidosis, he will lose Ca^{++} from his bones (bones serve as a buffer source with chronic acidosis). This Ca^{++} will be excreted by the kidneys. However, the alkaline urine pH leads to Ca^{++} precipitation and thus stone formation.

CHAPTER 9

1. Approximately two thirds of Ca^{++} reabsorption across the proximal tubule occurs by solvent drag, a process that depends on Na^+ reabsorption. Mannitol would inhibit Ca^{++} reabsorption by blocking solvent drag in the proximal tubule and thereby increase urinary Ca^{++} excretion.

2. Furosemide would inhibit the Na^+-K^+-$2Cl^-$ symporter and reduce the lumen-positive transepithelial voltage to 0. This, in turn, would inhibit passive Ca^{++} reabsorption by the paracellular pathway.

3. A rise in plasma $[P_i]$ increases the amount of P_i filtered by the glomeruli. Because the amount of P_i normally filtered is equal to the reabsorptive capacity of the kidneys, an increase in the amount of P_i filtered will increase urinary P_i excretion and reduce plasma $[P_i]$.

CHAPTER 10

1. Nephrogenic diabetes insipidus is a condition in which the late portion of the distal tubule and collecting duct does not respond to AVP. As a result, water reabsorption is impaired and a large volume of dilute urine is excreted. Long-term administration of thiazide diuretics provides symptomatic relief by reducing the volume of urine excreted. This occurs by two mechanisms. First, the diuretic-induced natriuresis reduces the volume of the ECF. This in turn reduces the

GFR and enhances proximal tubule reabsorption (see Chapter 6 for details). As a result, less fluid is delivered to Henle's loop and ultimately to the distal tubule and collecting duct, where water reabsorption is impaired. The net effect is that urine volume is decreased. Second, thiazide diuretics increase the abundance of aquaporin-2 in the principal cells of the late portion of the distal tubule and collecting duct (at least in the form of nephrogenic diabetes insipidus associated with Li^+ ingestion). The increased expression of aquaporin-2 would thus allow increased water reabsorption and thereby reduce urine output.

2. **a.** The long-term effect of diuretic therapy is a reduction in the volume of the ECF. With such a decrease, the blood volume and thus cardiac output are reduced. Because blood pressure is equal to cardiac output multiplied by the total peripheral vascular resistance, a decrease in cardiac output therefore reduces blood pressure (cardiovascular reflexes activate sympathetic outflow so as to increase peripheral vascular resistance and thereby try to maintain blood pressure). In addition, diuretics may cause some degree of vascular smooth muscle vasodilation, although the mechanism by which this occurs is not fully understood. This vasodilation reduces total peripheral vascular resistance, thereby decreasing blood pressure.

   b. Hypokalemia is a side effect of all diuretics acting proximal to the K^+ secretory site (late portion of the distal tubule and the cortical collecting duct). The most common diuretics given for the treatment of hypertension are thiazides. However, the loop diuretics, osmotic diuretics, and carbonic anhydrase inhibitors can also lead to hypokalemia. By their action, tubular fluid flow rate to the K^+ secretory site is enhanced, which stimulates K^+ secretion. In addition, the diuretic-induced decrease in ECF volume leads to stimulation of aldosterone and AVP, both of which stimulate K^+ secretion by the late portion of the distal tubule and cortical collecting duct.

   c. Treatment of the hypokalemia could involve supplementation of the diet with foods containing high levels of K^+ or with KCl tablets. Alternatively, a K^+-sparing diuretic could be given in combination with the thiazide diuretic.

3. Thiazide diuretics are secreted into the lumen of the proximal tubule by the same organic anion transport system that secretes penicillin. Competitive inhibition of secretion of the thiazide could decrease the effective concentration of the diuretic in the tubular field. Because thiazides act from the lumen, a reduction in their concentration at this site could reduce their effectiveness.

4. **a.** To maintain Na^+ balance, both individuals will excrete approximately 100 mEq/day of Na^+. Normally the kidneys excrete 99%+ of the daily ingested Na^+ load. The remainder is lost in the feces and in sweat. When individuals are treated chronically with a diuretic, they do not exhibit a sustained natriuresis. This is the diuretic braking phenomenon. After a relatively short period of negative Na^+ balance (i.e., intake < excretion), they again come into steady-state balance (i.e., intake = excretion). The ability to reestablish steady-state balance results from the diuretic-induced decrease in ECF volume and increased expression and function of Na^+ transporters. The decrease in ECF volume results in a decrease in the GFR and increased proximal tubule reabsorption. This in turn delivers less Na^+ to the portions of the nephron where the diuretic is acting. In addition, increased expression of Na^+ transporters in the segments where the diuretics act, as well as in other nephron segments, contributes to this response. Together, these modifications in renal Na^+ handling allow a new steady state to be reached where once again Na^+ excretion equals Na^+ ingestion.

   b. Individual A was treated with a loop diuretic. With inhibition of NaCl reabsorption by the thick ascending limb, less NaCl is deposited in the medullary interstitium. As a result, the osmolality of the interstitium declines, and water reabsorption from the collecting duct in the presence of AVP is reduced. Thus the loop diuretic inhibits the reabsorption of solute-free water. Individual B was treated with a thiazide diuretic, which, in contrast, inhibits NaCl reabsorption in the early distal tubule. Because this segment is located in the cortex of the kidney, medullary interstitial osmolality is not affected. Thus, when AVP is present, the urine can be concentrated. Thus thiazide diuretics do not impair solute-free water reabsorption.

c. Individual A is treated with a loop diuretic. Because the thick ascending limb has the highest rate of solute reabsorption of all the water-impermeable segments of the nephron (i.e., thin ascending limb, thick ascending limb, and early distal tubule), inhibition of solute transport at this site will greatly impair the kidneys' ability to dilute the urine. As a result, the urine osmolality will approach that of plasma (300 mOsm/kg H_2O), which is the osmolality of the glomerular filtrate as well as that of the tubular fluid exiting the proximal tubule. Individual B is treated with a thiazide diuretic, which acts only on cortical nephron segments (early distal tubule). This will impair urine dilution, but not as significantly because the thick ascending limb is still intact.

APPENDIX E

ANSWERS TO INTEGRATIVE CASE STUDIES

CASE 1

1a. The ECF volume of this man is increased above normal. The presence of edema, distention of the neck veins, and rales (sounds related to fluid in the lungs) is evidence of this increased volume. Additional evidence could be obtained by measuring weight gain because accumulation of each liter of extracellular fluid would increase body weight by 1 kg.

1b. The ECV in this man would be decreased from normal. With damage to the myocardium, cardiac output and therefore tissue perfusion would be reduced. This decreased cardiac performance will be sensed by the vascular baroreceptors as a decrease in the ECV.

1c. As noted previously, the reduced cardiac performance would be sensed by the vascular baroreceptors in the body as a decreased ECV. This will activate the sympathetic nervous system and the renin-angiotensin-aldosterone system and stimulate AVP secretion. Because ANP and BNP are secreted from the cardiac myocytes in response to stretch and because the heart is dilated (expanded ECF and vascular volume), ANP and BNP secretion will be stimulated.

1d. The kidneys would be avidly retaining Na^+. With a decrease in ECV, vascular volume sensors, especially in the high-pressure (juxtaglomerular apparatus, aortic arch, and carotid sinus) side of the circulation, would be activated and signals sent to the kidneys to retain Na^+.

- Sympathetic nerves innervating the afferent and efferent arterioles of the glomeruli would cause vasoconstriction. The net result would be to reduce the GFR. This in turn would reduce the filtered load of Na^+.

- Sympathetic innervation of the proximal tubule, thick ascending limb of Henle's loop, and collecting duct will also increase Na^+ reabsorption at these sites. This response is mediated by α_1-adrenoceptors on the cells.

- Increased sympathetic nerve activity, together with decreased perfusion pressure at the afferent arteriole, will result in the secretion of renin. This activation of the renin-angiotensin-aldosterone system will further stimulate Na^+ reabsorption because angiotensin II increases both proximal and distal tubule Na^+ reabsorption, and aldosterone increases Na^+ reabsorption in the late distal tubule and collecting duct. Angiotensin II acts directly on the cells of the proximal tubule to stimulate Na^+ reabsorption.

- With the decreased ECV, the GFR decreases and the filtration fraction increases. This in turn decreases the hydrostatic pressure and increases the oncotic pressure in the peritubular capillaries and thereby enhances overall reabsorption of fluid by the proximal tubule.

- With the increases in the ECF and vascular volumes, the heart dilates and ANP and BNP levels are elevated. However, the effect of these natriuretic peptides (inhibition of renin secretion and natriuresis) appears to be blunted by the effect of the other factors, all of which act to reduce Na$^+$ excretion. The net effect of these responses is retention of Na$^+$ by the kidneys. As a result of this Na$^+$ retention (positive Na$^+$ balance), the ECF volume will increase, leading to the formation of edema as seen in the physical examination of this man.

1e. The development of hyponatremia indicates that this man is in positive water balance. In this case the ingestion of water has exceeded the capacity of the kidneys to excrete solute-free water. There are several reasons why solute-free water excretion is impaired in this man.

- AVP secretion is stimulated because of the decreased ECV. As a consequence, the collecting duct reabsorbs more solute-free water.
- The decreased ECV results in a reduction in the filtered load of solute (NaCl) and water and an increase in fractional reabsorption by the proximal tubule (see earlier). As a result, there is decreased delivery of solute and water to the thick ascending limb, the primary site where solute-free water is generated.

1f. Hypokalemia in this man is the result of increased renal K$^+$ excretion. The major reason for increased K$^+$ excretion is related to the elevated levels of aldosterone in this man (secondary to decreased ECV). Aldosterone then acts on the late distal tubule and collecting duct to stimulate K$^+$ secretion. The enhanced secretion of K$^+$ by the late distal tubule and cortical collecting duct will result in increased K$^+$ excretion and the development of hypokalemia. Because delivery of Na$^+$ to the collecting duct is reduced in this man (see earlier), the hypokalemia will be mild. It is likely that extrarenal factors will also contribute to the development of hypokalemia because aldosterone causes K$^+$ to move into cells.

1g. In order to get an appropriate response to a loop diuretic, there needs to be adequate delivery of NaCl to the loop of Henle. As outlined before, GFR is reduced in congestive heart failure, which reduces the filtered load of NaCl. In addition, proximal tubule reabsorption is enhanced. The net result is a significant reduction in the delivery of NaCl to the thick ascending limb and thus a blunted response to the diuretic.

1h. As noted, the diuretic is given to prevent NaCl retention by the kidneys and thus reduce his edema. The additional NaCl lost from the ECF by the action of the diuretic will further reduce his ECV. As a result, the sympathetic nervous system will be further activated, as will the renin-angiotensin-aldosterone system. AVP secretion will also be stimulated.

1i. Loop diuretics increase the excretion of K$^+$ and thus can lead to the development of hypokalemia. Two important effects contribute to this response. First, the thick ascending limb of Henle's loop reabsorbs approximately 20% of the filtered load of K$^+$. Loop diuretics inhibit this process. K$^+$ is reabsorbed by the Na$^+$-K$^+$-2Cl$^-$ symporter in the apical membrane and by the paracellular pathway driven by the lumen-positive transepithelial voltage (inhibition of the symporter results in a reduction in the lumen-positive voltage). Second, the loop diuretic will cause increased delivery of Na$^+$ and fluid to the distal tubule and cortical collecting duct and thereby stimulate K$^+$ secretion. Because aldosterone levels are also elevated (secondary to decreased ECV), K$^+$ secretion is further stimulated. Together, these effects will enhance K$^+$ secretion and thus renal K$^+$ excretion, leading to a worsening of the hypokalemia.

1j. Creatinine is excreted from the body primarily by glomerular filtration Therefore, the amount of creatinine excreted is determined primarily by its filtered load. With a reduction in the ECV, the glomerular filtration rate is reduced. The reduced filtration rate will decrease the filtered load of creatinine and thus its excretion. As a result, the serum [creatinine] will increase. With the added decrement in the ECV caused by the loop diuretic, the glomerular filtration rate will fall further and thereby cause the serum [creatinine] to increase even more.

CASE 2

2a. This woman's symptoms and the electrolyte disturbances are most characteristic of decreased levels of adrenal cortical steroids and especially the mineralocorticoid hormone aldosterone. This is a patient with Addison's disease. The presence of hyperpigmentation suggests that the primary problem is at the level of the adrenal gland (i.e., nonresponsive to ACTH). ACTH levels are elevated in response to the decreased circulating levels of adrenal cortical steroids. (ACTH is synthesized as preproopiomelanocortin (POMC), and when this molecule is processed to ACTH several of the cleavage products have melanocyte-stimulating properties). These cleavage products act on the epidermal melanocytes leading to the hyperpigmentation of the gums and skin.

2b. Normally, the kidneys would respond to the decreased ECF volume present in this woman by dramatically reducing the excretion of Na^+. The urine $[Na^+]$ is unexpectedly high in this woman because of the reduced ability of her kidneys to reabsorb Na^+ in the thick ascending limb, distal tubule, and collecting duct (the distal tubule and collecting duct are especially important). This "Na^+ wasting" is a result of the low levels of aldosterone. Although the angiotensin II levels would be elevated in this woman, her adrenal glands are not secreting aldosterone in response to the angiotensin II. The hypotension is a result of the negative Na^+ balance present in this woman, which in turn reflects the decreased circulating levels of aldosterone. Because of the negative Na^+ balance, ECF volume will be decreased. Because plasma is a component of the ECF, vascular volume and hence blood pressure will be decreased.

2c. Hyponatremia indicates a problem in water balance. Thus, the ability of this woman's kidneys to excrete solute-free water is impaired, and she is in positive water balance (solute-free water ingestion > solute-free water excretion). There are several reasons for the decreased ability of this woman's kidneys to excrete solute-free water. Because of her decreased ECF and vascular volumes, her vascular baroreceptors are activated. As a result, the sympathetic nervous system and the renin-angiotensin-aldosterone system are activated. Nonosmotic release of AVP also occurs because of a fall in the ECF volume. As a

consequence of the elevated AVP levels, solute-free water is reabsorbed by the late portion of the distal tubule and collecting duct. In addition, the decreased ECF volume results in a decrease in the filtered load of solute (NaCl) and water and an increase in fractional reabsorption by the proximal tubule. As a result, there is decreased delivery of solute and water to the thick ascending limb, the primary site where solute-free water is generated.

2d. Urinary K^+ excretion is determined in large part by the amount of K^+ secreted into tubular fluid by the late distal tubule and cortical collecting duct. K^+ secretion at these nephron sites is reduced by the low levels of plasma aldosterone in this woman. In addition, aldosterone causes the uptake of K^+ into cells (e.g., skeletal muscle). In the absence of aldosterone, there will be less cellular uptake of K^+. This will also contribute to the development of hyperkalemia.

2e. This woman has a metabolic acidosis as evidenced by her low serum $[HCO_3^-]$. This is a result of the inability of her kidneys to excrete sufficient net acid to balance the nonvolatile acids produced each day through metabolism. The defect in her kidneys is reduced H^+ secretion by the α-intercalated cells of the late portion of the distal tubule and the collecting duct. H^+ secretion by these cells is dependent on aldosterone. This is both a direct and indirect effect. Aldosterone directly stimulates the α-intercalated cells to secrete H^+. It is also responsible for stimulating Na^+ reabsorption by the principal cells in these segments. This reabsorption of Na^+ generates a lumen-negative transepithelial voltage that facilitates H^+ secretion by the intercalated cell. Therefore, in the absence of aldosterone, H^+ secretion is impaired. This will reduce HCO_3^- reabsorption, the excretion of H^+ with urinary buffers, and the excretion of NH_4^+. Thus, net acid excretion is reduced.

CASE 3

3a. Na^+ excretion is determined by diet and ECF volume status. In a euvolemic individual, the amount of Na^+ excreted in the urine each day is approximately equal to the amount ingested in the diet. Because the man appears to be euvolemic, his daily Na^+ intake would be approximately 80 mEq/day. The hyponatremia in this man reflects a disorder of water balance. Specifically, the unregulated secretion of AVP prevents his kidneys from excreting solute-free water. As a result, his water intake exceeds the ability of his kidneys to excrete solute-free water and he is in positive water balance.

3b. Infusion of 1 L of isotonic saline will add 300 mOsm of NaCl (150 mmoles of NaCl = 300 mOsm) to his ECF together with 1 L of water. This will transiently increase the ECF volume and raise the plasma osmolality and $[Na^+]$. However, over time the entire amount of NaCl will be excreted because he is in steady-state Na^+ balance (excretion = intake). However, because of the inappropriate secretion of AVP, he will not be able to excrete the water. With a U_{osm} of 600 mOsm/kg H_2O, he will excrete the infused NaCl (300 mOsm) in 0.5 L of urine. Thus 0.5 L of solute-free water will remain in the body, and the plasma $[Na^+]$ will decrease. For this man, the addition of 0.5 L of solute-free water to his body fluid will reduce the plasma $[Na^+]$ to 119 mEq/L:

Total body osmoles (unchanged)	= 240 mOsm/L × 42 L = 10,080 mOsm
New total body water	= 42 L + 0.5 L = 42.5 L
New plasma osmolality	= 10,080 mOsm/42.5 L = 237 mOsm/kg H_2O
New plasma $[Na^+]$	= 237 mOsm/kg H_2O/2 = 119 mEq/L

3c. A 3% saline solution contains 513 mmol/L of NaCl (MW = 58.5 g/mole), which is 1026 mOsm/L. Thus 1 L of fluid and 1026 mOsm of solute are added to the body fluids. With the establishment of a new steady state, the infused NaCl will be excreted with 1.7 L of urine:

$$\frac{1026\ mOsm}{600\ mOsm/kg\ H_2O} = 1.7\ L$$

U_{osm} = 600 mOsm/kg H_2O because of the unregulated secretion of AVP. Therefore 1 L of infused water is excreted together with an additional 0.7 L of solute-free water. This will result in a new plasma $[Na^+]$ of 122 mEq/L:

Total body osmoles (unchanged)	= 240 mOsm/L × 42 L = 10,080 mOsm
New total body water	= 42 L − 0.7 L = 41.3 L
New plasma osmolality	= 10,080 mOsm/41.3 L = 244 mOsm/kg H_2O
New plasma $[Na^+]$	= 244 mOsm/kg H_2O/2 = 122 mEq/L

3d. The simplest treatment option would be to restrict his intake of fluids so that intake does not exceed the ability of his kidneys to excrete solute-free water (i.e., he should drink only in response to thirst). Another treatment option would be to block the effect of AVP on the collecting duct. Currently, AVP receptor antagonists (aquaretics) are available for this purpose.

CASE 4

4a. The acid-base disorder of this man is a metabolic acidosis. In the absence of insulin, the metabolism of fats and carbohydrates is altered such that nonvolatile acids (keto acids) are produced. The nonvolatile acids are rapidly buffered by cellular and extracellular buffers. Buffering in the extracellular fluid results in a decrease in the plasma $[HCO_3^-]$, which lowers the pH. The deep rapid breathing reflects the respiratory compensation (Pco_2 is lowered). The plasma anion gap is calculated using the following formula (normal value is 8 to 16 mEq/L):

$$Anion\ gap = [Na^+] - ([Cl^-] + [HCO_3^-])$$
$$or\ 130 - (95 + 7) = 28\ mEq/L$$

The plasma anion gap is elevated because of the presence of unmeasured anions; in this case the anions would be the keto acids such as acetoacetate and β-hydroxybutyrate.

4b. Despite the hyperkalemia in this man, he is probably K^+ depleted. The K^+ depletion is a result of K^+ shift out of the cells (see later) and enhanced K^+ excretion by the kidneys because of the glucose-induced osmotic diuresis (i.e., the increased urinary flow rate increases K^+ secretion in the late distal tubule and collecting duct). Hyperkalemia is a result of a shift of K^+ out of cells (e.g., skeletal muscle) into the extracellular fluid. This shift occurs because of the lack of insulin and the hypertonicity of the ECF secondary to the elevated [glucose]. The acidosis is probably not a major contributing factor to the development of hyperkalemia in this situation. When acidosis is induced by mineral acids (e.g., HCl), movement of H^+ into cells during the process of intracellular buffering results in a shift of K^+ out of the cells into the ECF. However, with organic acidosis, as occurs in this situation, the cellular buffering of the organic acids does not result in a significant shift of K^+ out of the cell. The polyuria is a result of an osmotic diuresis induced by glucose (also the keto acids). Normally, all of the filtered load of glucose is reabsorbed by the proximal tubule. However, in this man the filtered load of glucose exceeds the reabsorptive capacity of the proximal tubule. Consequently, the nonreabsorbed glucose will remain in the lumen of the proximal tubule, where it will act as an osmotically active particle. This will establish an osmotic gradient opposite to that generated by the NaCl reabsorptive processes. This glucose-induced osmotic diuresis will increase the delivery of NaCl and water to the distal tubule and cortical collecting duct, which stimulates K^+ secretion at these sites. As a result, K^+ excretion from the body will be increased. In addition, keto acids (anions) are excreted with a cation (Na^+ and K^+). Thus, some additional K^+ will be excreted because of the high excretion rate of the keto acids. Increased K^+ excretion together with the shift of K^+ from the ICF to the ECF noted previously (secondary to the insulin deficiency and hyperosmolality) will lead to progressive whole-body K^+ depletion. Accordingly, an increase in serum $[K^+]$ is not always indicative of positive K^+ balance. This man is in negative K^+ balance and is at risk for the development of hypokalemia when insulin is administered and the metabolic abnormalities are corrected.

4c. The serum $[K^+]$ fell for several reasons. Insulin causes K^+ to move into cells. The mechanism responsible for this effect of insulin is related to stimulation of the Na^+-K^+-ATPase. With increased activity of the Na^+-K^+-ATPase, K^+ uptake into the cell is enhanced. In addition, insulin's effect on glucose metabolism will lower the serum [glucose]. As a consequence, the osmolality of the ECF will decrease and cause additional K^+ to move into cells. Finally, administration of fluids will reexpand the ECF and dilute the K^+ in this compartment. For all of these reasons, K^+ is usually administered during the course of treatment so as not to induce hypokalemia.

CASE 5

5a. This is a metabolic acidosis with a normal anion gap (anion gap = 13 mEq/L). The two most frequent causes of nonanion gap acidosis are defects in renal acid excretion (renal tubular acidosis) and loss of HCO_3^- from the body (e.g., diarrhea). In this case, the relatively alkaline urine pH in the presence of systemic acidosis suggests a defect in renal acid excretion. Normally, the urine should be maximally acidic with this degree of systemic acidosis. The most likely diagnosis is distal renal tubular acidosis (i.e., a defect in H^+ secretion or H^+ permeability of the late distal tubule and collecting duct). The renal stone that brought this man to the physician is probably a calcium-containing stone because the solubility of calcium is reduced in alkaline urine. His filtered load of Ca^{++} is also elevated, reflecting the loss of Ca^{++} from his bones because of buffering of the acidosis.

5b. Normally, the kidneys respond to a metabolic acidosis by increasing net acid excretion. This typically occurs with a urine pH of less than 5.5. Thus, the urine pH of 6.4 indicates some defect in renal acid excretion. As noted, this is a case of distal renal tubular acidosis, where the defect is an inability of the distal nephron to acidify the urine maximally. Because of this defect, there is impaired HCO_3^- reabsorption, decreased excretion of titratable acid, and decreased excretion of NH_4^+. Therefore renal net acid excretion is less than net endogenous acid production, and metabolic acidosis (nonanion gap) develops.

5c. Urinary net charge should be negative under normal conditions, reflecting the excretion of NH_4^+ in the urine. The positive value confirms the fact that the kidney is the cause of the acidosis because insufficient amounts of NH_4^+ are being excreted.

CASE 6

6a. This is a mixed acid-base disorder because the P_{CO_2} is elevated and the serum $[HCO_3^-]$ is decreased. There is a component related to respiratory acidosis caused by poor gas exchange in the lungs. In addition, her hypoxia (low P_{O_2}) has resulted in anaerobic metabolism by her tissues with the generation of lactic acid. Buffering of the lactic acid has resulted in a decrease in her serum $[HCO_3^-]$.

6b. This girl was given an injection of epinephrine by the paramedics to dilate her airways. Epinephrine is a β-selective agonist that not only acts to relax her constricted airways but also stimulates the Na^+-K^+-ATPase, causing enhanced K^+ uptake into cells (e.g., skeletal muscle).

CASE 7

	Initial	After Day 2
Total body water (L)	18 L	16 L
ECF volume (L)	6 L	4 L
ICF volume (L)	12 L	12 L
Total body osmoles (mOsm)	5040 mOsm	4480 mOsm
ECF osmoles (mOsm)	1680 mOsm	1120 mOsm
ICF osmoles (mOsm)	3360 mOsm	3360 mOsm

Points to consider:

1. It is assumed that the 2-kg weight loss reflects only the loss of body fluids (i.e., 2 L) and not tissue mass. Given the short time period involved, this is a reasonable assumption.

2. Because the plasma $[Na^+]$ has not changed this is isotonic loss of fluid. Consequently, all of the fluid loss will occur from the ECF (there is no

osmotic gradient to cause fluid to leave the ICF). This is a simplification, but again reasonable.

3. All of the osmole loss will occur from the ECF, essentially as NaCl.

4. Calculations:
   Initial Conditions
   Total body water = 30 kg × 0.6 = 18 L
   ECF volume = 18 L × 1/3 = 6 L
   ICF volume = 18 L − 6 L = 12 L
   Total body osmoles = 140 × 2 × 18 L = 5040 mOsm
   ECF osmoles = 6 L × 2 × 140 = 1680 mOsm
   ICF osmoles = 5040 − 1680 = 3360 mOsm
   Day 2
   Total body water = 18 L − 2 L = 16 L
   ECF volume = 6 L − 2 L = 4 L
   ICF volume = 12 L
   Total body osmoles = 140 × 2 × 16 L = 4480 mOsm
   ECF osmoles = 4 L × 2 × 140 = 1120 mOsm
   ICF osmoles = 4480 − 1120 = 3360 mOsm

CASE 8

	Initial	After Day 2
Total body water (L)	18 L	16 L
ECF volume (L)	6 L	2 L
ICF volume (L)	12 L	14 L
Total body osmoles (mOsm)	5040 mOsm	3840 mOsm
ECF osmoles (mOsm)	1680 mOsm	480 mOsm
ICF osmoles (mOsm)	3360 mOsm	3360 mOsm

Points to consider:

1. Compared with the child in Case 7, this child is in much more serious condition. This child has lost 2 L of fluid with excess NaCl from the ECF. As a result he has become hyponatremic.

2. Because of the hyponatremia there is now a driving force to cause water to move from the ECF to the ICF. This movement will further reduce the volume of the ECF (of which the vascular volume is a component). This child is very near vascular collapse.

3. Calculations:

    Initial Conditions
    Total body water = 30 kg × 0.6 = 18 L
    ECF volume = 18 L × 1/3 = 6 L
    ICF volume = 18 L − 6 L = 12 L
    Total body osmoles = 140 × 2 × 18 L = 5040 mOsm
    ECF osmoles = 6 L × 2 × 140 = 1680 mOsm
    ICF osmoles = 5040 − 1680 = 3360 mOsm

    Day 2
    Total body water = 18 L − 2 L = 16 L
    ECF volume = 480 mOsm/240 mOsm/kg H_2O = 2 L
    ICF volume = 16 L − 2 L = 14 L
    Total body osmoles = 120 × 2 × 16 L = 3840 mOsm
    ECF osmoles = 3840 − 3360 = 480 mOsm
    ICF osmoles = 3360 mOsm

Isotonic dehydration (Case 7) is most common in pediatric patients, but hyponatremic dehydration (Case 8) is more common than hypernatremic dehydration (Case 9) in young pediatric patients (i.e., ~10 kg)—as more often than not their parents are trying to keep them hydrated with hypotonic solutions (e.g., juice, electrolyte replacement drinks). This results in "partial" rehydration with free water, which results in their sodium/solute losses exceeding water losses relatively speaking.

The children in Cases 7 and 8 need 2 L of water and some NaCl. For Case 7 this can be accomplished by infusing 2 L of isotonic saline (0.9% NaCl). However, the child in Case 8 needs additional NaCl. For this child infusion of an appropriate combination of isotonic and hypertonic saline would be required. In practice only isotonic saline is administered, and the kidneys reabsorb sufficient quantities of Na^+ to correct the deficit.

CASE 9

	Initial	After Day 2
Total body water (L)	18 L	16 L
ECF volume (L)	6 L	5.5 L
ICF volume (L)	12 L	10.5 L
Total body osmoles (mOsm)	5040 mOsm	5120 mOsm
ECF osmoles (mOsm)	1680 mOsm	1760 mOsm
ICF osmoles (mOsm)	3360 mOsm	3360 mOsm

Points to consider:

1. This child has lost 2 L of fluid but has a net loss of water. As a result he has become hypernatremic and the plasma osmolality is 320 mOsm/kg H_2O.

2. Because of the hypernatremia there is now a driving force to cause water to move from the ICF to the ECF.

3. Calculations:

    Initial Conditions
    Total body water = 30 kg × 0.6 = 18 L
    ECF volume = 18 L × 1/3 = 6 L
    ICF volume = 18 L − 6 L = 12 L
    Total body osmoles = 140 × 2 × 18 L = 5040 mOsm
    ECF osmoles = 6 L × 2 × 140 = 1680 mOsm
    ICF osmoles = 5040 − 1680 = 3360 mOsm

    Day 2
    Total body water = 18 L − 2 L = 16 L
    ICF osmoles = 3360 mOsm
    ICF volume = 3360 mOsm/320 mOsm/kg H_2O = 10.5 L
    ECF volume = 16 L − 10.5 L = 5.5 L
    Total body osmoles = 160 × 2 × 16 L = 5120 mOsm
    ECF osmoles = 5.5 L × 320 mOsm/kg H_2O = 1760 mOsm

4. This child needs 2 L of water and some NaCl. Infusion of hypotonic saline would be appropriate. However, fluid replacement should be accomplished slowly (i.e., over 48-72 hours), and the serum $[Na^+]$ should decrease by no more than 10 mEq/L in 24 hours.

CASE 10

1. The initial acid-base disorder is a respiratory alkalosis. This results from tachypnea secondary to hypoxia. The increased respiratory rate in response to hypoxia results in a decrease in the Pco_2, and therefore the development of a respiratory alkalosis.

2. After therapy the acid-base disorder is a respiratory acidosis, which reflects inadequate ventilation.

3. The girl remains hypoxic five hours after the initial presentation despite therapy (note that the

Po_2 remains 60 mm Hg despite therapy with 40% oxygen). After a period of tachypnea and labored breathing that lead to respiratory alkalosis she became fatigued due to hypoxia. Consequently, her respiratory effort decreased and breathing became slow and shallow. The hypoventilation caused respiratory acidosis. The decreased breath sounds and decreased wheezing on auscultation reflect decreased air movement from hypoventilation. It is an ominous sign in a patient with hypoxia and requires immediate intervention. Note that decreased wheezing in an asthmatic patient would be a sign of improvement only in the presence of normal breath sounds and improving arterial Po_2.

APPENDIX F

CHAPTER 2

1. Which of the following structures is a barrier to the filtration of proteins across the glomerulus?
   a. Capillary endothelial cells
   b. Basement membrane
   c. Lacis cells
   d. Parietal epithelial cells
   e. Mesangial cells

2. The macula densa is part of which of the following structures in the kidney?
   a. Extraglomerular matrix
   b. Vasa recta
   c. Afferent arteriole
   d. Juxtamedullary nephron
   e. Juxtaglomerular apparatus

3. The efferent arteriole of some juxtamedullary nephrons enters the renal medulla and becomes which of the following vessels?
   a. Interlobular artery
   b. Arcuate artery
   c. Vasa recta
   d. Glomerular capillary
   e. Interlobar artery

4. The function of the vasa recta is to:
   a. Concentrate the urine
   b. Exclude proteins from Bowman's space
   c. Secrete renin
   d. Regulate tubuloglomerular feedback
   e. Deliver oxygen and nutrients to the renal medulla

5. Podocin is mutated in what renal disease?
   a. Nephrotic syndrome
   b. Alports disease
   c. Polycystic kidney disease
   d. Nephrogenic diabetes insipidus
   e. SIADH

6. What is the order of blood flow through the renal vasculature?
   a. Renal artery–interlobular artery–arcuate artery–interlobar artery–afferent arteriole
   b. Renal artery–interlobar artery–arcuate artery–interlobular artery–afferent arteriole
   c. Afferent arteriole–glomerular capillaries–peritubular capillary–efferent arteriole
   d. Renal artery–interlobar artery–arcuate artery–interlobular artery–peritubular capillary
   e. Renal artery–interlobar artery–arcuate artery–interlobular artery–vasa recta

7. The renal corpuscle consists of:
   a. Afferent arteriole and glomerular capillaries
   b. Afferent arteriole, glomerular capillaries, and efferent arteriole
   c. Glomerular capillaries and Bowman's capsule
   d. Macula densa and the juxtaglomerular apparatus
   e. Glomerular capillaries and mesangial cells

8. Mutations in PKD1 cause polycystic kidney disease. Polycystin has what function?
   a. It transports potassium.
   b. It transports calcium.
   c. It transports water.
   d. It is an adhesion molecule.
   e. It transports sodium.

9. The nephrotic syndrome:
   a. Is characterized by a decrease in the permeability of the glomerular capillaries to proteins

213

b. Is characterized by a change in podocyte structure, including a thickening of foot processes

c. Is characterized by a decrease in extracellular volume depletion.

d. Is characterized by an increase in the permeability of the glomerular capillaries to proteins

e. Is caused by a decrease in renal blood flow

10. Mesangial cells:
   a. Are specialized cells in the afferent arteriole
   b. Secrete antiinflammatory cytokines
   c. Secrete renin
   d. Are located in the renal medulla
   e. Have phagocytic activity

CHAPTER 3

1. According to the tubuloglomerular feedback theory, an increase in tubular fluid NaCl concentration near the macula densa will result in which of the following?
   a. A decrease in the glomerular filtration rate of the same nephron
   b. An increase in renal blood flow to the glomerulus of the same nephron
   c. Activation of the renal sympathetic nerves
   d. An increase in proximal tubule solute and water reabsorption
   e. An increase in renin secretion

2. Which of the following structures is a barrier to the filtration of proteins across the glomerulus?
   a. Capillary endothelial cells
   b. Basement membrane
   c. Lacis cells
   d. Parietal epithelial cells
   e. Mesangial cells

3. Starling forces determine fluid movement across glomerular capillaries. An increase in the GFR would be caused by?
   a. A decrease in Kf
   b. An increase in P_{BS}
   c. A derease in π_{GC}
   d. A decrease in P_{GC}
   e. A decrease in π_{bs}

4. A 56-year-old man was admitted to the hospital with a myocardial infarction. At admission, his serum creatinine was 1.2 mg/dL, and his creatinine clearance was 100 mL/min. Over the next 3 days, he had several periods of hypotension, and his serum creatinine increased to 3.6 mg/dL. Assuming that he is in steady-state balance for creatinine (i.e., amount excreted = amounted produced), what is his predicted creatinine clearance?
   a. 10 mL/min
   b. 33 mL/min
   c. 50 mL/min
   d. 66 mL/min
   e. 100 mL/min

5. Which of the following statements regarding the GFR is true?
   a. Plasma oncotic pressure is constant along the length of the glomerular capillary
   b. Net filtration pressure decreases from the afferent to the efferent end of the capillary
   c. Net filtration pressure increases from the afferent to the efferent end of the capillary
   d. Filtration occurs at the afferent end and reabsorption at the efferent end of the capillary
   e. Plasma oncotic pressure decreases along the length of the glomerular capillary

6. Which of the following responses to a fall in arterial pressure accounts for the ability of the kidneys to autoregulate GFR?
   a. Decreased resistance of the efferent arteriole
   b. Increased delivery of fluid to the end of the proximal tubule
   c. Increase resistance of the afferent arteriole
   d. Increased [NaCl] in tubular fluid at the macula densa
   e. Decreased in resistance of the afferent arteriole

7. GFR will decrease in which of the following conditions?
   a. Dilation of the afferent arteriole
   b. Decrease in renal nerve activity
   c. Decrease in plasma oncotic pressure
   d. Increase in hydrostatic pressure in Bowman's space
   e. Increase in renal blood flow

8. A healthy 25-year-old woman donates a kidney to her identical twin, who has chronic renal failure. Her serum [creatinine] before removal of the kidney is 1.0 mg/dL. After donating her kidney, her serum [creatinine] increases to 2.0 mg/dL. One month later her serum [creatinine] has decreased to 1.5 mg/dL. Which of the following accounts for the fact that her serum [creatinine] fell from 2.0 to 1.5 mg/dL?
   a. Decreased production of creatinine by skeletal muscle
   b. Enhanced secretion of creatinine by the proximal tubule
   c. Increase in the GFR of each of the remaining nephrons
   d. Expansion of her ECF volume

9. The woman described in question 8 has not modified her diet since removal of her kidney. What is the change in renal handling of Na^+ now that she has only one kidney?

Urinary Na^+ Excretion/24 h	Fractional Excretion of Na^+
a. No change	No change
b. No change	↑
c. ↑	↑
d. ↓	↓
e. ↓	↑

10. A substance (Y) is found in the plasma at a concentration of 2 mg/dL. A 24-hour urine collection is done to determine the renal clearance of Y. The following data are obtained:
    Urine volume: 1.44 L
    Urine [Y]: 500 mg/L
    What is the renal clearance of Y?
    a. 5 mL/min
    b. 25 mL/min
    c. 36 mL/min
    d. 100 mL/min
    e. 250 mL/min

11. Starling forces are measured across a capillary wall, and the following values are obtained:
    Capillary hydrostatic pressure: 30 mmHg
    Capillary oncotic pressure: 25 mmHg
    Interstitial hydrostatic pressure: 0 mmHg
    Interstitial oncotic pressure: 15 mmHg

If the reflection coefficient for protein across this capillary wall is 0.5, what is the pressure and direction of fluid flow across the capillary wall?

	Net Pressure	Direction of Fluid Flow
a.	5 mm Hg	Into capillary
b.	10 mm Hg	Out of capillary
c.	15 mm Hg	Out of capillary
d.	20 mm Hg	Out of capillary
e.	25 mm Hg	Out of capillary

12. Urine albumin is measured to evaluate:
    a. Acid-base status
    b. Renal disease
    c. Renal blood flow
    d. GFR
    e. The concentrating ability of the kidneys

CHAPTER 4

1. A portion of Na^+ reabsorption in the late portion of the proximal tubule is passive through the paracellular pathway. What is the primary driving force for this passive reabsorption of Na^+?
   a. A lower luminal than peritubular hydrostatic pressure
   b. A higher luminal than peritubular [Na^+]
   c. A lumen-positive transepithelial voltage
   d. A lower interstitial fluid pressure than luminal fluid oncotic pressure

2. Na^+ reabsorption by the thick ascending limb of Henle's loop is:
   a. Inhibited by a decrease in peritubular capillary hydrostatic pressure
   b. Inhibited by angiotensin II
   c. Increased with increased delivered load of Na^+
   d. Inhibited by K^+-sparing diuretics
   e. Increased by natriuretic peptides

3. Starling forces regulate sodium and water reabsorption by the proximal tubule. Which of the following changes in Starling forces would increase reabsorption?
   a. Increase in capillary hydrostatic pressure
   b. Increase in capillary oncotic pressure
   c. Decrease in capillary oncotic pressure
   d. Decrease in the permeability of the peritubular capillary to sodium and water

4. Which of the following increases the reabsorption of sodium and chloride in the distal tubule and collecting duct?
   a. Uroguanylin
   b. Peritubular Starling forces
   c. Natriuretic peptides
   d. Aldosterone
   e. Urodilatin

5. The tubuloglomerular feedback mechanism regulates:
   a. Blood pressure
   b. Sodium excretion
   c. GFR and RBF
   d. Potassium excretion
   e. Urine osmolality

6. An increase in which of the following would result in a decrease in net proximal tubular fluid reabsorption?
   a. Peritubular capillary hydrostatic pressure
   b. Glomerular capillary hydrostatic pressure
   c. Renal medullary interstitial oncotic pressure
   d. Peritubular capillary oncotic pressure
   e. Filtration fraction

7. Which hormone increases the urinary excretion of sodium and water?
   a. Epinephrine
   b. Aldosterone
   c. Angiotensin
   d. ANP
   e. Insulin

8. The proximal tubule reabsorbs what percent of the filtered NaCl and water?
   a. 100%
   b. 67%
   c. 50%
   d. 25%
   e. 10%

9. An increase in the osmolality of the medullary interstitial fluid would directly:
   a. Stimulate urea reabsorption by the proximal tubule
   b. Stimulate sodium reabsorption by the distal tubule
   c. Stimulate water reabsorption by the descending limb of Henle's loop
   d. Stimulate sodium reabsorption by the ascending limb of Henle's loop
   e. Stimulate water secretion by the medullary collecting duct

10. Normally at least 99% of the filtered load of which of the following substances is reabsorbed in the proximal tubule:
    a. Chloride
    b. Albumin
    c. Water
    d. Bicarbonate
    e. Urea

CHAPTER 5

1. The daily excretion rate of total osmoles for an individual is 900 mOsm. If this individual has a urine-concentrating defect and can produce urine having a maximum osmolality of only 300 mOsm/kg H_2O, what is the minimum volume of water that must be ingested in order to prevent a rise in the osmolality of the body fluids? (Assume that insensible water loss is 1.5 L/day.)
   a. 1.5 L/day
   b. 3.0 L/day
   c. 4.5 L/day
   d. 6.0 L/day
   e. 7.5 L/day

2. An individual is stricken with an illness characterized by nausea, vomiting, and diarrhea. Over a 2-day period, this individual experiences a 3-kg loss in weight without a change in the plasma $[Na^+]$. What can be concluded about body fluid volumes and composition in this individual?
   a. The volume of ICF is increased
   b. The volume of the ECF is decreased
   c. The total body osmoles increased
   d. The plasma osmolality is decreased

3. Which of the following maneuvers would be expected to stimulate AVP secretion?
   a. Infusion of 1 L hypertonic NaCl
   b. Infusion of 1 L of an isoosmotic urea solution
   c. 5% expansion of the ECV
   d. Infusion of 1 L of D5W
   e. An acute increase in blood pressure

4. An individual has no urine output over a 2-day period. During this time, body weight increases by 2 kg. Plasma [Na^+] is unchanged. What can be concluded about the volumes and composition of the body fluids?
   a. The volume of the ICF is decreased
   b. The volume of the ECF is increased
   c. The total body water is normal
   d. The plasma osmolality is decreased

5. AVP has which of the following actions?
   a. Increases the water permeability of the thick ascending limb of Henle's loop
   b. Increases the urea permeability of the cortical portion of the collecting duct
   c. Increases the water permeability of the collecting duct
   d. Decreases the GFR
   e. Increases the water permeability of the proximal tubule

6. A patient has polyuria and polydipsia, and the urine osmolality is 100 mOsm/kg H_2O. After an intravenous injection of AVP, urine volume decreases and urine osmolality increases. What is the most likely disorder in this patient?
   a. SIADH
   b. Osmotic diuresis
   c. Central diabetes insipidus
   d. Nephrogenic diabetes insipidus
   e. Nephrolithiasis (renal stone)

7. An individual with polyuria resulting from nephrogenic diabetes insipidus is treated with a thiazide diuretic, which inhibits NaCl reabsorption by the distal tubule. After several weeks of therapy, daily urine output has decreased. What is the most likely explanation for the ability of the thiazide diuretic to reduce urine output in this individual?
   a. Stimulation of AVP secretion
   b. Decrease in ECF volume
   c. Decreased water permeability of the collecting duct
   d. Decreased expression of V_2 receptors by collecting duct cells
   e. Stimulation of NaCl reabsorption by the thick ascending limb of Henle's loop

8. Hyponatremia can sometimes be seen in individuals whose ECF volume is decreased by more than 10%. Which of the following factors contributes to the development of hyponatremia in this situation?
   a. Decreased levels of AVP
   b. Elevated levels of natriuretic peptides
   c. Increased excretion of Na^+ by the kidneys
   d. Reduced excretion of solute-free water by the kidneys
   e. Development of positive Na^+ balance

9. A 20-year-old woman runs a marathon in 90° F weather. If she replaces all volume lost in sweat by drinking distilled water, what would happen to the volume and composition of her body fluids? (Note: Sweat is a hypotonic NaCl solution.)
   a. Total body water would be decreased
   b. Hematocrit would be decreased
   c. ICF volume would be decreased
   d. ECF volume would be increased
   e. Plasma osmolality would be decreased

10. If an individual loses 2 kg of body weight in a 48-hour period, with no change in P_{osm}, it means that the individual has:
    a. Lost 2 kg of NaCl
    b. Lost 2 liter of ECF
    c. Lost 2 kg of muscle mass
    d. Lost 2 kg of adipose tissue
    e. Hyponatremia

CHAPTER 6

1. Three individuals, each weighing 55 kg and each having a plasma [Na^+] of 145 mEq/L, are infused with different solutions. Individual A is infused with 1 L of isotonic NaCl (290 mOsm/kg H_2O); individual B is infused with 1 L of a mannitol solution (290 mOsm/kg H_2O); and individual C is infused with 1 L of a D5W (5% dextrose) solution (290 mOsm/kg H_2O). Assuming that there is no urine output, and after complete equilibration of the ECF and ICF, which of these individuals will have a lower plasma [Na^+]?
   a. Individual A
   b. Individual B

c. Individual C
d. Individuals A, B, and C will have the same plasma [Na$^+$]

2. Which of the following will occur with a decrease in the ECF volume?
   a. Increase in GFR
   b. Increase in angiotensin II levels
   c. Increase in natriuretic peptide levels
   d. Increase in free water clearance
   e. Increase in fractional excretion of Na$^+$

3. A 56-year-old woman has congestive heart failure with generalized edema. Which of the following plays an important role in the formation of edema in this woman?
   a. Increased interstitial hydrostatic pressure
   b. Decreased interstitial oncotic pressure
   c. Increased plasma oncotic pressure
   d. Decreased renal excretion of Na$^+$
   e. Decreased venous pressure

4. A 78-year-old woman with congestive heart failure develops pitting edema of her legs. Compared with a healthy (i.e., euvolemic individual), what set of parameters would be expected in this woman?

	Plasma Volume	ECF Volume	ECV
a.	↓	↓	↓
b.	↓	↑	↓
c.	↑	↑	↓
d.	↑	↑	↑
e.	↑	↓	↓

5. Hyponatremia can sometimes be seen in individuals whose ECF volume is decreased by more than 10%. Which of the following factors contributes to the development of hyponatremia in this situation?
   a. Decreased levels of AVP
   b. Elevated levels of natriuretic peptides
   c. Increased excretion of Na$^+$ by the kidneys
   d. Reduced excretion of solute-free water by the kidneys
   e. Development of positive Na$^+$ balance

6. A 45-year-old woman has a blood pressure of 140/90 mm Hg. Her doctor recommends a low-salt diet. What would you predict her plasma [Na$^+$] and ECF volume would be compared with their values on her previous diet? (Note: Assume she has reached a new steady state on her new diet.)

	Plasma [Na$^+$]	ECF Volume
a.	No change	↓
b.	No change	No change
c.	No change	↑
d.	↓	No change
e.	↓	↓

7. A 20-year-old woman runs a marathon in 90° F weather. If she replaces all volume lost in sweat by drinking a sports drink that also contains 30 mEq/L of Na$^+$, what would happen to the volume and composition of her body fluids? (Note: Sweat is a hypotonic NaCl solution.)
   a. Total body water would be decreased
   b. Hematocrit would be decreased
   c. ICF volume would be decreased
   d. ECF volume would be increased
   e. Plasma osmolality would be decreased

8. Low-pressure vascular circuit volume receptors (baroreceptors) are located in which of the following vascular structures?
   a. Aortic arch
   b. Cardiac atria
   c. Carotid sinus
   d. Juxtaglomerular apparatus of the kidney
   e. Renal veins

9. What would be the expected neural and hormonal profile in a person whose ECF volume was decreased? (Note: Changes are in comparison to the euvolemic state.)

	Sympathetic Nerve Activity	Aldosterone Levels	ANP Levels
a.	No change	↑	↑
b.	↑	↑	↓
c.	↑	↑	No change
d.	No change	↑	↓
f.	↓	↓	↑

10. A 42-year-old woman is recovering in the hospital after removal of a benign brain tumor. She develops SIADH, and her plasma [Na$^+$] falls from 142 mEq/L to 128 mEq/L. Urine osmolality is 600 mOsm/kg H$_2$O. Administration of 1 L of isotonic saline to this woman would result in

which of the following changes in her plasma [Na$^+$] and urinary Na$^+$ excretion?

	Plasma [Na$^+$]	Urinary Na$^+$ Excretion/24 h
a.	No change	↑
b.	↑	↑
c.	↓	↑
d.	↑	No change
e.	↓	↓

11. The kidneys maintain a constant plasma [Na$^+$] by regulating the excretion of?
   a. Urea
   b. Water
   c. Creatinine
   d. Protein
   e. Albumin

12. Hypernatremia is seen is patients with a "defect" in the ability to regulate the urinary excretion of:
   a. Sodium
   b. Potassium
   c. Urea
   d. Protein
   e. Water

13. A patient develops gastroenteritis with vomiting and diarrhea. He is admitted to the hospital and at admission his plasma [Na$^+$] is 135 mEq/L. Over the next 2-day period he loses 2 kg of weight and his plasma [Na$^+$] decreases to 115 mEq/L. Compared with arrival in the hospital, what are the P$_{osm}$ and ECF volume 2 days after admission?

	P$_{osm}$	ECFV
a.	↓	No change
b.	No change	↑
c.	↑	↑
d.	↓	↓
e.	No change	No change

14. A child (body weight = 30 kg) develops gastroenteritis with vomiting and diarrhea. He is admitted to the hospital, and at admission his plasma [Na] is 140 mEq/L. Over a 2-day period he loses 2 kg of weight; however, his plasma [Na$^+$] has not changed. Compared with arrival in the hospital what are the P$_{osm}$, ECF volume, and ICF volume 2 days after admission?

	P$_{osm}$	ECFV	ICFV
a.	↓	No change	↓
b.	No change	↓	No change
c.	↑	↑	↑
d.	↓	↓	↓
e.	No change	No change	↓

15. Extracellular fluid volume is normally what percent of body weight?
   a. 60%
   b. 40%
   c. 20%
   d. 10%
   e. 75%

CHAPTER 7

1. A reduction in dietary K$^+$ intake would be expected to alter K$^+$ transport in which segment of the nephron?
   a. Proximal convoluted tubule
   b. Descending limb of Henle's loop
   c. Proximal straight tubule
   d. Collecting duct
   e. Thick ascending limb of Henle's loop

2. Which of the following enhances urinary potassium excretion?
   a. An osmotic diuresis
   b. Acute metabolic acidosis
   c. Hypoaldosteronism
   d. Decreased tubular flow rate
   e. A water diuresis

3. Which of the following hormones plays an important role in keeping the plasma concentration of potassium within normal limits?
   a. Calcitriol
   b. Arginine vasopressin
   c. PTH
   d. Insulin
   e. Glucagon

4. A healthy individual weighing 60 kg is infused with 1 L of isotonic saline to which 20 mEq of K$^+$ has been added. Following the infusion, the plasma [K$^+$] of this individual has increased from 3.5 mEq/L to 7.8 mEq/L. What is the most likely explanation for the development of hyperkalemia in this individual?

a. Shift of K^+ from the ICF into the ECF
b. Impaired renal excretion of K^+
c. The increase in plasma $[K^+]$ of 4.3 mEq/L is what is expected from the addition of 20 mEq/L of K^+ to the ECF
d. Contraction of the ECF volume
e. Development of hyperosmolality

5. A 35-year-old man is diagnosed with an aldosterone-secreting adrenal tumor. What effect would the elevated levels of aldosterone have on his serum $[K^+]$ and plasma renin levels? (Note: Changes are indicated compared with a state of normal aldosterone levels.)

	Serum $[K^+]$	Plasma Renin Levels
a.	↑	↑
b.	↑	↓
c.	↓	No change
d.	↓	↑
e.	↓	↓

6. A 45-year-old man is placed on an angiotensin-converting enzyme inhibitor as part of his therapy for hypertension. If he does not change his diet, what changes in his serum $[Na^+]$ and serum $[K^+]$ would you expect?

	Serum $[Na^+]$	Serum $[K^+]$
a.	No change	↓
b.	No change	↑
c.	↓	No change
d.	↑	↑
e.	↓	↓

7. Aldosterone:
a. Reduces urinary potassium excretion
b. Stimulates sodium reabsorption by the proximal tubule
c. Increases water reabsorption by the TAL of Henle's loop
d. Causes hyperkalemia
e. Secretion is stimulated by angiotensin II

8. Which of the following acutely causes hyperkalemia?
a. Increased plasma epinephrine
b. Increased plasma insulin
c. Increased plasma aldosterone
d. Increased P_{osm}
e. Organic acidosis

9. Pseudohyperkalemia is due to:
a. Lysis of red blood cells
b. Increased plasma epinephrine
c. Increased plasma insulin
d. Increased plasma aldosterone
e. Increased plasma angiotensin II

10. Which segment of the nephron regulates how much K^+ is excreted in the urine?
a. Proximal tubule
b. Descending limb of Henle's loop
c. Ascending limb of Henle's loop
d. Macula densa
e. Collecting duct

CHAPTER 8

Match the acid-base disturbance with the clinical scenario and arterial blood gases described in questions 1 through 5.

a. Metabolic acidosis with respiratory compensation
b. Metabolic alkalosis with respiratory compensation
c. Respiratory acidosis with renal compensation (chronic respiratory acidosis)
d. Respiratory acidosis without renal compensation (acute respiratory acidosis)
e. Metabolic acidosis and respiratory acidosis

1. An individual with an asthma attack:

$$pH = 7.32; \; [HCO_3^-] = 25 \text{ mEq/L};$$
$$P_{CO_2} = 50 \text{ mm Hg}$$

2. An individual with diabetes mellitus, who forgets to take insulin:

$$pH = 7.29; \; [HCO_3^-] = 12 \text{ mEq/L};$$
$$P_{CO_2} = 26 \text{ mm Hg}$$

3. An individual with cardiopulmonary arrest:

$$pH = 6.85; \; [HCO_3^-] = 10 \text{ mEq/L};$$
$$P_{CO_2} = 60 \text{ mmHg}$$

4. An individual with a gastric ulcer who ingests large quantities of antacids:

$$pH = 7.45; \; [HCO_3^-] = 30 \text{ mEq/L};$$
$$P_{CO_2} = 45 \text{ mm Hg}$$

5. An individual with a 20-year history of smoking 3 packs/day who has emphysema:

$$pH = 7.37; \ [HCO_3^-] = 28 \ mEq/L;$$
$$P_{CO_2} = 50 \ mm \ Hg$$

6. During a 24-hour period, an individual excretes in the urine 60 mmol of NH_4^+, 40 mmol of titratable acid, and 10 mmol of HCO_3^-. If this individual is in acid-base balance, how much nonvolatile acid was produced from metabolism?
   a. 80 mmol/day
   b. 90 mmol/day
   c. 100 mmol/day
   d. 110 mmol/day
   e. 120 mmol/day

7. In response to a metabolic acidosis, the kidneys increase the excretion of net acid. Which of the following is the most important component of this compensatory response?
   a. Increased filtered load of HCO_3^-
   b. Enhanced reabsorption of HCO_3^- by the proximal tubule
   c. Increased synthesis and excretion of NH_4^+
   d. Reduced H^+ secretion by the distal tubule and collecting duct
   e. Reduced secretion of HCO_3^- by the collecting duct

8. A 6-year-old boy presents to the emergency department with fever, abdominal cramps, and diarrhea. Arterial blood gases are as follows:

   pH : 7.28 (normal: 7.35-7.45)

   P_{CO_2}: 24 mm Hg (normal: 33-44 mm Hg)

   HCO_3^- : 11 mEq/L (normal: 22-28 mEq/L)

   What is the acid-base disorder?
   a. Metabolic acidosis with respiratory compensation
   b. Metabolic acidosis with respiratory acidosis
   c. Acute respiratory acidosis
   d. Chronic respiratory acidosis

9. A mechanism that dampens the acute (minutes) effect of respiratory acidosis on blood pH is:
   a. Stimulation of carotid/aortic body chemoreceptors
   b. Buffering by extracellular proteins

   c. Buffering by extracellular HCO_3^-
   d. Buffering in cells
   e. Reduced renal HCO_3^- reabsorption

Match the portion of the nephron to the function described in questions 10 and 11.
   a. Proximal tubule
   b. Descending limb of Henle's loop
   c. Ascending limb of Henle's loop
   d. Distal tuble
   e. Collecting duct

10. Urine pH is the most acidic at this site.

11. NH_4^+ is reabsorbed from the tubular fluid at this site.

12. A 60-year-old woman comes to the emergency department with shortness of breath. An arterial blood sample is obtained.
    P_{O_2}: 75 mm Hg (normal: 75-100 mm Hg)
    P_{CO_2}: 58 mm Hg (normal: 33-44 mm Hg)
    HCO_3^-: 24 mEq/L (normal: 22-28 mEq/L)
    pH: 7.24 (normal: 7.35-7.45)

    What is this woman's acid-base disorder?
    a. Metabolic acidosis
    b. Metabolic alkalosis
    c. Acute respiratory acidosis
    d. Acute respiratory alkalosis
    e. Chronic respiratory acidosis

13. Which of the following sets of arterial blood values represents a combined metabolic and respiratory acidosis?

	pH	P_{CO_2} (mm Hg)	$[HCO_3^-]$ (mEq/L)
a.	7.32	28	14
b.	7.47	20	14
c.	7.08	49	14
d.	7.51	49	38
e.	6.98	13	3

14. The plasma anion gap is calculated to:
    a. Distinguish between metabolic and respiratory disturbances
    b. Distinguish between acute and chronic metabolic acidosis
    c. Distinguish between acute and chronic respiratory acidosis
    d. Determine if organic acids are accumulating in the blood
    e. Assess the severity of chronic renal failure

15. Renal tubular acidosis is:
    a. Caused by hyperventilation
    b. Caused by excessive H^+ ion secretion by the distal tubule
    c. A mechanism to reduce the loss of HCO_3^- in the urine
    d. A disease characterized by reduced renal H^+ ion secretion
    e. Caused by loop diuretics

CHAPTER 9

Match the portion of the nephron to the function described in questions 1 and 2.
    a. Proximal tubule
    b. Descending limb of Henle's loop
    c. Ascending limb of Henle's loop
    d. Distal tuble
    e. Collecting duct

1. Site where calcitriol is synthesized

2. Site where parathyroid hormone (PTH) stimulates Ca^{++} reabsorption

3. A 65-year-old man has chronic renal failure. What are the expected changes in his plasma Ca^{++}, P_i, and calcitriol levels? (Note: Changes are those expected compared with an individual with normal renal function.)

	Serum [Ca^{++}]	Serum [P_i]	Calcitriol Level
a.	↓	↑	↓
b.	↑	↑	↑
c.	↑	↓	↓
d.	↓	↓	↓
e.	↑	↑	↓

4. Which of the following conditions would be expected to reduce the free (i.e., ionized) [Ca^{++}] in the plasma?
    a. Metabolic acidosis
    b. Reduced dietary intake of phosphate
    c. A tumor secreting parathyroid hormone–like peptide
    d. Ingestion of calcitriol
    e. Acute respiratory alkalosis

5. The nephron segment that is most important in the regulation of phosphate excretion is:
    a. The proximal tubule
    b. The descending thin loop of Henle

c. The distal tubule
d. The cortical collecting duct
e. The inner medullary collecting duct

6. PTH:
    a. Decreases intestinal calcium absorption.
    b. Stimulates renal phosphate reabsorption.
    c. Decreases renal calcium excretion.
    d. Decreases calcitriol production.
    e. Decreases plasma calcium concentration.

7. Expansion of the extracellular fluid volume will:
    a. Stimulate P_i reabsorption in the thick ascending limb
    b. Decrease P_i reabsorption in the proximal tubule
    c. Increase the secretion of P_i in the distal tubule
    d. Inhibit P_i reabsorption in the medullary collecting duct
    e. Increase Ca^{++} secretion in the collecting ducts.

8. Hypercalcemia:
    a. Increases (more negative) the threshold potential in nerves
    b. Increases plasma PTH levels
    c. Causes tetany
    d. Decreases plasma calcitriol levels
    e. Directly decreases intestinal P_i absorption

9. PTHRP is a hormone secreted by:
    a. Proximal tubule cells
    b. Brain cells
    c. Cancer cells
    d. Heart cells
    e. Intestinal cells

10. Urinary phosphate excretion will increase:
    a. During a decrease in extracellular fluid volume
    b. If AVP levels are high
    c. During hyperphosphatemia
    d. Following the administration of a potassium-sparing diuretic
    e. During hypoglycemia

CHAPTER 10

For questions 1 through 4, match the appropriate diuretic with the statement.
    a. Carbonic anhydrase inhibitor
    b. Loop diuretic

c. Thiazide diuretic

d. Potassium-sparing diuretic

1. Administration of this diuretic leads to an increase in the kidneys' ability to excrete solute-free water (C_{H2O}).

2. Administration of this diuretic may lead to the development of hyperkalemia.

3. Administration of this diuretic impairs the kidneys' ability to reabsorb solute-free water ($T^c_{H_2O}$).

4. Administration of this diuretic results in a decrease in renal Ca^{++} excretion.

5. An individual weighs 60 kg and ingests a diet containing 100 mEq/day of Na^+. This individual is placed on a thiazide diuretic. After 2 weeks of taking this diuretic and with no change in diet, what can be concluded about Na^+ balance in this individual?
   a. Total body Na^+ content is increased
   b. Urine Na^+ excretion is greater than 100 mEq/day
   c. Na^+ content of the ECF is reduced
   d. The plasma $[Na^+]$ is increased
   e. The Na^+ content of the ICF is increased

6. An individual is treated with a thiazide diuretic for mild hypertension. After 3 months of therapy, the plasma $[Na^+]$ has decreased from 143 mEq/L to 135 mEq/L. Which of the following factors plays a role in the development of hyponatremia in this individual?
   a. Enhanced reabsorption of solute-free water by the early distal tubule
   b. Reduced excretion of solute-free water
   c. Shift of water from the ICF to the ECF
   d. Diuretic-induced stimulation of the thirst center
   e. Reduced effect of AVP on the collecting duct

7. The use of a thiazide diuretic that inhibits NaCl reabsorption in the distal tubule does which of the following?
   a. Decreases the ability of the kidneys to excrete solute-free water
   b. Decreases the urinary excretion of NaCl
   c. Decreases the urinary excretion of K^+
   d. Increases the ability of the kidneys to excrete a concentrated urine
   e. Increases plasma $[K^+]$

8. Diuretics that inhibit NaCl reabsorption by the thick ascending limb of Henle's loop do which of the following?
   a. Stimulate calcium reabsorption by the thick ascending limb
   b. Decrease urine flow rate
   c. Stimulate urinary excretion of K^+
   d. Stimulate countercurrent multiplication
   e. Increase the osmolality of the medullary interstitial fluid

9. An individual with polyuria resulting from nephrogenic diabetes insipidus is treated with a thiazide diuretic. After several weeks of therapy, daily urine output has decreased. What is the most likely explanation for the ability of the thiazide diuretic to reduce urine output in this individual?
   a. Stimulation of AVP secretion
   b. Decrease in ECF volume
   c. Decreased water permeability of the collecting duct
   d. Decreased expression of V_2 receptors by collecting duct cells
   e. Stimulation of NaCl reabsorption by the thick ascending limb of Henle's loop

10. A 35-year-old man is placed on a thiazide diuretic for hypertension. If his urine was measured within the first 24 hours after starting the diuretic, what might you expect would happen to his excretion of Na^+, K^+, and Ca^{++}?

	Na^+	K^+	Ca^{++}
a.	↑	↑	↑
b.	↑	↓	↑
c.	↓	↑	↑
d.	↓	↓	↓
e.	↑	↑	↓

11. Administration of a loop diuretic to a healthy individual for several weeks would be expected to have which of the following effects on body fluid composition and volume?

	P_{osm}	ECF Volume	ICF Volume
a.	↑	↓	↓
b.	No change	↓	No change
c.	↓	No change	↑
d.	↓	↑	↓
e.	No change	No change	No change

12. A healthy 21-year-old man participates in a clinical trial of a new loop diuretic. Before administration of this new diuretic, his urine osmolality is 600 mOsm/kg H_2O and his urine output is 1.5 L/day. Which of the following values for urine osmolality and urine output would you predict as a result of the diuretic's action on his thick ascending limb of Henle's loop?

Urine Osmolality (mOsm/kg H_2O)	Urine Output (L/day)
a. 1200	0.75
b. 1000	0.9
c. 600	1.5
d. 300	3.0
e. 200	4.5

13. Which of the following could be characterized as a calcium-sparing diuretic?
    a. Mannitol
    b. A carbonic anhydrase inhibitor
    c. A loop diuretic
    d. A thiazide diuretic
    e. An AVP antagonist

14. Which class of diuretics is the most effective in promoting urinary HCO_3^- excretion?
    a. Carbonic anhydrase inhibitor
    b. Aquaretics
    c. Thiazide diuretic
    d. Aldosterone antagonist
    e. Loop diuretics

15. A potassium sparing diuretic (e.g., amiloride) given alone would be expected to:
    a. Decrease urinary sodium excretion
    b. Increase the ECF volume
    c. Increase plasma $[K^+]$
    d. Decrease plasma $[Na^+]$
    e. Decrease urinary HCO_3^- excretion

ANSWERS TO REVIEW EXAMINATION

CHAPTER 2

1. b	3. c	5. a	7. c	9. d
2. e	4. e	6. b	8. b	10. e

CHAPTER 3

1. a	4. b	7. d	9. b	11. e
2. b	5. b	8. c	10. b	12. b
3. c	6. e			

CHAPTER 4

1. c	3. b	5. c	7. d	9. c
2. c	4. d	6. a	8. b	10. b

CHAPTER 5

1. c	3. a	5. c	7. b	9. e
2. b	4. b	6. c	8. d	10. b

CHAPTER 6

1. b	4. c	7. e	10. c	13. d
2. b	5. d	8. b	11. b	14. b
3. d	6. a	9. b	12. e	15. c

CHAPTER 7

1. d	3. d	5. e	7. e	9. a
2. a	4. a	6. b	8. d	10. e

CHAPTER 8

1. d	4. b	7. c	10. e	13. c
2. a	5. c	8. a	11. c	14. d
3. e	6. b	9. d	12. c	15. d

CHAPTER 9

1. a	3. a	5. a	7. b	9. c
2. d	4. e	6. c	8. d	10. c

CHAPTER 10

1. a	4. c	7. a	10. e	13. d
2. d	5. c	8. c	11. b	14. a
3. b	6. b	9. b	12. d	15. c

INDEX

Page numbers followed by *f* indicate figures; *t*, tables; *b*, boxes.